LEADERSHIP IN HEALTH CARE

⑤SAGE | 50 YEARS

LEADERSHIP IN HEALTH CARE

THIRD EDITION

JILL BARR AND LESLEY DOWDING

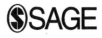

Los Angeles | London | New Delhi
Singapore | Washington DC

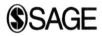

Los Angeles | London | New Delhi
Singapore | Washington DC

SAGE Publications Ltd
1 Oliver's Yard
55 City Road
London EC1Y 1SP

SAGE Publications Inc.
2455 Teller Road
Thousand Oaks, California 91320

SAGE Publications India Pvt Ltd
B 1/I 1 Mohan Cooperative Industrial Area
Mathura Road
New Delhi 110 044

SAGE Publications Asia-Pacific Pte Ltd
3 Church Street
#10-04 Samsung Hub
Singapore 049483

Editor: Becky Taylor
Associate editor: Emma Milman
Production editor: Katie Forsythe
Copyeditor: Mary Dalton
Proofreader: Thea Watson
Indexer: Gary Kirby
Marketing manager: Tamara Navaratnam
Cover design: Wendy Scott
Typeset by: C&M Digitals (P) Ltd, Chennai, India
Printed in Great Britain by
CPI Group (UK) Ltd, Croydon, CR0 4YY

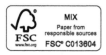

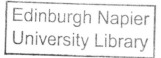

Library of Congress Control Number: 2014959181

British Library Cataloguing in Publication data

A catalogue record for this book is available from
the British Library

ISBN 978-1-4739-0455-2
ISBN 978-1-4739-0456-9 (pbk)

At SAGE we take sustainability seriously. Most of our products are printed in the UK using FSC papers and boards.
When we print overseas we ensure sustainable papers are used as measured by the Egmont grading system.
We undertake an annual audit to monitor our sustainability.

CONTENTS

ABOUT THE AUTHORS

Jill is a Principal Lecturer at the University of Wolverhampton, leading a Community team in a number of awards from pre-registration return to practice, prescribing to Masters Awards in community and public health nursing. Her own professional career has been exciting, varied and totally integrated with personal development including writing with Lesley Dowding for nearly 15 years. Jill qualified as a nurse, midwife and health visitor working in all these areas as well as gaining her nursing licence in Michigan, USA. With a breadth of practice experiences in the acute, community and industry, the patients, women, families and communities that have been served have been important to this personal development.

Lesley's career has encompassed a number of differing experiences since qualification, as a nurse and midwife, ranging from General Theatres, Midwifery, Gynaecology, Nanny in the USA, Veterinary Assistant, Anaesthetics & Recovery Sister, and as Nurse Tutor within Schools of Nursing and Universities. Lesley teaches a variety of subjects for Pre-Registration Nursing students including management studies and has a passion for effective management techniques, endeavouring to make what might be considered dry theory applicable to clinical practice. To do this Lesley and Jill have written two books related to management theory and practice in health care: *Managing in Health Care: A Guide for Nurses, Midwives and Health Visitors* (2002) Pearson Education; and *Leadership in Health Care* (2008; 2012) Sage.

Sue Saillet, a longtime friend of Lesley's, is the artist responsible for the cartoons to lighten the subject area. The reason we chose the fish theme was because of their tendency to swim together in a shoal following their leader – but unfortunately on occasion with little or no thought! Sue gained an honours degree in Illustration from Plymouth University in 2007.

FOREWORD

Recognition of the need to develop strong leaders is widespread. This need is amplified when applied to the health care setting. Much of the received wisdom on how to develop effective leaders and efficient managers is drawn from business and industry. Whilst helpful and transportable, this wisdom requires even further interpretation when applied to caring for vulnerable people.

This book provides such an interpretation with its focus on contemporary health care and the critical responsibility of leaders; it provides something of a leadership companion. In an era where the consequences of failure in leadership have never been more prominent, nor tragic, leadership development assumes significant importance.

Investment in leadership development, whilst critical for both the health care workforce and those being cared for, is being eroded. Budgets can no longer be stretched to include comprehensive and often prohibitively expensive leadership development for all of those who occupy leader positions. This book will provide the opportunity for leaders and aspiring leaders to evaluate leadership practices and employ evidence-based strategies for ensuring strong clinical leadership results in high quality care delivery.

In an era now referred to as post-Francis, the text has developed through addition of some key features around the '6 Cs' and patient safety and human factors. Following scrutiny of professional conduct, there is additional focus on professional regulation and interprofessional working.

Finally, with migration and employment mobility continuing to be shaped by new ways of working, global leadership is also considered.

Jill Barr and Lesley Dowding have combined their significant clinical and education experience and expertise to provide a comprehensive guide which clinical leaders can follow to enhance leadership. Included within the book is a mixed approach to support the leader repertoire, taking account of team and personal development. This book is a must-have for aspiring, new and developing leaders in health care settings.

Dr Alexandra Hopkins

Dean

University of Wolverhampton

PREFACE

WHY THIS BOOK?

Effective leadership underpins the efficient and safe running of any clinical practice. Indeed in everyday life it may be necessary to use leadership skills in our family life in getting children to school in time, managing the domestic chores and planning for future holidays. The way in which we do it, and the effects it has on others, is important. Leadership is a topic that concerns policy through to practice in health care. The 'modernisation' agenda highlights the importance of leadership in clinical practice. The NHS Leadership Centre exemplifies the importance of leadership through a range of initiatives. Being able to give skilled and evidence-based care is important, but it is also about working in a performance-measured health service to meet the expectations of society.

Leadership is a vital part of today's health care practice. Therefore, it is useful to have an understanding of the variety of theories supporting actions and applied to leadership practice in the UK. One view may be that leadership comes from within and is something that is with you from birth. Contrary to this is the idea that leadership skills can be learned or developed. It is our belief that an ability to lead people in delivering a quality health service relies on developing these skills.

To this end, this book explores the underpinning theories of leadership and applies them to the health care scenario wherever it is practised. It debates the nature of leadership by examining diversity, individual values, the idea of team as 'hero', and the variety of skills required to achieve effective and efficient health care delivery.

WHO IS IT FOR?

This book supports the health care professional (HCP) in identifying the application of leadership theory to their own clinical practice. It is applicable to all professions allied to medicine including students of adult, mental health, children's nursing, midwifery, health visiting, operating department practitioners, paramedic sciences, and more. Theories offer the 'bones' for exploring the nature of leadership; the difficulty comes in applying those theories to practice.

Recognising the theory–practice gap is important because each informs the other when searching and developing more effective ways of delivering health care to a demanding public. Pre- and post-registration courses usually include aspects of leadership theory but it has been noted that some students experience difficulty in application; as such this book is for them.

HOW DO I USE IT?

The chapters are designed to direct you as a health care professional, through a structured approach, starting with leading as an individual, through to team working and on to the organisational perspective, reflecting both micro and macro levels of health care systems.

Each chapter commences with a list of Learning Outcomes; followed by an Introduction outlining the content of the chapter. Within each chapter there will be a variety of activities with questions related to the content, self-knowledge, literature application, review questions, 'stop and think' activities and preferred styles. Each chapter will conclude with a Summary of Key Points, highlighting the ways in which the learning outcomes have been met and some suggested further reading.

Throughout the book the words patient or client will be used interchangeably to indicate the care user, patient or client depending on the context of care.

We hope that you will find this book – used in conjunction with other texts – a useful tool to aid you in interpreting and using effective leadership skills in your professional and personal lives.

Jill Barr and Lesley Dowding

PUBLISHER'S ACKNOWLEDGEMENTS

The authors and publisher would like to thank the following for their kind permission to republish material.

Figure 2.2 Johns' Model of Reflection is republished with permission of John Wiley and Sons.

Figure 4.4 Good to Great by Jim Collins © 2001. Used by permission of Curtis Brown, Ltd. All rights reserved.

Figure 7.1 The 6Cs © Crown copyright. Available at: www.england.nhs.uk/nursing vision

Figure 8.1 Bounded Problems and Figure 8.2 Unbounded Problems © The Open University. Reproduced with kind permission of The Open University.

Figure 12.1 EFQM Excellence Model © EFQM 2014. Available at: www.efqm.org/the-efqm-excellence-model

Figure 13.3 Denison's model of cultural change is reproduced with kind permission of Denison Consulting www.DenisonCulture.com

Myers-Briggs Type Indicator®, Myer-Briggs®, MBTI® and the MBTI logo® are all registered trademarks of the Myers-Briggs Type Indicator Trust in the United States and other countries.

We would like to thank the reviewers for their invaluable feedback on the initial proposal for a third edition and draft chapters from the text. We would also like to thank Emma, Becky and Katie for their ongoing support.

We would also like to thank the students who provided scenarios which informed the companion website video discussions.

HOW TO USE THE COMPANION WEBSITE

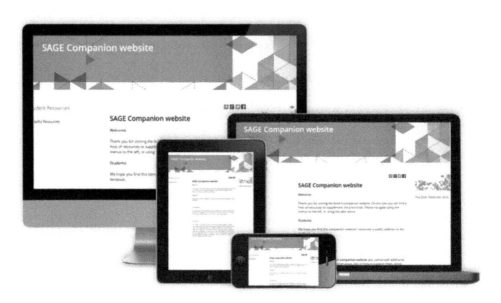

Visit https://study.sagepub.com/barr for access to a wealth of resources to support your studies if you are a student and teaching if you are a lecturer. Look out for the web icon in the chapters to see where web material is available.

The companion website includes:

- **For Students**
    - Weblinks to further resources and to activities to test your own leadership and management styles
    - Additional documents to deepen your understanding of some of the key concepts introduced in the book
    - Activities and exercises to help you apply theory to practice
    - A video introduction to the authors and their experience as leaders in nursing.

- **For Lecturers**
    - Author videos and a podcasts explaining key concepts and areas that students commonly find difficult, for you to use in your seminars or to set for 'flipped classroom' preparation work.

PART 1

THE INDIVIDUAL

1 THE NATURE OF LEADERSHIP

Learning Outcomes

By the end of this chapter you will have had the opportunity to:

- Discuss the notions of leadership and followership
- Define leadership
- Discuss the importance of the changing context related to health care
- Compare leadership and management
- Debate the art and science of leadership.

INTRODUCTION

So you want to find out about leadership, but what does this mean exactly? How do you know that you are not already a leader? You may be thinking that you have only just started your career in one of the many health care professions and that the leadership issue will not raise its head for some years, but you could assume some leadership roles early on. Similarly, you may have been a qualified practitioner for some time and are about to move into a position that has a formal, recognised leadership role. Whatever the reason, this chapter will allow you to start to think about leadership and its role in your life and career.

The concept and theories of leadership have evolved and are continuing to do so, but how can a book on leadership help you to be a better leader? Daft (2008: 24) reminds us that it is important to bear in mind that leadership is both an art and a science. Leadership is an art because many of the leadership skills and qualities required cannot be learned and a science because there is a growing body of knowledge that describes the leadership process. By keeping this in mind we can understand how a variety of leadership skills can be used to attain the best possible care for our patients. Jeffrey (2013) talked of the term *'nurse leader'* as being a misnomer because in the English language we place adjectives in front of nouns (e.g. blue car, not the car blue); the term *nurse leader* would therefore imply that this person is a leader who just happens to be a nurse. I am convinced that this is not the case; nurse leaders are certainly nurses at their core and become nurses who lead.

When first thinking about leaders in health care, we may identify people like Florence Nightingale (1820–1910), famous for her work at Scutari Hospital in the Crimea, collecting data (the beginnings of research in nursing) in order to improve practice. Mary Seacole (1805–1881), another nurse, was refused an interview to go to the Crimea. Such was her belief that there was a real need for her talents there, she paid for herself to go and went on to be known as 'Mother Seacole'. She is now held up as one of the first black women leaders. Dr E.L.M. Millar highlighted the need for effective training within the Ambulance Service of the 1960s, which ultimately led to the current technician training and paramedic degree (Kilner, 2004). These people did much for caring, through their pursuit of improved standards and acting as role models in the health care work they did. In today's society you might think of John F. Kennedy (1917–1963), Nelson Mandela (1918–2014), Barack Obama (1961–), Benazir Bhutto (1953–2007), Indira Gandhi (1917–1984) or even Tony Blair (1953–) as being renowned leaders. Beverley Malone (1948–) is currently the chief executive officer of the National League for Nursing in the United States. Prior to assuming this position in February 2007 she served as general secretary of the Royal College of Nursing for six years. I heard her speak at a National Association of Theatre Nurses conference – she was inspirational and so enthusiastic about nursing today that everyone left with the intention of being a nurse who has the power to strongly advocate for their patients. Whoever you think of as an influential leader, they must be enthusiastic and love their chosen profession in order to command such respect and to be able to infuse others with energy and enthusiasm. Leadership involves people being led, so there must be those who are happy to be followers. We must, therefore, remember that effective leaders and effective followers may sometimes be the same people playing different roles at different times. This book will try to engender this verve for effective leadership. In order to address the identified learning outcomes, this chapter will introduce the nature of leadership, comparing management and leadership, and the art and science of leadership.

THE IMPORTANCE OF LEADERSHIP IN PATIENT AND CLIENT CARE OUTCOMES

Recently there have been a number of high profile system failures where patient/client care has been affected through poor and ineffective leadership. Following the Francis Report (2013) the Prime Minister David Cameron asked Professor Don Berwick, a leading expert in patient safety, to look at what needs to be done 'to make zero harm a reality in our NHS'. The Berwick Report (2013) 'A promise to learn – a commitment to act' identified a number of existing problems such as a lack of leadership in risk management systems. The executive summary made ten recommendations which are:

1. The NHS should continually and forever reduce patient harm by embracing wholeheartedly an ethic of learning.
2. All leaders concerned with NHS healthcare – political, regulatory, governance, executive, clinical and advocacy – should place quality of care in general, and patient safety in particular, at the top of their priorities for investment, inquiry, improvement, regular reporting, encouragement and support.
3. Patients and their carers should be present, powerful and involved at all levels of health care organisations from wards to the boards of Trusts.
4. Government, Health Education England and NHS England should assure that sufficient staff are available to meet the NHS's needs now and in the future. Healthcare organisations should ensure that staff are present in appropriate numbers to provide safe care at all times and are well-supported.
5. Mastery of quality and patient safety sciences and practices should be part of initial preparation and lifelong education of all health care professionals, including managers and executives.
6. The NHS should become a learning organisation. Its leaders should create and support the capability for learning, and therefore change, at scale, within the NHS.
7. Transparency should be complete, timely and unequivocal. All data on quality and safety, whether assembled by government, organisations, or professional societies, should be shared in a timely fashion with all parties who want it, including, in accessible form, with the public.
8. All organisations should seek out the patient and carer voice as an essential asset in monitoring the safety and quality of care.

9. Supervisory and regulatory systems should be simple and clear. They should avoid diffusion of responsibility. They should be respectful of the goodwill and sound intention of the vast majority of staff. All incentives should point in the same direction.
10. We support responsive regulation of organisations, with a hierarchy of responses. Recourse to criminal sanctions should be extremely rare, and should function primarily as a deterrent to wilful or reckless neglect or mistreatment.

The need for quality in the delivery of care is vital, and failings were highlighted in a variety of instances where this has clearly not been the case e.g. Bristol Royal Infirmary (2001), Baby P (2007), the Mid-Staffordshire NHS Foundation Trust scandal (2013), and Gosport Hospital (2013) to name a few; this will be further discussed in Chapter 12. All these events have changed the landscape of how we look at the duty of care; in all these situations the failure of effective leadership and management strategies were shown to be complicit in the failure of care provision and workers seemed to have become complacent about their roles. They have reminded us of the importance of raising concerns and acting on them before it is too late, and of developing a workplace culture which enables staff to have the confidence to speak out (UNISON, 2011). All is not doom and gloom though; the Royal Colleges, National Institute of Clinical Excellence (NICE) and Care Quality Commission (CQC) highlight areas of good care provision and there are lessons to be learned from those papers in order to ensure high quality care for all.

In the light of the findings from the various reports it can be seen that the need for effective leadership is vital. These leaders, whatever their background, must demonstrate 'best practice' in their clinical areas and dedicate themselves to supporting, marketing, and 'driving through' an innovation (Greenhalgh et al. 2004: 182). They have become known as Champion Nurses and practise at a level that encourages others to better themselves to ensure all patients receive first class, evidence-based care at all times. Stoddart et al. (2014) highlighted a project that suggested systematic 'Care Comfort Rounds' for 'in-patients' whether this be in hospital or care/nursing homes; the project led to proactive rather than reactive nursing care delivery and the number of falls and the use of all buzzers were reduced. Active nursing rounds – variously known as 'intentional' or 'care and comfort' rounds – are still relatively new in their present format; what is important is that it is patient- rather than task-focused: every hour, a nurse checks in with the patient, not to 'do something' but to find out if s/he is comfortable and if there is anything s/he needs. Whilst this might be thought to be a regressive move (in that it was commonplace in the 1950s, 1960s and 1970s) it means that the patients' health and welfare are assessed at regular (hourly) intervals during the day so leading to safer, effective patient-centred practice. The current notion of care comfort rounds started in the United States and has been adopted in some UK hospitals, including some hospital Trusts participating in The Kings Fund Hospital Pathways Programme (Kings Fund, 2012). In acute settings key aspects that are usually checked during Care Comfort/Active Nursing/Intentional rounds include the 'Four Ps':

    i. Positioning: Making sure the patient is comfortable and assessing the risk of pressure ulcers.

    ii. Personal needs: Scheduling patient trips to the bathroom to avoid risk of falls.

    iii. Pain: Asking patients to describe their pain level on a scale of 0–10.

    iv. Placement: Making sure the items a patient needs are within easy reach.

During each round the following behaviours (which may be summarised on a prompt card) are undertaken by the nurse:

- Use an opening phrase to introduce themselves and put the patient at ease
- Perform scheduled tasks
- Ask about the 'Four P's' (described above)
- Assess the care environment (e.g. fall hazards, temperature of the room)
- Use closing key words e.g. 'is there anything else I can do for you before I go?'
- Explain when the patient will be checked on again
- Document the round

Structured methods of intentional rounding are underpinned by leadership support, e.g. regular staff meetings to review activities and progress. Staff training and accountability structures are used to 'hardwire' the required behaviours and competencies into routine practice (Studer Group, 2007). In the USA it is deemed part of the daily care to conduct a full health assessment on all patients by the registered nurse. In order to ensure that this is not just a paper exercise, NHS Trusts need to identify suitable registered nurses whose responsibility it is to implement this systematic care standard as a change in practice. These leaders need to ensure an effective implementation of this strategy (both day, night, and at weekends, i.e. 24 hours a day, 7 days a week) in order to improve patient outcomes.

Activity

- In your experience, have you observed a similar activity to Care Comfort Rounds?
- Consider your clinical environment and list the pros and cons in implementing a system such as Care Comfort Rounds.

You might have thought of the time consuming element of filling in yet another form but Stoddart's project has shown that not only was all-round patient care improved but staff satisfaction in care delivery was also increased (Stoddart et al., 2014: 22); as with any change the implementation of a 'new' work practice has to be considered with a great deal of communication, planning and education for it to succeed (Chapter 13).

Employees have rights just as patients and patient/clients have rights, similarly employers have a duty of care (Department of Health (DH), 1974, 1999a, 2005b); under the *Management of Health and Safety at Work Regulations* (Department of Health, 1999b) employers are obliged to assess the nature and scale of risks to health and safety in the workplace and base their control measures on it. We have to accept that as humans we are all able to make mistakes but learning from the failure of others is imperative; the Department of Health (2000b) paper *An Organisation with Memory* highlights that failure is almost always unintentional and comes about through a variety of small omissions/errors rather than via a single colossal one. It set out to understand what was known about the scale and nature of serious failures in the United Kingdom's National Health Service (NHS) system, examine how the NHS might learn from those failures, and recommend methods to minimise future failures. Despite the valuable information contained within the document the NHS continues to struggle with implementation of the recommendations.

RELATIONSHIPS BETWEEN LEADERSHIP AND FOLLOWERSHIP

Owen (2011: xvii) postulates that one barrier in the definition of leadership is the belief that leadership is related to seniority. However, he goes on to state that leadership is not about position but about behaviour. Think about the following situation in relation to leadership:

> Sue Potter is a third year student on placement in the clinical area. During the course of the day, she notices that a second year student in the same placement area often comes to ask her for advice related to patient/client care for a given situation. Sue happily explains the procedure to the other student, highlighting the current research supporting the action. A qualified member of staff also approaches Sue for information related to the research, as it was an area of care he had not been involved with for some time. Sue was happy to tell the qualified person what she knew and then started to reflect on her own abilities in leading and teaching. She then started to examine why people felt that they could come to her for information and support.

Although Sue was not yet qualified, she was clearly seen as a leader within that situation. The skills Sue demonstrated – being approachable and teaching others willingly – are those of leadership. Sue's example of supporting and sharing her knowledge can be applied to any field of health care provision.

It is important, then, to examine some of the variety of definitions of leadership available. Daft (2005: 4) states that: 'scholars and other writers have offered more than 350 definitions of the term leadership' and concludes that leadership 'is one of the most observed and least understood phenomena on earth'.

Tappen et al. (2004: 5) suggest that there are a number of primary tasks involved with being a leader:

1. Set direction: mission, goals, vision and purpose
2. Build commitment: motivation, spirit, teamwork
3. Confront challenges: innovation, change, and turbulence.

So leadership would appear to be a people activity and occurs within group life; it is not something done to people. Leaders are seen to be effective because they have charisma which allows them to articulate a vision for a given group of followers and generate enthusiasm for that vision (Haslam and Reicher, 2011: 5). Without followers there cannot be leaders and without leaders there cannot be followers, so being an effective follower is as important to the health care professional as being an effective leader.

> ### ▶ Activity
>
> Can you identify situations when you have been a leader and when you have been a follower?

You might have been a leader during your time at school, as a prefect, sports team captain; or outside school as a Girl Guide, Boy Scout, youth club leader; or even a member of a parent–teacher association. Conversely, you might also have identified those same situations as being times when you were a follower. Similarly, there may be times in your clinical area when you were a follower due to being unsure of yourself; but other times when you were a leader like Sue. 'Followership' is not a passive, unthinking activity. On the contrary, the most valuable follower is a skilled, self-directed team member who participates actively in setting the team direction; invests his/her time and energy in the work of the team; thinks critically and advocates for new ideas (Grossman and Valiga, 2012). Tappen et al. (2004: 5–6) suggest that there are a number of things you can do to become a better follower:

1. If you discover a problem, clearly you would inform your team leader of the problem but you might also offer a suggestion as to how it might be rectified
2. Freely invest your interest and energy in your work
3. Be supportive of new ideas and new directions suggested by others
4. When you disagree with the ideas explain why
5. Listen carefully and reflect on what your leader or manager says
6. Continue to learn as much as you can about your speciality area
7. Share what you learn with others.

If you are to be an effective leader, it is vital that you recognise the opportunities for leadership all around you and that in these situations you act like a leader, influencing others in order to bring about change for a better quality of care provision. Leaders have to face some hard decisions in their work, remembering at all times that managing scarce resources – such as equipment, pharmaceuticals and transport – may not be easy, and that managing people is much more complex.

DEFINING LEADERSHIP

Leadership can be defined in a number of ways but it is still an elusive concept. Indeed, key authors cannot agree on the nature or essential characteristics of leadership but offer a variety of perspectives. This indicates that leadership is thought to be about relationships. Leadership is a discipline that is evolving, indeed Alvesson and Spicer (2010: 4) note the understanding, interpretation and response to leadership is variable and complex. On the one hand, distrust and control are seen as features while, on the other, support and close contact may be dominant. Alongside this, on a more positive note, Rafferty (1993: 3–4) offers up the leadership notion that:

> vision is driven from an emotional front with some practical ability to achieve that vision; leaders inspire you, and others will follow and trust you. They will trust in your integrity. Leaders care for the people they are leading/serving. Leaders try to strengthen and promote these people. They facilitate and help and encourage and praise.

However, Bernhard and Walsh (1995: 17) identify leadership as a process that is 'used to move a group towards goal setting and goal achievement … and can be learned'. Stewart (1996: 3) recognises leadership as discovering the way ahead and encouraging and inspiring others to follow. She agrees with the idea that leadership involves '… *the spirit, personality and vision*'. Rafferty (1993: 3–4) thinks of leaders as people who *'have that combination of conceptual ability'* whilst Daft (2008) expands on this by indicating that leaders allow room for others to grow and change themselves in the process; they also act as facilitators, coaches and servants. Sayle (1993 in Sadler 2003: 33) takes a less dramatic view of leadership – the working leader. A case for the working leader is presented; that is the person who makes the organisation work to the maximum effect. Leadership skills are needed to overcome the bureaucratic contradictions of organisational life.

> ◢ Activity
>
> Can you find a definition that fits in with clinical leadership?

Clinical leadership is a relatively recent term and is seen as being about facilitating evidence-based practice and improved patient outcomes through local care (Millward and Bryan, 2005: xv; Stanley and Sherratt, 2010: 115–121; Anonson et al. 2014: 127–136). Working with common definitions can lead into concept analysis: a deeper process involving antecedents, attributes and consequences being unpacked (Walker and Avant, 2010). At a deeper level, leadership could be seen from various perspectives as being:

- A characteristic trait – based in trait theory
- A position – based in the functional approach
- A quality – based in trait theory
- A process – based in functional approaches
- A power relationship – style, or the effect on group behaviour.

These perspectives will be developed further in Chapter 4. How you view leadership will influence your clinical beliefs, values and behaviours. Leadership must be a part of caring. Patients and patient/clients deserve care that is well led at all levels of the NHS or health industry organisations.

HEALTH CARE – A CHANGING CONTEXT

Due to the driving technological forces and rising expectations, our health service has expanded to encompass a much greater provision than that envisaged when the NHS was set up in 1948. The NHS has its history in a liberal socialist ideology of health being a right for all, regardless of ability to pay. Its current complexity and philosophy has put great emphasis on leadership at all levels. It could also be said that the health service of today is seen by the public almost as a religion or a system of belief. This may be due to the expectation that the health service can cure all ills. The view that health is a much more sought after and accessible commodity is stronger than it was in the past. Sofarelli and Brown (1998) conducted a leadership literature review and then strongly argued for the need to move from the previous bureaucratic NHS management model to a model of a leadership-focused health service. This new model is useful in order to cope with the apparent dramatic change and uncertainty in the health service today. Bishop (2009: xii) noted the emergence of significant policy changes. The Darzi 'Next Stage Review' (DH, 2008a) highlighted the emergence of more clinician-led services, and the critical and main leadership role of clinicians drawn from nursing and allied health professionals. In 2010 the Coalition Government NHS Policy supported this continued perspective (DH, 2010a, 2010b, 2010c). Storey and Holti (2013: 8) advocate a new NHS leadership model that encourages high staff involvement and engagement focusing on meeting service user needs. They highlight the need to manage and improve care with openness to a variety of perspectives including 'soft' intelligence rather than the narrow range of hierarchical imposed targets.

In support of this, nurses and health care practitioners today need specific leadership skills and clinical development in order to help them deal with this rapidly changing situation in clinical care (Barr and Dowding, 2012; Gopee and Galloway, 2014). Indeed, this can relate to all health care professionals as changes are occurring rapidly everywhere. Rippon (2001), however, argued that leadership training per se will not produce the quality of leaders required to bring through change. A more sustainable solution lies with the development of what he terms 'growth cultures' in order to develop leaders with emotional intelligence (Chapter 10). It is emphasised that leaders need to focus on inward rather than outward bound experiences, enabling a spiritual growth based on relationships and awareness (Wright, 2000). 'Inward' could mean greater self-awareness and need for learning whereas 'outward' could relate to expected behaviours. The notion of growth cultures, emotional intelligence and change will be discussed further in Chapters 10, 11 and 13.

GLOBAL LEADERSHIP

The notion of global leadership is a relatively new term which developed in the 1990s (Lobel, 1990; Kets de Vries and Mead, 1992; Pucik et al., 1992; Rhinesmith, 1993; Moran and Riesenberger, 1994; Brake, 1997). The term global encompasses more than simple *geographic reach* in terms of business operations; it can be about the world but is generally thought to be about having '*helicopter vision*', or being '*across*' a number of areas i.e. when a helicopter is on the ground, if the pilot looks down s/he can see only a small circular surface area below the helicopter and has virtually little or no information about the surroundings. The more it goes up the more surface it covers, meaning that the pilot gradually starts to get a clear picture of the ground and surroundings; s/he can see every detail of the area s/he is covering at this stage. The further up it goes, the more information the pilot can get about the area.

Global leadership also includes the notion of *cultural reach* in terms of people and *intellectual reach* in the development of a global mindset (Osland et al., 2006). It can be suggested that it is concerned with the interaction of people and ideas among cultures rather than the efficacy of particular leadership styles demonstrated by particular leaders in their home countries. Global leadership differs from domestic leadership in terms of issues related to connectedness; boundary spanning; complexity; ethical challenges; dealing with tensions and paradoxes; pattern recognition; building learning environments in towns and communities; and leading large scale efforts – across diverse cultures (Osland et al., 2006). You may think of the World Health Organization (WHO) as one organisation that leads on health globally.

> ◆ Activity
>
> Can you think of any situations where a leader might have had a global effect within health care provision?

In terms of world influence you might have thought of Gandhi (political influence), Alexander the Great (military influence), Mother Theresa (spiritual influence) or within health care there are many to consider – Waterlow (2005) and the development of the pressure sore risk assessment tool that is used globally; Roper, Logan and Tierney (1980; 2000) who identified the activities of daily living used for the basis of assessment within the majority of health care provision in the acute sector; or further back in nursing history Florence Nightingale, who worked so hard to get basic nursing practice recognised for the good it did. Within the ambulance service it could have been Dr Millar who introduced the standardisation of training, which again is the foundation for all training within the service and is an idea used to underpin training throughout the world. Today, global health leaders may not be famous but locally there may be Unit Leaders you can think of who have helped generate better practice by *'borrowing'* ideas from other areas in the world to implement in their own practice. Sharing best practice is a very global health activity.

Freshwater (2014: 93–7) distinguishes that leaders need to anticipate challenges, contest the status quo, work towards creativity and diversity, make decisions and learn through reflection and feedback. However 'a really formidable leader is the person who can balance and integrate the caring heart with the global mind'. This perspective highlights that leaders need to attune or resonate with patients and clients who ultimately will be able to receive the outcome of good leadership.

HOW WE SEE OURSELVES AND HOW OTHERS SEE US

In order to move forward in considering our readiness for leadership it might be useful to consider how we see ourselves and more importantly how others see us. The 'Johari Window' (Luft and Ingham, 1955) allows us to see how much the perceptions and knowledge we have about ourselves are also seen by others. The 'Window' has four areas:

Known to self/known to others (Arena)	Not known to self/known to others (Blind Spot)
Known to self/not known to others (Facade)	Not known to self/not known to others (Unknown)

Figure 1.1   Johari Window – the four areas

What is interesting about this is that if you ask your friends or colleagues what they think your characteristics are they often see differing elements to you. By understanding who we are and how others see us we can begin to adapt our behaviours at work to get the best from our teams. Remember this is about you and so there are no correct answers. As we receive feedback from friends we might be able to change any negative elements and also recognise the positive elements of our personalities and adapt to meet the role of leadership, so improving relationships with others within the team.

Recently I met with a student who displayed a lovely disposition, a keenness to learn, who engaged well with reflection but presented with a constant frown on her face, portraying her anxiety to her team and clients. On discussing this perception, which may be seen as her blind spot, the student thought about it and noted that it had come as no surprise; she relayed her daughter had commented on her *'scary face'* in the past. This arena then enabled her to attempt to adjust her persona.

An example of the façade could be that I am basically quite shy but because my role as a leader requires me to speak at meetings, conferences and in class I can overcome the shyness so that the world at large sees me as an ebullient, jovial person. Often when a person puts on their uniform or work clothes they also 'put on' their altered persona.

COMPARING LEADERSHIP AND MANAGEMENT

There appears to be some ambiguity between the notions of leadership and management. Currently the terms *leadership* and *management* may be used interchangeably because the differences between them may not always be straightforward. Most of us think we can recognise leadership but we may not find it easy to find in ourselves.

> ### ➤ Activity
>
> Jot down your ideas of the differences between a manager and leader in health care.

Current thinking indicates that managers have formal authority to direct the work of a given set of employees; they are formally responsible for the quality of that work and what it costs to achieve it. Neither of these elements is necessary to be a leader. Leaders are an essential part of management but the reverse is not true: you do not have to be a manager to be a leader but you do need to be a good leader to be an effective manager. Table 1.1 reflects the differences between leadership and management.

Table 1.1 Differences between leadership and management

Leadership	Management
• Based on influence and sharing	• Based on authority and influence
• An informal role	• A formally designated role
• An achieved position	• An assigned position
• Part of every health care professional's responsibility	• Usually responsible for budgets, hiring and firing people
• Initiative	• Improved by the use of effective leadership skills
• Independent thinking	

The amount of time taken up in leadership activities might differ from person to person (Sadler, 2003). Cunningham (1986, in Sadler, 2003) noted that leadership is an 'integral part' of the management role and as such may not be seen as a separate entity (Figure 1.2). However, Bennis and Nanus (2004) indicate that there are two other models to be considered. They are where leadership is seen as half-and-half of the same concept (Figure 1.3) and where there is partial overlap (Figure 1.4).

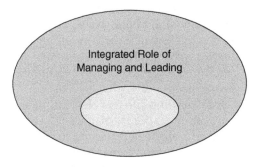

Figure 1.2   Leadership within management

Source: Adapted from Sadler, 2003

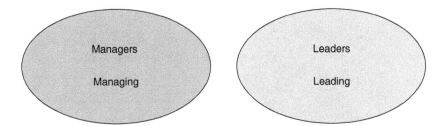

Figure 1.3   Leadership alongside management

Source: Adapted from Sadler, 2003

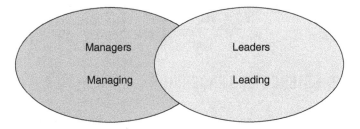

Figure 1.4   Leadership overlapping with management

Source: Adapted from Sadler, 2003

In each case the time taken up by leadership functions will differ. Overall, manage-ment is defined in relation to the achievement of organisational goals in an effective and efficient way. This means that planning, vision, staffing, direction and resources are the main concerns that need to be managed. Managers often seem to have a bad press as *'us and them'* with the *'them'* controlling the *'us'*. It should be remembered that management and leadership should work together to achieve a common aim of effective quality patient care. Dowding and Barr (2002) discuss the potential effects of a wide variety of management approaches on practice. Examining these individually – or in some detail – is not the remit of this book. However, if you consider the history of management approaches, it is evident that the way in which leaders and managers function within the health care system is greatly influenced by the overall management philosophy in place. Miner (2005) suggested that organisational knowledge goes hand in hand with effective management.

Therefore, it is necessary to view the different elements of an organisation in order to understand why it functions in a specific manner (Chapter 11). It can also help to clarify or structure how you might be expected to behave in a given situation in order to uphold the reputation of that organisation. Similarly, it may help us to adopt management practices which, while considered 'old', might be the most appro-priate for a given situation.

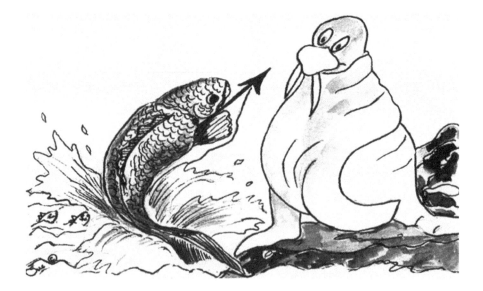

THE ART AND SCIENCE OF LEADERSHIP

Donahue (2011) indicated that nursing has been called the oldest of the arts and the youngest of the professions. Stewart (1918, in Donahue, 2011) goes further to state that the science, spirit and skill of nursing was beginning to develop as it became apparent that love and caring alone could not ensure health or overcome disease.

Nursing education, in the past, has concentrated on the science element or *'medical model'*, whereby nurses were told what to learn and when to learn it in relation to the disease and the disease process. More recently, it was recognised that the patient is unique and not just a collection of symptoms. Nursing then became more 'art' focused concentrating on holism rather than being medical/science focused, concentrating on the disease process. This has now changed to include a holistic approach, not only to deliver care in relation to a specific condition but also to include the family and regular carers. However, health care professionals need to recognise the strength of their medical knowledge as health technology advances in order to provide health education to the patients and their families. For leadership, the notion of science and art must go hand in hand in order to respect the uniqueness of the patient and their health condition.

The concept of leadership has evolved over the last century and continues to change. That isn't to say that the old ways of doing things are not good but that in today's health business society there are different ways of getting things done; ways that enable 'management' and 'leadership' to work together. Leadership is both an art and a science. It is an art because of the many skills and qualities that cannot be learned via a textbook; a science because of the growing body of knowledge that describes the leadership process, leadership skills and the application of these elements within a given practice area. Knowing about leadership theories allows us to analyse situations from a variety of perspectives, to understand the importance of leading an organisation to success and to suggest well-thought-out alternatives to enhance a quality practice. Studying leadership gives you skills that can be applied not only within the workplace but also in your everyday life. This book will lead you through a variety of situations as an individual and a member of a corporate body.

Summary of Key Points

This chapter has briefly looked at various aspects of leadership in order to meet the identified learning outcomes. These were:

- **Discuss the notions of leadership and followership** This was achieved by examining how you might already be a leader in some situations and a follower in others. Also, we examined how a variety of writers have described leadership, so that you can select the definition that comes closest to your own perception of the role. The use of the Johari Window will help you to recognise your attributes and weaknesses so making you a better leader.
- **Define leadership** By selecting and understanding the multifaceted nature of leadership the benefits of effective leadership were examined: as Daft (2005: 4–5) said, 'leadership is an emerging discipline that will evolve'. Don't expect to get it right

(Continued)

(Continued)

every time but with knowledge of the leadership theory you might get it right some of the time.

- **Discuss the importance of the changing context related to health care** The National Health Service (NHS) emerged due to a socialist ideology of health being a right for all, regardless of ability to pay. Leadership within the health service has always been seen as important because of the size of the NHS and the changing policy and practices. Global leadership as a notion has also been explored.
- **Compare leadership and management** This perennial argument related to the differences (or not) between leaders and managers. Much of the problem in understanding the concepts relates to the fact that the two philosophies are so closely linked and the words used are interchangeable, hence the possible lack of differentiation when we think and speak of leaders.
- **Debate the art and science of leadership** Stewart (1918) highlights that the science, spirit and skill of health practice was beginning to develop as it became apparent that love and caring alone could not ensure health or overcome disease.

FURTHER READING

Adair, J. (2010a) *Effective Leadership: Masterclass*. London: Kogan Page.

Adair, J. (2010b) *Effective Strategic Leadership*. London: Pan Books.

Adair, J. (2011) *Effective Leadership: How to be a Successful Leader*. London: Pan Books.

Adair, J. (2013) *Confucius on Leadership*. London: Macmillan.

Bower, F. (2000) *Nurses Taking the Lead: Personal Qualities of Leadership*. Philadelphia, PA: WB Saunders Company.

Cook, M.J. (2001) 'The attributes of effective clinical nurse leaders', *Nursing Standard*, 15 (35): 33–6.

Cook, M.J. and Leathard, H. (2004) 'Learning for clinical leadership', *Journal of Nursing Management*, 12 (6): 436–44.

Elias, R. (2010) 'How personality affects leadership', *Independent Nurse*, 22: 40–1.

Mahoney, J. (2001) 'Leadership skills for the 21st century', *Journal of Nursing Management*, 9: 269–71.

Northouse, P.G. (2012) *Leadership Theory and Practice* (6th edn). London: Sage.

Sadler, P. (2003) *Leadership MBA Masterclass* (2nd edn). London: Kogan Page.

Stanley, D. and Sherratt, A. (2010) 'Lamp light on leadership: clinical leadership and Florence Nightingale', *Journal of Nursing Management*, 18: 115–21.

Visit the companion website at https://study.sagepub.com/barr3e for more resources.

2 WHAT MAKES A LEADER?

Learning Outcomes

By the end of this chapter you will have had the opportunity to:

- Recognise the importance of clinical leaders in health care
- Reflect on personal experiences of leaders in clinical practice
- Develop self-awareness
- Develop practice mastery through evidence-based practice.

INTRODUCTION

In Chapter 1, the concept of leadership was examined. It is now appropriate to scrutinise some of the experiences related to some of the leaders we have met in clinical practice. Highlighting the ideology related to clinical leaders in health care will lead us into the characteristics of a leader. Discussion related to leaders met in practice will lead on to a consideration of the possible reasons for their actions. In order to investigate one's own abilities, various tools are provided which you may use; these tools will be available and the results discussed prior to conclusions being drawn. The notion of practice mastery and the need for evidence-based practice will be addressed as the chapter concludes.

CLINICAL LEADERS IN HEALTH CARE

Globally, health care has the same complex issues whether it is in a developed, developing or underdeveloped country. In Britain, the NHS has been led by a succession of governments, with manifestos which addressed their vision for improving the health service.

Historically, health care was built on a system of vocational leaders such as doctors, nurses, midwives and ambulance technicians who used 'care and cure' methods to help people get better. Leadership has more recently been seen as important because of the size of the NHS. It was the largest European employer with 1.3 million employees (NHS Jobs, 2014) and was hailed as the third largest world industry after the Red Army in China and the Indian Railway. However it is now in fifth position (with 1.7 million employees) after McDonalds, Walmart/Asda and the Chinese military with the US Department of Defence at the top (BBC, 2012).

The current economic climate requires public services to be managed more efficiently – especially in the area of staffing and in the light of the ongoing burden of pensions in the UK. The context of public service effectiveness however is paramount. Clinical leadership, as well as educational and research leadership, is required in the health service to respond to the demands of society for the future. Thompson and Hyrkas (2014) have gone further to promote the need for *global leadership* strategies for high quality health services in terms of empowerment, competency development and excellent leadership including patient and workforce safety issues in the context of globalisation. Excellent leadership is often perceived in the skills and characteristics of those who lead teams.

CHARACTERISTICS OF A LEADER

Maxwell (1999) maintains that there are 21 indispensable qualities of a leader. They are listed in Table 2.1.

> ## Activity
> • Rank these qualities in the order you think most important.
> • Justify why you believe in their importance.

Table 2.1 Indispensable qualities of a leader (Maxwell, 1999)

Character	Charisma	Commitment
Communication	Competence	Courage
Discernment	Focus	Generosity
Initiative	Listening	Passion
Positive Attitude	Problem Solving	Relationships
Responsibility	Security	Self-discipline
Servanthood	Teachability	Vision

Although it can be seen that the skills required are far reaching, they need a great deal of thought and discussion from a personal perspective. The following can be highlighted:

- *Character:* The disposition, quality or calibre of ability a person has is important. For instance, the way an individual handles a clinical emergency will either create respect or distrust for future events. Maxwell (1999: 5) highlights a saying that states: 'If you think you are leading and no one is following you, then you're only taking a walk.'
- *Charisma:* This is about making others feel good about themselves by trying to see the best in others rather than concentrating on their faults. Napoleon Bonaparte called leaders 'dealers in hope' (Maxwell, 1999: 11). Whenever you meet someone new, try to make a good impression by doing things like remembering their name. Do it every day and it will increase your charisma, as people will recognise that you care about their feelings.
- *Communication:* This element is vital, as good leaders must be able to share their knowledge and ideas with others in order to achieve organisational goals. Getting people to work together requires good communication, so without good communication you travel alone. Be clear in your writing and speaking but also be aware of the need for active listening. Giuliani (2002) (New York Mayor at the time of the 9/11 attacks) describes a successful leader as someone who is able to develop and communicate strong beliefs, accept responsibility, surround themselves with strong people but also to study, read and learn independently. Sullivan and Garland (2010: 23) concur with this, noting 'the leader is anyone who uses interpersonal skills to influence others to accomplish a specific goal'. It can be seen then that the position a member of staff holds in the organisational structure is associated with a particular pattern of expected behaviour and may be related to others' expectations of that role.
- *Passion:* If, as Nightingale, Seacole and Millar demonstrated, you have a passion for your profession it is usually met with a positive response. The impossible might become possible. Passion is contagious; I recall hearing Beverly Malone, General Secretary of the Royal College of Nursing (2001–2006), speaking about the power to care in nursing at a theatre nurses' conference, and how much

power nurses hold even if they think they don't. The passion for nursing she imparted was terrific; I became excited about my profession again (as did most of the audience).

- *Servanthood:* Maxwell (1999: 133) asserts that you have to love your people more than your position, thus being a servant leader. This is not a low skilled activity – it is about attitude. A true leader serves people by ensuring that their best interests are maintained. Maxwell (1999: 138) further states that effective servanthood will be attained if the leader can:

Stop lording it over people and *start* listening to them;

Stop role-playing for advancement and *start* risking for others' benefit;

Stop seeking your own way and *start* serving others.

It seems that today you cannot open a journal related to any industry without leadership, in some context, leaping out at you. This is because we are currently in a state of change, which is moving the business of organisations from the 'old style' management approach, emphasising stability and control, to a more rational approach which purports to encourage effective leadership that values change, empowerment and relationships. The management of change is another subject area to consider in order to understand how effective leadership can enhance the change process (Chapter 13).

There is more recent debate about which of these characteristics are seen as innate personality traits, which are seen as learned skills and the processes and outcomes involved in leadership (Northouse, 2012) which will be discussed later. The characteristics of a good leader also include the ability to use interpersonal skills to engender trust among the team members as they address and work through change. In an organisation without a clear mindset a leader will not have the ability to be effective; John F. Kennedy intimated that you cannot know you have arrived if you don't know where you are going, which indicates that planning, passion and vision are vital.

EXPERIENCES OF LEADERS IN CLINICAL PRACTICE

When we think about our own clinical experiences in the context of leaders, we may think about role models and people we aspire to become. Qualitative research through in-depth personal interviews in Canada by Anonson et al. (2014) on perceptions of frontline staff regarding exemplary nurse leadership found the key common characteristics were:

- a passion for nursing
- a sense of optimism
- the ability to form personal connections with their staff
- excellent role modelling and mentorship
- an ability to manage a crisis while guided by a set of moral principles.

On reflection, we remembered three particular people in our own professional experience and they were all quite different.

1. *Charge Nurse A* 'ran' the medical ward and linked to a CCU. It was my first nursing experience and I had nothing else to compare it with. He was a quiet but very efficient manager. I have to say I do not remember his presence very much, but there was a very happy team spirit, with each part of the hierarchy supporting and teaching others. There was a sense of belonging because individuals were able to contribute their ideas of how tasks might be completed; also they were able to suggest how things might be 'done better'. From memory, the care on the ward was excellent and he set and monitored the standards. In those days it was task-driven duties. There were constant emergencies but the team felt a sense of achievement at the end of the long shifts.

2. *Sister B* ran a surgical ward. Again the mode of working was that of task allocation but the ward was run with precision, in a military style. Everyone knew their allocated job, what was expected of them and the time frame in which they had to function. I recall being quite scared by Sister and would never dream of speaking to her unless she spoke to me first. Although this placement was very intimidating at times, it was happy and the patients all felt that they were getting the best care possible in a very efficient and effective way; and the staff felt that they had done a 'good' job when they completed their shifts, however difficult it might have been.

3. *Sister C* by comparison was quite disorganised; nobody knew what was going on, what they were supposed to be doing and often there were panic situations where something had to be done all of a rush. Sister used to shout a lot when things were not done but, unless we were at 'panic stage', didn't tell us what we were supposed to be doing. Many people work in a frenzied panicky way because that is how their mind works, but in a leadership situation it is imperative that all members of the team know what is going on and so it is vital that there is a degree of organisation.

Each of these leaders, in their own way, demonstrated their own style. Two were far more effective than the third but each presented communication skills at differing levels. Indeed, Starns (2000) highlights the militarisation policy adopted in early British nursing history. Dame Katherine Jones, the first Matron-in-Chief, wanted to link the registered nurse with the military 'officer classes'; she felt that the registered nurse status would be further secured by imposing the Army framework and style on civilian nursing. This might reflect the actions and leadership style of Sister B.

Lewin et al. (1939) originally identified three main leadership styles:

- Laissez-faire – little direction or facilitation approach (Sullivan and Garland, 2010: 60)
- Autocratic – directive and controlling (Tappen et al., 2004: 7)
- Democratic – participative and encouraging collaborative teamwork (Gopee and Galloway, 2009: 55).

> ### ◆ Activity
>
> What style of leadership do you think Charge Nurse A and Sister C used?

Charge Nurse A appeared to be rather participative or democratic, while Sister C used a laissez-faire style.

Lewin's categories have been used extensively since 1939. Wider categorisation of leadership styles are diverse and may include:

- **Coercive:** using many sanctions and few rewards; gives directives rather than directions; useful for simple, straightforward tasks.
- **Authoritative:** has clear vision and provides long-term direction; is prepared to justify and take responsibility for the direction; useful where there is a clear aim and people are buying into it.
- **Affiliative:** aims to avoid conflict and develop harmony; avoids confrontation; useful for getting to know people and how things are done around the organisation.
- **Democratic:** encourages participation and seeks consensus; aims to seek commitment through ownership; sometimes useful when the leader is not clear about the most appropriate direction.
- **Pacesetting:** focuses on task accomplishment to a high level of excellence; tends to take the lead; useful in managing change.
- **Coaching:** encourages the development of others; identifies strengths and weaknesses; useful for long-term development of people and the organization (Chapter 10). (National Professional Qualification for Headship (NPQH), 2005)

It is perceived that the most effective leadership style is that exhibited by democratic leaders. However, it should be remembered that one style will not be adopted for all occasions but that a mixture of styles will be required, depending on the situation.

LEADERSHIP AND FOLLOWERSHIP STYLES

Having noted that there are a variety of clinical leadership styles, it would be useful to analyse one's own ability as a leader but also as a follower. Daft (2010) suggests that leaders who demonstrate an awareness of their rationality as well as their emotion-driven impulses learn to trust their instincts and realise that these feelings can provide useful information about difficult leadership decisions. So in order to be successful, leaders must also look inwards to their hopes and dreams. Part of preparedness for leadership might be to test what sort of style you prefer as a leader by taking a Leadership and Followership Test of the type described by Frew (1977).

This test helps you understand how and why both you and your colleagues react within a particular situation. As a potential leader, this information can help you to develop and become more effective.

ASSESSING YOUR ABILITIES/SKILLS

As well as using the Leadership and Followership Style Test set out on the companion website there are other ways of identifying your own abilities. One of these is SWOT analysis; this is a technique attributed to Ansoff (1987) but may have originated from the work of Albert Humphrey in the 1960s. It has long been thought of as an admirable way of identifying both individual and organisational Strengths, Weaknesses, Opportunities and Threats (SWOT) (Table 2.2). Tappen et al. (2004) indicate that, on an individual level, borrowing the SWOT tool from the corporate world can guide you through your own internal strengths and weaknesses, providing an analysis of external opportunities and threats that might help you in your job search or career planning.

SWOT analysis is always a useful exercise to undertake and even keep within your professional portfolio. It can be used when applying for a new position or course as it clearly highlights your attributes and how they can be matched against the criteria for the position or course entry. It can also be a basis for the additional information requested during your annual Development and Performance Review (DPR). Together with identifying internal individual strengths and weaknesses, an external situational analysis can identify how threats might be changed to opportunities in order to enhance individual and organisational performance.

Table 2.2 SWOT analysis

Strengths	Weaknesses
• Skills • Qualifications • Life experiences • Professional experiences • Punctual • Hardworking • 'Fit' with the job description	• Age • Gender • Skills; Experience • Time keeping • Planning/organisation • Narrow/broad focus
Opportunities	**Threats**
To be able to rectify: • Insufficient appropriate skills • Insufficient appropriate experience • Insufficient appropriate knowledge	• 'Fit' with the job description • Training • Career development • New courses • New experience

On a wider institutional/organisational level this tool can also be used to identify where weaknesses might be addressed in order to increase the efficiency and economy of an organisation. As we hear of some NHS Trusts getting into financial, staffing and environmental difficulties, the thought given to SWOT analysis may assist in changing practices in significant areas.

PROBLEM SOLVING STYLES: THE MYERS-BRIGGS TYPE INDICATOR® (MBTI®)

Another point for consideration when leaders are being appointed relates to problem-solving styles. For many, the Myers-Briggs Type Indicator® (1995) is one tool for identifying ways in which individuals differ in gathering and evaluating information for problem solving and making decisions. (Myers-Briggs Type Indicator®, Myer-Briggs®, MBTI® and the MBTI logo® are all trademarks or registered trademarks of the Myer-Briggs Type Indicator Trust in the United States and other countries.)

Four dimensions are considered within the tool, each of which has two polar aspects.

1. **Introvert (I) – Extrovert (E):** This dimension focuses on where people gain interpersonal strength and mental energy. Extroverts gain energy from being around and interacting with others, whereas introverts gain energy by focusing on personal thoughts and feelings.

Table 2.3 Extrovert/introvert dimensions

	Positive Impact	Negative Impact
Extrovert	Spreads energy, enthusiasm	Loud mouth, does not include other people
Introvert	Thoughtful, gives space to others	Nothing worth saying? Uneasy networker

2. **Sensing (S) – Intuition (N):** This identifies how a person absorbs information. Those with a sensing preference gather and absorb information through the five senses, whereas intuitive people rely on less direct perceptions. Intuitivists, for example, focus more on patterns, relationships and hunches than on direct perception of facts and details.

Table 2.4 Sensing/intuition dimensions

	Positive Impact	Negative Impact
Sensing	Practical, concrete, detailed	Dull, unimaginative
Intuition	Creative, imaginative	Flighty, impractical, unrealistic

3. **Thinking (T) – Feeling (F):** This dimension relates to how much consideration a person gives to emotions in making a decision. Feeling types tend to rely more on their values and sense of what is right and wrong, and they consider how a specific decision will affect other's feelings. Thinking types tend to rely more on logic and are very objective in the decision making process.

Table 2.5 Thinking/feeling dimensions

	Positive Impact	Negative Impact
Thinking	Logical, rational, intellectual	Cold and heartless
Feeling	Empathetic, understanding	Soft-headed, fuzzy thinker, bleeding heart

4. **Judging (J) – Perceiving (P):** This dimension concerns an individual's attitudes toward ambiguity and how quickly a person can make a decision. People with a judging preference like certainty and closure. They enjoy having goals and deadlines and tend to make decisions quickly based on available data. Perceiving people, conversely, enjoy ambiguity, dislike deadlines and may change their minds several times before making a final decision. Perceiving types like to gather a large amount of data information before making a decision.

Table 2.6 Judging/perceiving dimensions

	Positive Impact	Negative Impact
Judging	High work ethic, focused and reliable	Compulsive neat freak, uptight, rigid, rule bound
Perceiving	Work–life balance, enjoys work	Lazy, messy, aimless and unreliable

Clearly from these four dimensions 16 unique personality types can be identified. Owen (2009: 4) suggests that there is no 'leader type' but there are tentative suggestions that leaders are equally divided between extrovert and introvert types. Leaders – in the main – are intuitive, feeling and judging (that is, ENFJ or INFJ).

Activity

- Try the *example personality test* to see what sort of personality you or your colleagues might exhibit.
- You may want to compare the results with the Jung and Myers-Briggs typology test found on the internet site www.humanmetrics.com/cgi-win/jtypes2.asp (accessed 28 August 14).
- Consider what these results tell you about how you are perceived.
- Do you think your personality type is correct?

Lesley remembers completing a personality assessment and thinking how accurate the assessment was (she was ISTJ), even though she hadn't given the questions much thought. Within clinical practice she found that knowledge of her personality type gave her a greater insight into how she interacted with both patients and colleagues. It made her more aware of how other people worked so that when they were asked to complete a job they went about it in their own way and not necessarily the way she would have done. "*I was probably using my 'emotional intelligence' before it became a leadership construct*" she said. Greater discussion related to EI (Goleman, 1995) takes place in Chapter 10.

More recently she undertook the Jung/Myers-Briggs test which provided an SJTI result. Jill on the other hand has an ENFJ Myers-Briggs (MBTI®) test result. Interestingly, in terms of writing this book, one author sees themself as a linear thinker and the other thinks in circles, arrows and flamboyant diagrams; we see that each style is valued and feel we complement each other's strengths and weaknesses by being able to see and work from different creative perspectives. Effective teams need a variety of personality types otherwise conflict, complacency and apathy might occur.

REFLECTIVE PRACTITIONER

Increasingly, we are asked to maintain a personal professional profile (Nursing and Midwifery Council (NMC), 2008; Health and Care Professions Council (HCPC) (2013a)), the purpose of this record usually being to fulfil Post Registration Education and Practice (PREP) (NMC, 2008; HCPC, 2013a) requirements by providing evidence of activities undertaken to update knowledge and practice. In order to do this effectively we should utilise a model of reflection. There are many identified within the literature; however, the one selected must be understandable, useable, effective and fit for the intended purpose. Schön (1987) differentiated between reflection-in-action and reflection-on-action; in later literature he also talks of reflection-before-action. Each of these indicates when reflection should take place, that is, before, in or on action. It is thought that reflection-before-action is likely when the practitioner has met a specific situation before and draws on past memories and records in order to influence the way in which the current situation is handled. In-action, on the other hand, is normally limited as the need to act quickly in complex situations is paramount; by comparison on-action takes place once the incident has been dealt with and assists the practitioner to gain insights and make amendments as necessary.

The simplest of reflective cyclical models linked to experiential learning has been proposed by Driscoll (2007) based on ideas by Borton (1970) which identified three simple questions that can be related to healthcare practice.

- What?
- So what?
- Now what?

Activity

Can you use Driscoll's model and explore a recent and significant health care episode or event in which you were involved? Write notes on each of the 'boxed' stages.

Another reflective model often used in health care is one that is described by Gibbs (1988) (Figure 2.1) wherein a series of similar but possibly more academic questions are posed; Johns' (1995) model (Figure 2.2) builds on the questions posed by Gibbs but adds other dimensions e.g. Influencing Factors and Learning.

Whatever model is used, by answering the questions in order one can work through an experience, learn by it and review it later. Reflection is an excellent process by which to learn and this is most certainly the case for the newly emerging leader. In order to become effective it is useful to analyse critically any situation, taking care to discover the parts that can be improved upon. Taylor (2010), when talking of the value of reflection, notes that there are three main kinds of reflection:

1. technical (based on scientific method and rationale)
2. practical (leads to interpretation, description and explanation of human interaction)
3. emancipatory (leads to transformative action)

which are categorised according to the kind of knowledge they involve and the work interests they represent. Each type is important in developing the effective practitioner within the clinical area.

Activity

- Think about what reflection means to you.
- To what extent does your definition agree with that of the authors mentioned here or in other books you have read?
- Keep a record of your thoughts to refer back to as you progress in your career.

I normally use a mixture of Gibbs' and John's models of reflection to consider the direction of my career, identifying what I want to change and what I am doing well. It is a way of moving forward. It does, however, feel a bit cumbersome at times but once you are used to using a model of reflection – and reflecting on action – it goes a long way to improving practice.

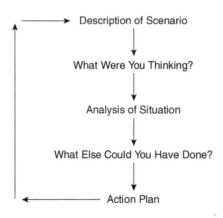

Description of Scenario

What Were You Thinking?

Analysis of Situation

What Else Could You Have Done?

Action Plan

Figure 2.1   Feedback loop as a model of reflection

Adapted from Gibbs, G. (1988) *Learning by Doing: A Guide to Teaching and Learning Methods.*
Further Education Unit: Oxford Polytechnic.

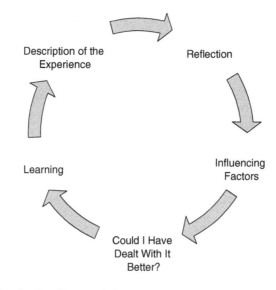

Description of the
Experience

Reflection

Influencing
Factors

Could I Have
Dealt With It
Better?

Learning

Figure 2.2   Johns' reflective model

Republished with permission of John Wiley and Sons

PRACTICE MASTERY – EVIDENCE-BASED PRACTICE

There is a need for evidence-based practice within nursing, midwifery and health care
generally (Pearson et al., 1997; Shorten and Wallace, 1997; Steffaleno and Carlson,
2010; NMC, 2015). This could be considered as saying that health care practice

should be based on effective research rather than rituals, traditions and whims. It is this evidence-based movement that is testing the validity of long-standing procedures, seeking to replace them with newer, research-based ones.

Being able to master your own specific professional practice may come after many years in a clinical area. On occasion time can be lost when you put yourself in the hands of others to direct your professional development. Often when people look back, they realise that they could have reached career fulfilment much earlier, if they had relied on their own determination. 'Self-mastery' is about empowering *yourself* to reach your own goals and dreams. This is related to the seminal work of the Harvard professor of business and nurse researcher Kanter (1983, 1991, 1993) which is still held as important in our world of health care practice. Kanter's theory of structural power in organisations suggested that knowing and realising an individual's full potential, rediscovering new ways and insights towards taking actions, will enable personal goals to be achieved. Laschinger (2010) used the work of Kanter to link the empowerment of the health professional to the empowerment of the patient for better health outcomes. Bennis et al. (1994) identified that we all have a large amount of untapped potential which can be used within the work situation to achieve personal growth and mastery. Self-mastery is about being driven by vision and also being able to act as a focaliser, a facilitator, a synergiser as well as a co-creator, learner and shaper.

In terms of professional practice, mastery is about continuously focusing on trying to improve your own skills and knowledge. What do you want to learn today?

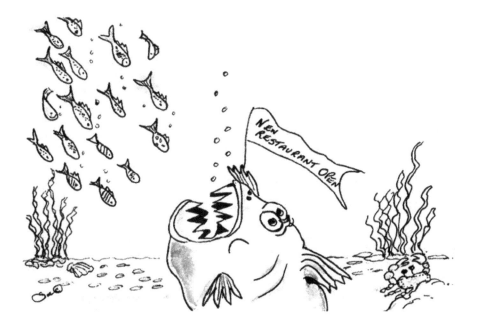

What skills do you want to gain this week, this month, this year? What achievements have you planned for the next five years? Being a 'master' in your particular practice means there is no chance to stay still. Along with new skills, the ability to critically understand how these skills benefit patients and clients, and how they can be improved, is all part of searching and mastering the evidence base underpinning practice.

Summary of Key Points

This chapter has briefly looked at various aspects of leadership in order to meet the identified learning outcomes. These were:

- **Recognise the importance of clinical leaders in health care** We all learn from observation of our role models.
- **Reflect on personal experiences of leaders in clinical practice** We will learn things that we will not wish to repeat in our practice setting and at the same time there will be elements that we would wish to carry forward.
- **Develop self-awareness** The development of self-awareness through the use of tools such as SWOT analysis and the leadership–followership tools can only serve to enhance the care you offer as well as your career prospects.
- **Develop practice mastery through evidence-based practice** In all professions it is important to ensure that the care offered is current and based on reliable evidence. It is only in this way that we can develop mastery of our individual professions.

FURTHER READING

Adams, C. (2010) 'What leadership skills will community nurses need to improve outcomes in the new NHS?', *Nursing Times*, 106 (48): 10–12.

Jasper, M., Rosser, M. and Mooney, G. (2013) *Professional Development, Reflection and Decision-Making in Nursing and Healthcare* (2nd edn). Chichester: Wiley-Blackwell.

Manion, J. (2011) *From Management to Leadership: Strategies for Transforming Health* (3rd edn). San Francisco, CA: Jossey-Bass.

Reynolds, J. and Rogers, A. (2002) 'Leadership styles and situations', *Nursing Management*, 9 (10): 27–30.

Rocchiccioli, J.T. and Tilbury, M.S. (1998) *Clinical Leadership in Nursing*. Philadelphia, PA: WB Saunders Co Ltd.

Silberman, M. (2007) *The Handbook of Experiential Learning*. San Francisco, CA: John Wiley and Sons Inc.

Tappen, R.M. (1995) *Nursing Leadership and Management* (3rd edn). Philadelphia, PA: F.A. Davis.

Taylor, B. (2010) *Reflective Practice for Health Care Professionals: A Practical Guide* (3rd edn). Maidenhead: Open University Press.

Wedderburn, T.C. (1999) *Leadership in Nursing*. London: Churchill Livingstone.

Visit the companion website at https://study.sagepub.com/barr3e for more resources.

3   CULTURE, DIVERSITY AND VALUES

Learning Outcomes

By the end of this chapter you will have had the opportunity to:

- Examine the breadth of the concept of culture
- Discuss the importance of cultural diversity influencing health and health care
- Discuss leadership in the context of cultural diversity
- Examine the theoretical models of transcultural care
- Critically reflect on personal transcultural care and leading the culturally diverse.

INTRODUCTION

It is essential that leaders recognise the importance of health care individuality; how it relates to the delivery of health care to patients and clients as well as to the uniqueness of staff team members. Health care professionals (and their leaders) bring a richness of individuality into the relationships they have with their patients. We will discuss the value of trait theory and the variety of personality characteristics that are valued in actual and potential leaders (Chapter 4 explores this further). In terms of your own self awareness, a number of self-evaluation exercises such as Myers-Briggs® (1995) can help to highlight differences. Whether we are more reserved or extrovert than others can help us recognise how these can be used as leadership strengths. The value of individuality, however, cannot be isolated from the roles and responsibilities required within an organisation such as the health service. Regardless of individual differences in staff, patients and clients will also want to understand what they can expect as a standard of care from the health care staff involved. This chapter will attempt to relate the notion of cultural diversity and values in the present climate of public accountability.

WHAT IS CULTURE?

Culture is an important aspect of diversity within the health service. For example, if people from foreign countries, who do not speak English, require health care there will be a barrier to accessing the correct services; this has implications for the health care professional in supporting these patients and clients. So what do we mean by culture, though? Sardar and Van Loon (1997: 4–5) noted several definitions of 'culture', such as one by anthropologist Tylor (1832–1917):

> Culture is that complex whole which includes knowledge, belief, art, morals, law, customs and other capabilities and habits acquired by man as a member of society. (Tylor, 1871: 1)

Another writer, Mead (1970 in Sardar and Van Loon, 1997), noted that 'culture is a learned behaviour of a society or a sub-group'; it is therefore difficult to agree a basic overall definition as culture encompasses many different things. Cultural concepts will vary according to where you live and work or whatever your social context is. This means that culture supports how individuals assemble into sub-groups within society. What kind of different cultures can we see represented in health service staff? Cortis (2003) points to diversity differences in a broad classification of ability, age, ethnicity, gender, religion and sexuality. At a deeper level, culture can be seen as not just group identity but also as a way of determining deeper notions of acceptable behaviour:

- Values
- Attitudes
- Beliefs
- Ideas
- Behaviours.

These factors are important for individual human development. The 'worldview' of different societal groups helps individuals in defining themselves to form values related to their lives and the world they live in. This gives a sense of identity, belonging and self-worth in order to be mutually supportive and to survive in society (Kagawa-Singer and Chung, 1994; Leininger, 1997). Kelly-Heidenthal (2004) identifies a model reflecting the ways people differ (Table 3.1).

Table 3.1 Characteristics of culture (Kelly-Heidenthal, 2004)

- Culture is both learned and taught
- Culture is shared
- Culture is social in nature
- Culture is dynamic and adaptive

The development of multiculturalism, for example eastern European, black and ethnic minority people living alongside a predominantly indigenous population, is a relatively recent feature in the UK. Many people describe a feeling of 'twoness', where they live in two worlds: one life at home and the other at work. They sometimes find themselves striving to adopt cultural behaviours and attitudes that will help them to be successful in a multicultural country, while at the same time maintaining ties to their racial and ethnic community and culture. This leads to the development of sociocultural skills and attitudes as they integrate both the dominant culture and their own (Daft, 2005: 446).

Culture and health are linked as a functional aspect in society and relate to the influence of the values, beliefs and practises of promoting one's own health and illness prevention. Culture thus gives reason for causation, detection and treatment/care of the ill and the well in order to determine social roles, expectations and relationships (Spector, 2002). Cultural behaviour can be recognised in our society through the various transparent dress codes, eating habits, music tastes or attendance at different social gatherings outside work such as the theatre, the mosque, the tennis or golf club, night club or, even, the hen/stag weekend. On the one hand, some of these exhibited behaviours can give an individual a sense of belonging; on the other hand, they may be seen as a superficial cultural identity that may lead to discrimination from outside groups.

Case 1

Paul is a 30-year-old man who is HIV positive. He lives with his partner at 23 Lee Street. Paul is dying from an AIDS-related illness. A community nurse has been asked to visit in order to provide support. Upon arrival at the flat, the nurse discovers Paul's partner is dressed up as a female, with lipstick and make-up. A group of gay friends are there, wearing gay pride T shirts, chanting songs, making speeches and playing music.

The nurse orders them to be quiet while she carries out an assessment. She becomes cross when they don't stop and asks them to have some respect for Paul while she tries to talk to him. Eventually she is able to proceed and finish her paperwork.

On her return to the health centre, she comments to her colleagues on what she describes as 'the nonsense' going on at 23 Lee Street, stating that 'these people have such weird behaviour'.

Case 2

Mrs Polaski is a 77-year-old lady who lives in her own three-bedroom, semi-detached house. All her relatives live outside the area and she only sees them when they come to visit on special occasions. Mrs Polaski's neighbour regularly visits to 'keep an eye' on her, doing her shopping and collecting her pension and helping her out generally.

Following a recent fall she was admitted to hospital. In planning for her discharge, the assessment team advised Mrs Polaski that she should really make arrangements to move into a residential home, where she would be safer. The patient responded by saying that she intended to stay at home as her neighbour was happy to look in and help her out. The Nurse advised Mrs Polaski that it was unfair to expect a neighbour to take on all that responsibility. Mrs Polaski then refused to discuss it further but the assessment team recorded that they recommended that the patient needed residential care.

Activity

- Identify and jot down issues that are unfair and hence discriminatory in these two case studies.
- Provide an alternative response that would help to promote anti-discriminatory practice in care delivery.
- You may wish to use these questions for discussion with colleagues.

You may have thought that in both cases scant regard was given to either Paul's or Mrs Polaski's right to live in the way they wished. Both of these people were regarded as different. While the nurse visiting Paul may have been quite correct in asking for – not ordering – some quiet, it was wrong of her to pass comments about 'the nonsense' when she got back to the health centre. Of course, one could say that it is human nature to discuss the 'unusual' with one's colleagues. It is important to recognise, though, that the way Paul's friends dress is irrelevant to the care offered. Similarly, while Mrs Polaski was made aware of the possible problems of her staying at home, and this could be documented, her personal views on her choices should also be aired, discussed and documented. It is easy to think that cultures are made up of people who are all the same and that they never change characteristics. However, it is important to see the diversity of deeper values even between people who have a common identity. The values and beliefs held by student nurses, the local Muslim community, members of an Elton John fan club, or members of a city football club may be quite different.

Activity

Write down the obvious differences between individuals in your present working team.

If you found this difficult, raise one of the following issues in your work group and then a social group and note the various perspectives:

- Terrorist laws
- Endemic Ebola
- Speed cameras
- The wearing of ethnic associated dress/behaviour
- Immigration controls at airports.

Think back to when your team discussed an issue raised on the radio or in the paper and try to identify the various value statements that individuals made and how they differed from one another. Usually these are very emotive issues and can highlight not only people's values but also their difficulties with other groups in society. Generational, class and gender differences will underpin the diversity of values. Religious and ethnic group beliefs and values will all change over time. For instance, ideas concerning international issues, such as the ideologies in some of the global war zones or various new reproductive technologies such as cloning, can vary considerably even in one cultural section of society. Despite noting the differences in various cultures, Mulholland (1995) highlights the mistake in thinking that differences in minority groups are more important than similarities with other minority groups. It is, therefore, useful actively to engage in looking for similarities between different cultures.

DIVERSITY OF VALUES IN HEALTH CARE

It was during the late 1980s that diversity research began to appear and influence management literature. Normally health care is delivered by a team of people engaged in a variety of professions. The make-up and ability of these teams to function well together depends on a good working relationship being built up. It poses the question – How similar and how different should the team members be? It could be argued that where there are more similarities than differences the team may function effectively but not be proactive; however, the wider diversity perspectives may, in time, offer a broader knowledge base potentially leading to greater innovation. Borrill et al. (2000) found that the greater the number of professional groups represented in the team, the higher the level of innovation in patient care. Jackson (1996) describes two differing diversities as being either task related (organisational position or specialised technical knowledge) or relations oriented (age, gender, social status and personality) whilst Mathieu et al. (2008) elaborates and offers three definitions of diversity as being functional, personality and demographic diversity.

Recognising diversity creates a tolerance for the richness of values in our society as a whole but, on the negative side, can lead to the development of stereotypical ideas of people who don't belong to our specific subgroup. It is important to recognise the main cultural groups where adverse reactions occur in relationships at work and particularly in the health service. The main cultural groups affected, as suggested by social research, are: ethnicity, age and gender. Leaders and teams therefore need always to be aware of the diversity of values in working relationships and should seek to be sensitive and responsive to that diversity (Marquis and Huston, 2014).

ETHNIC DIVERSITY

Ethnic diversity is a beautiful thing; it allows people to get to know one another and share cultural aspects and enhances tolerance between groups. It can reduce the chances of developing prejudice, racism and phobias depending on the level of exposure a person is receiving when venturing to different destinations and experiencing a variety of unique cultures. Ethnicity has been defined in many ways but is often equated with race or colour and is even confused with religion on a day-to-day basis. *Race* refers to the grouping of people based on biological similarities, such as genetic features (including skin colour), whereas *ethnicity* is seen as a generic term for how a group perceives its own identity (Kelly-Heidenthal, 2004). *Ethnocentrism* is the term for a belief that one's own culture is better than that of other groups, without considering the values of other groups, and is thus discriminatory. These issues raise concerns in our society as to how we can move cultural integration forward.

It is also important to identify other implications of culture for our health service. Harrison (2004) noted that around 13 per cent of NHS staff come from Black and ethnic minority groups. She highlights a *Nursing Standard* survey of diversity in the NHS. The response rate was similar to the racial breakdown in the NHS. Among the respondents were nurses from across the UK, working in a variety of settings and in all clinical grades. These were a few of the statements made by nurse respondents:

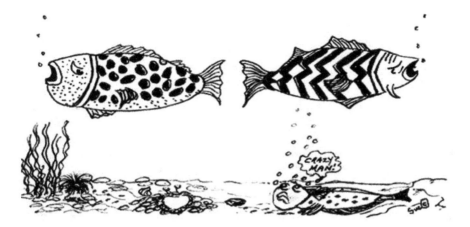

'Even I, as a senior nurse with a degree, am spoken to by my senior in a certain tone of voice.' (Asian, Grade G)

'I was left to take patients to the toilet and clean commodes all the time for 11 years because of my colour and ethnicity.'(Asian, Grade F)

'I hear racist comments on a daily basis from unqualified staff, such as health care assistants, boasting about joining or voting for the British National Party and ignorant comments are made on a frequent basis.' (White, Grade E)

'Each time you are on duty, for whatever reason, nobody else but you will remain on the ward until the end of the shift. Others are told to go early, which is unfair.' (Black, Grade D)

'One type of ethnic group of women will always make a fuss after surgery.' (Reported to have heard this by White, Grade D)

'Twenty years ago, as a newly qualified RGN, I was the only white nurse on the ward and I used to get called names because of my pale skin. In the canteen a coloured lady refused to serve me when I asked for black tea.' (White, Nursing Home Nurse)

'I find it is the patients, especially older people, who are racist. They often make racist comments.' (White, Grade E)

'Most black nurses have to fight for everything, unlike white staff.' (Black, Grade E)

'I find staff from BME backgrounds seem to get preferential treatment. This is not equal.' (White, Grade E)

'It is extremely difficult for people from ethnic minorities to progress. They always have to have more qualifications and work harder.' (Black, Grade F)

'I work with Indians, Filipinos, Africans, Norwegians and many other nation-
alities. Where else would you get that? I love it. Differences in culture exist. We
just have to recognise this and get on with the job.' (White, Grade E). (Harrison,
2004: 12–13)

These views, whilst dated, continue to highlight both remaining racism in the
NHS and the very real difficulty in changing institutional racism, despite professional codes of conduct and education. This, therefore, raises important implications for primary, secondary and higher education in our society today. The glass
ceiling is the invisible barrier, in ethnocentric organisations, that separates
minority groups – such as women, older staff and people with disabilities – from
progressing in their career; if members of such groups do achieve better positions, they are often paid unequally or are unequally valued. In 2009 research
was published by the NHS Institute of Innovation and Improvement (NHS III)
into access of Black and Minority Ethnic (BME) staff to senior positions in the
NHS. It noted:

47% of registrars and 25% of consultants were from non-white backgrounds.
This compares with 14% of the total NHS workforce being from a non-white
background. This indicates the need for further investigation because of the
steep reduction of non-white registrars becoming consultants. It also indicates that the medical route (and indeed the nursing route), offers opportunities for BME staff to obtain clinical director and subsequently board level
positions as medical and nursing directors. However, anecdotal evidence
would suggest that relatively few are currently achieving board position.
(NHS III, 2009a: 14)

The report provides further data reflecting underrepresentation of BME staff in
NHS middle management but indicates a glass ceiling between middle and senior
NHS management. Eight recommendations relating to building capacity of leadership in the NHS were set out. All health care leaders and managers should work
positively to enable all NHS staff to have equal opportunities (EO) in the workplace,
regardless of their gender, ethnicity or sexual orientation (DH, 2001a). EO focuses
on compliance with legislation whilst diversity is concerned with celebrating the
characteristics of the group and is driven by a business case for EO.

AGE DIVERSITY

Marquis and Huston (2011) raise the point that different generations exhibit different value systems from each other, which influence health care (Martin, 2003;
McNeese-Smith and Crook, 2003; Hill, 2004) (Table 3.2). There is a view that the
older generations of health workers are very respectful of authority, supportive of

Table 3.2 Different generation value systems

Year of Birth	Generation
1925–1942	Silent Generation or Veteran Generation
1943–1960	Baby Boomers
Early 1960–1980	Generation X
1980–1995	Generation Y, Echo Boomers or Millennium Generation
1995 onwards	Generation Z

hierarchy and disciplined (the Silent Generation; Veteran/War Generation; Traditionalists). A younger generation (Baby Boomers) have similar traditional work values and ethics, but are seen as more materialistic and willing to work long hours ('live to work'). They have been taught to think more as creative individuals, and fit well with independent and flexible roles. Generation X, in contrast, defines success differently. They tend to lack an interest in one lifetime career in one place, and value flexible contracts and 12-hour shifts, which give them more scope for other activities during the rest of the week ('work to live'). Generation Y is seen as the first group that is globally aware, seeking roles that will push their limits. They are seen as self-confident, optimistic, team dependant, techno-savvy and socially conscious (Nexters or Internet Gen). Generation Z is seen to be more tolerant than Generation Y of racial, sexual and generational diversity, and less likely to subscribe to traditional gender roles.

> ## ◆ Activity
>
> • How do you think all these generations can work together in a clinical environment?
> • Do you think it can cause conflict?

You may observe from your clinical practice that all these generations can work effectively together as long as they respect where others are coming from and what their individual expectations of team working are. Of course, there may be conflict at times but this is all part of team working. Stanley (2010) conducted a literature review of the four generational categories in the nursing workforce and highlighted the different needs and attitudes that these groups bring to the workforce. This resulted in implications for recruiting and retaining staff from these different generations, particularly in the context of nursing shortages. The research also highlighted the emergence of Generation Z which appears to have the following features: their lifestyle integrates easily with media technology and digital communication and they were born into the postmodern and globalisation era.

GENDER DIVERSITY

It has been identified that 77 per cent of NHS staff are women and 23 per cent are men; however, of all the NHS staff only 7 per cent of female staff are doctors or dentists and 28 per cent of male staff are doctors or dentists (see Table 3.3) (NHS Employers, 2014). There are proportionally fewer women in senior management posts and NHS managerial culture is still controlled by a transactional leadership style (Markham, 2005). Differences in leadership style can be linked to gender as highlighted in research by Rosener (1990), which concluded that men were more likely to be transactional leaders while women had a preference for transformational styles. This has to be seen within the context of the late 1980s and may not necessarily reflect the current position. Gender has also been seen to influence communication. Grohar-Murray et al. (2010) suggest that men and women communicate differently in groups. Women tend to be more passive in groups and, as new leaders or managers, are more hesitant in speaking to groups, though this may not necessarily be so true now.

Table 3.3   Gender balance in the NHS

	Doctors or Dentists	Other Occupations in NHS
Men (23% NHS total)	28% of the total 23%	72% of total for men
Women (77% NHS total)	7% of the total 77%	93% of total for women

Espenshade and Radford (2009) found that although women are more likely to do better overall, men are more likely to gain the highest degrees. They noted that women's confidence in their own academic abilities erodes faster than men's over their time at university and that they are more hesitant about speaking up in class. The language of men and women also differs and the notion that women have less self-belief than men may help to explain why men are more likely to take the lead. Ford's (2006) research using an in-depth narrative approach found four themes emerging which reflected a masculine model of leadership through the need for:

- Macho-management
- Post-heroic leadership
- Influences from outside
- Career paths.

The emerging need for talent management in the context of coaching (Chapter 10) and mentoring is now developing within the scope of leadership courses to influence and address gender inequities.

> ### ◆ Activity
>
> - How do you feel when having to speak to small groups of peers?
> - How do you feel when having to speak to large groups of peers?
> - How do you feel when having to speak in groups of people you do not know very well?

Initially I was quite worried about having to talk to group peers because I had always felt that I had nothing of interest to say; they would all know far more than I did about any given subject. Once I got over my initial lack of confidence and found I could contribute to discussions, raise issues and make a reasonable attempt at getting my point of view or experiences over to others, I felt more at ease with this activity. Like all things, it's difficult getting over that initial barrier. It is, however, much easier to speak to a group of people you do not know as you have fewer preconceived ideas of their expectations of you, or your view of them.

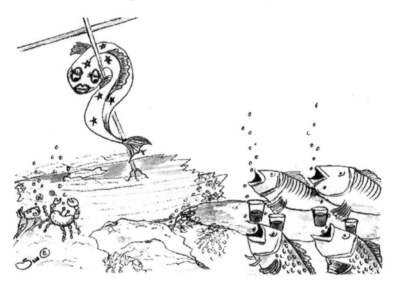

Although men and women work alongside each other in the NHS, they are socialised quite differently (Grohar-Murray and DiCroce, 2002). It has been suggested that:

> Women tend to use communication in a personal manner to maintain or establish relationships, share ideas and learn about others and go about it in a quieter and more tentative manner whereas men, on the other hand, tend to use communication in an instrumental way to reach their goals. They also appear to be rather more direct and forceful. (Wood, 2012)

Recognition of these differences in leadership matters because communication styles are an important element of getting messages through to people, as well as of understanding the needs of people in a team. Chapter 7 will further develop the notion of diversity of communication styles. Managing and leading health care teams involves an underpinning philosophy of the importance of individuals and developing teams who can manage diversity in their everyday work. It is useful to get teams to develop awareness of some of the models of transcultural care and to try and work towards a fully integrated transcultural operational delivery in the health service.

Equality in the workforce is vital as not only does it improve the corporate image and attract ethical investors but it is also a much better use of human resources. This notion of equity comes, as does much of the management and leadership theory, from North America where there is a plethora of published material related to diversity and equality. The values, beliefs and material objects surrounding each person are said to constitute their culture, so when any young person comes to train for work in the health service that move may engender a culture shock as they have to become accustomed to a new set of 'norms' – this is known as cultural entry gate. As the new student becomes experienced s/he will pass their experiences on to the next generation – known as cultural transmission.

Multiculturalism is another workforce phenomenon. New staff may have challenges as they start to be integrated into their professional role. Some identify with their own traditional culture initially and find difficulty in absorbing the professional expectations, e.g. some staff may be expected to deliver intimate care to the opposite sex giving rise to dissonance and anxiety. Cultural lag may be an issue for leadership; this is the notion related to a changing cultural context driven by technology which may give rise to social problems and team conflict as staff work to keep up with the speed of technological and cultural changes e.g. the emergence of fertility treatments, organ donation and potentially some legislation related to end of life care.

ABILITY DIVERSITY

The Disability Discrimination Act (DDA 1995, extended in 2005) said that it was unlawful for organisations to discriminate in employment. Since 2010 the DDA has been replaced by The Equality Act (2010) which continues to protect the interests of disabled people.

Increasingly, in the delivery of health care, we meet with individuals who have unseen disabilities e.g. Dyslexia, Dyspraxia, Dyscalculia, Asthma, Deafness ... Reasonable adjustments have to be made to enable these people to function in the workplace and within their chosen profession. I remember a student who was quite severely dyslexic: he had a laptop that had a programme suited to his needs and he used this, both as a student and as a qualified nurse, to record patient assessments; clearly these were all downloaded at the completion of his shift in order to maintain confidentiality.

Prior to 1999 it was impossible for a person with hearing loss to train to become a registered nurse but following the DDA these students were accepted into training, were offered help – e.g. interpreters for British Sign Language; note takers in lectures and electronic stethoscopes in order to listen for manual blood pressure recording, in order to enable them to study effectively (University of Salford, 2009).

Following qualification employers must also make effective working adjustments to ensure the safety of the employee and of course his/her patients. One nurse talks of being involved with a cardiac arrest procedure (Weaver, 2013)

> 'I offered to do CPR and asked one of the anaesthetists if he could lift his hand each time I had to stop and start, which he did, therefore allowing me to fully participate in a life-saving event.'

She needed the hand signal because, for Ms Manning, fast-paced moments like these are silent ones. Profoundly deaf, she relies on observation and training to keep up with the unpredictable nature of her profession.

This worked well and the patient survived; it just takes teamwork and an understanding of each other's needs (emotional intelligence plays a part here) in order to make the whole experience work.

MODELS OF TRANSCULTURAL CARE

Leininger (1997) offers a model underpinned by the notion that one's cultural background affects the reactions generated by any given situation. The value of a culturally diverse workforce is that patients and clients perceive that health service delivery involves a transculturally sensitive openness. First, the importance of *care as a concept*, within all cultures, should be recognised. However, what is defined as *caring* can be different in different cultures. Second, each culture identifies what it considers to be adequate and necessary care. Transcultural care requires an acute awareness of each culture's:

- lifestyle patterns
- values
- beliefs and norms
- symbols and rituals
- verbal and nonverbal communication
- caring behaviours
- shared meanings
- rituals of health, wellness and illness.

For example, a few weeks ago when I was looking after an older Asian man with prostate cancer, his son and daughter-in-law asked whether there was any possibility of him being moved to a single room. They were concerned about their mother, who was sleeping in a chair by their father's bed, with limited privacy in the three-bedded men's ward. Some of the staff felt the request was unreasonable and wondered why the mother did not go home to bed as the father 'had been admitted for symptom control not for terminal care'.

> ◆ Activity
>
> Jot down what you think about the issues of this ethical dilemma.

It is difficult getting single rooms for all families. However, the caring behaviours within this family needed to be understood. The gentleman expected his wife to look after him and be with him at night, even while he was in a hospice. They had been married for 34 years. Their caring, sharing, togetherness and closeness behaviours were ingrained within this family unit. Neither spoke good English and both pre-ferred to have their children bring them a familiar diet from home. This left them feeling isolated from the majority of other families. The mother found sleeping dif-ficult with other men in the room. The outcome was that a single room was eventually found for them until an early discharge plan was organised.

Giger and Davidhizar's (2004) transcultural care model consists of five central concepts underpinning care:

- Transcultural nursing and provision of culturally diverse nursing care
- Culturally competent care
- Cultural uniqueness of individuals
- Culturally sensitive environments
- Culturally specific illness and wellness behaviours.

When undertaking a culturally competent assessment of patients, professionals should recognise the following attributes of every cultural group:

- Communication
- Personal space/touch and closeness
- Social organisation
- Time
- Environmental control
- Biological variations.

Diversity of values and beliefs is to be welcomed, but how does this fit with what the public expect from health care staff as a whole? Patients and clients expect some consistency of action and advice from health care professionals. There are now a plethora of academic, professional standards and benchmarks associated with each professional health care group. These professional qualifications, codes of conduct and policy drivers invariably influence and shape specific roles in health care.

Bennett's (1986) model highlighted a staged development of diversity awareness leading to more competent care in health care practice. These stages are:

- Denial (incompetent)
- Defence
- Minimising differences

- Acceptance
- Adaption
- Integration (competent).

Diversity of values and beliefs are to be welcomed in health care teams, but how does this fit with what the public expect from health care staff as a whole? Patients and clients expect some consistency of action and advice from health care professionals. Excellent patient communication skills are essential. There are now a plethora of academic, professional standards and benchmarks associated with each professional health care group. These professional qualifications, codes of conduct and policy drivers invariably influence and shape specific roles in health care.

LEADING A CULTURALLY DIVERSE TEAM

A health care team featuring diversity of race, culture, age, ability and sexual orientation will be one that reflects the breadth of patient diversity, resulting in a beneficial, culturally mirrored partnership of staff and patients. In order to work effectively as a team, leaders could reflect on the following recommendations:

- When problem solving, be sure to examine the diversity of the workgroup so you can get diverse perspectives for the solutions to be more widely accepted
- Understand how team members respond to conflict and their expectations
- Work towards understanding the benefits of diversity and appreciate all contributions
- Avoid assumptions that cultural groups act and respond in the same way
- Avoid labelling
- Value everyone's differences and recognise similarities. Seek out different experiences from the majority
- Pay close attention to both verbal and non-verbal communication for cultural cues
- Ask for clarification to avoid assumptions, *and*
- Assist those in minority groups to be successful. Include them in informal networking within the team culture.

Summary of Key Points

This chapter has examined the issues related to diversity, values and professional care in order to meet the identified learning outcomes. These were:

- **Examine the breadth of the concept of culture** This was examined in relation to the uniqueness of individuals and the norms, values and beliefs of various cultures.
- **Discuss the importance of cultural diversity, influencing health and health care** This was also explored within the context of the health service.

(Continued)

(Continued)

- **Discuss leadership in the context of cultural diversity** Leading culturally diverse teams was examined in the context of diversity and recommendations were made.
- **Examine the theoretical models of transcultural care** These were discussed in order to manage anti-discriminatory and anti-oppressive behaviour in the health service.
- **Critically reflect on personal transcultural care** This was examined and related to leading the culturally diverse team.

FURTHER READING

Bolam vs Friern Hospital Management Committee (1957), 1 WLR 582; (1957) 2 All ER 118.

Fletcher, L. and Buka, P. (1999) *A Legal Framework for Caring.* Basingstoke: Macmillan.

Francis, R. (2013) *Report of the Mid-Staffordshire NHS Foundation Trust Public Inquiry.* London. The Stationery Office.

Haddad, A.M. (1992) 'Ethical problems in healthcare', *Journal of Advanced Nursing,* 22 (3): 46–51.

Harvey, C. and Allard, M.J. (2011) *Understanding and Managing Diversity* (5th edn). Harlow: Prentice Hall.

Sin, C.H. and Fong, J. (2008) '"Do no harm"? Professional regulation of disabled nursing students and nurses in Great Britain', *Journal of Advanced Nursing.* 62 (6): 642–52, June.

Thompson, V. (2009) Salford Student Becomes the First Deaf Male Nurse. www.nursing-times.net (accessed 29 August 2014).

Walsh, M. (2000) *Nursing Frontiers: Accountability and Boundaries of Care.* Oxford: Butterworth-Heinemann.

Weaver, H. (2013) Determined and Dedicated. www.nursingtimes.net (accessed 30 August 2014).

Visit the companion website at https://study.sagepub.com/barr3e for more resources.

4 THEORIES OF LEADERSHIP

Learning Outcomes

By the end of this chapter you will have had the opportunity to:

- Identify the evolution of leadership theories
- Compare and contrast the various leadership theories
- Critically discuss the application of these theories in relation to health care.

INTRODUCTION

This chapter highlights the evolution of some of the work of the main leadership writers and the context in which their ideas surfaced. Despite the discipline of leadership being comparatively young and relatively unchallenged, the main theories noted here still have influence and hold ground today within health care. Attempts will be made to link the theories to the practice setting. It must be recognised that the most effective leaders adjust their style and approach to the prevailing situation. This means that the suggestions made here are just that, suggestions, and not a recipe for immediate success.

EVOLVING THEORIES OF LEADERSHIP

The concept of leadership can mean different things to different people depending on their various perspectives. There has been a range of ways identified to classify leadership theories (Rafferty, 1993; Mullins, 1999, 2005; Daft, 2005, 2008; Northouse, 2012) but it may be useful to look at leadership in the following forms:

- as a collection of personal characteristics or traits
- as a function within an organisation
- as an effect on group behaviour
- as an influence on forming an organisational culture.

Most of the ideas contained in the above theories can be seen as evolutionary. The emerging research data are seen to contribute to the greater knowledge base in the area of leadership. It could be argued that some of the ideas are not always based on good quality evidence – particularly the older research where we would now consider the research biases to be transparent. Hewison and Stanton (2003) examined the development of management theory, in order to compare it to emerging nursing theory and to identify the implications for health care. They concluded that health care management was based on the 'fads and fashions' of the prevailing theory at the time and questioned whether many ideas were scientifically valid. The complex development of management/leadership theories has been influenced by the prevailing psychological or sociological theories of the time. More specifically, the school of behaviourism within the psychology discipline and the school of functionalism within the discipline of social science underpin some of the leadership theories. Therefore, most of these ideas and theories relate to both social science and psychology as relevant perspectives.

The basis of psychology is the study of how individual people attempt to make sense, through cognitive processes, of their social world; how their social contexts affect their social behaviours; and how individuals share their representation of the social world with others (Cardwell et al., 1996). Social science relates to the study of how social groups in society behave. There is an overlap of the two disciplines but the former focuses more on individuality and the latter on group processes. For the purpose of this chapter, four simple perspectives of how leadership is classed have been mapped against the various disciplines and ideas (Table 4.1).

Table 4.1 Comparative classifications of developing leadership theories (Van Seters and Field, 1990; Crainer, 1996; Sadler, 2003)

Leadership Classification	Development of Leadership Theories
1 Leadership as a collection of personal characteristics or traits	• Personality era
2 Leadership as a function within an organisation	• Influence era • Situational era
3 Leadership as an effect on group behaviour	• Behavioural era • Contingency era • Transactional era • Role development
4 Leadership as an influence on forming an organisational culture	• Organisational cultural era • Transformational era • New leadership era

LEADERSHIP AS A COLLECTION OF PERSONAL CHARACTERISTICS OR TRAITS

Trait or 'Great Man' theory was popularised around the 1900s and focused on the idea of some universal traits of leaders. 'Great Man' theory is based on the belief that leaders possess exceptional qualities. It has been argued that trait theory was born out of the philosophy of Aristotle (384–322 BC), who believed that some are *born to lead* and others are *born to be led*, thus linking back to the notion of leadership and followership (Chapter 2). It also raises the assumption that some people have specific leadership qualities and others do not. This assumption could be seen as a way to identify potential leaders for the future.

Activity

- So what do you think about effective leaders?
- What characteristics do you think they need?
- Are they different now from those that were needed in the last century?
- Write down any other leadership characteristics that you think are important from what you have experienced or have heard about.

You may have a list that includes the following:

- Someone who knows what's got to be done
- Someone who gets things done
- Good communicator
- Admirable
- Good persuader
- Good at bringing about change.

You may have found this difficult, as the way some people lead others varies in time and place; sometimes it is hard to identify characteristics that they all share. This may be because in different contexts, leaders require different attributes. You are not alone in your difficulties. The literature is still confusing and there is much debate about the value of trait theory in the world of work today. Leadership traits seem to become more noticeable in retrospect, alongside recognition of a significant achievement. Bennis (1999) highlighted that past research showed that there were seven attributes essential to leadership:

1. Technical competence in one's own field
2. Conceptual, abstract or strategic thinking
3. Track record
4. People skills
5. Taste to cultivate talent
6. Judgement
7. Character.

Marquis and Huston (2006: 50) identified certain characteristics of leaders in terms of their intelligence, personality and abilities (Table 4.2).

Table 4.2 Characteristics of leaders (Marquis and Huston, 2006: 50)

Intelligence	Personality	Abilities
Knowledge	Adaptability	Able to enlist cooperation
Judgement	Creativity	Interpersonal skills and tact
Decisiveness	Cooperativeness	Diplomacy
Oral fluency	Alertness	Prestige
	Self confidence	Social participation
	Personal integrity	
	Emotional balance and control	
	Non-conformity	
	Independence	

Source: Adapted from Marquis, B.L. and Huston, C.J. (2006) *Leadership Roles and Management Functions in Nursing: Theory and Application* (8th International edn). Philadelphia, PA: Lippincott

However, in the mid-1940s trait theory was challenged as the research was found to be inconclusive and contradictory, especially as the relationship between leaders and the context of the situation were seen as more important. Trait theory has also been criticised because it does not seem to take account of organisational culture, and may even negate the part that social class, gender and race inequalities play in maintaining the status quo in leadership positions. Indeed, Bennis and Nanus (1985) identified the following myths about leadership:

- Leadership is a rare skill
- Leaders are born not made
- Leaders are charismatic.

Senge (1990), Gardner (1990) and recent NHS leadership policy agree that leadership qualities and skills can be developed and are not inherited. This then leads us to ask a number of questions pertinent to the style you might adopt in your quest to become an effective leader.

Activity

- Do you believe you have inherited leadership qualities?
- Do you believe you have developed your present leadership qualities from experience?
- Do you believe you could develop further leadership skills?

The answers you reached in the above Activity will depend on your individual views of what leadership is about and the results you got from the leadership/followership test you completed in Chapter 2. In terms of developing present leadership qualities, for instance, you may have included such influences as observing and emulating senior colleagues in the way they have dealt with specific situations. Similarly, reading about leadership theory may help you to develop; you may feel that you learn more through leadership workshops and exercises, that is, 'learning whilst doing'.

You may subscribe to 'Great Man' theory first suggested by Carlyle in 1841, who said that 'the history of the world is but the biography of great men and that great leaders emerge to deal with specific situations'. However, Great Man theory has largely gone out of fashion today in favour of other theories which discuss the development of leaders through study and experience. As such, the nature/nurture debate is still ongoing. More recently leadership has been linked to the intelligence debate; studies that correlate family IQ suggest reasoning and spacial ability are more linked to the nature argument. In more recent times the emergence of the 'Flynn' effect (Flynn, 2009) has been noted. This theory highlights that IQ has been seen to be increasing in all countries over time, predominately due to environmental effects; this and the Bell Curve notion of intelligence (Lynn, 2008) makes IQ a complex area in research. Lynn's work relates to the social stratification of global race to IQ and thus genetic predisposition. This is hugely controversial but has implications for leadership selection involving trait theory. There is evidence that trait theory is also still valued. In trying to set desirable attributes and competencies for job positions in the health service, you will see that essential and desirable criteria for the roles are based on trait assumptions.

These position/role attributes give rise to questions such as, 'Are leaders born or made?' and 'Is leadership an art or a science?' Whatever you decide, in the first instance, if you are being interviewed for a clinical leadership post you can argue both ways. If you believe leaders are born you could argue for inherited trait theory based on your leadership experience. However, if you think leaders are made you could discuss developmental training which could enhance deficits in attributes you have for the post.

◆ Activity

Write 50 words to reflect on how trait theory influences practice in health care today.

You may have considered the fact that potential leaders go 'on courses' to teach them how to lead, but how many of them actually come back and deliver what they have been taught? According to Marquis and Huston (2006) this may be because they are not the sort of person who likes to make decisions and direct people, indicating that they may not have the trait required to be an effective leader.

I remember well a colleague who was promoted into a post that had 'leader' in its title. However, she would have been unable to lead the rats out of Hamelin – even with the help of the pied piper! She simply didn't know how to lead effectively.

When you are in the clinical area, look to see which person you would be most likely to ask for advice. This may not be the person with leader in their title but someone who is seen to be approachable, knowledgeable and willing to impart knowledge – the traits, according to Bennis (1999), of a good leader.

LEADERSHIP AS A FUNCTION WITHIN AN ORGANISATION

The theories connected with this category relate to social functionalism. These theories relate to how social organisation is maintained and how it functions. The nature of social structures, their integration, harmony and evolutional stability towards the organisation as a whole underpin these theories (Weitz et al., 2011). Ideas within this category centre on the nature and consequences of these structures and how leadership as a structure supports the function of the organisation to carry out its work with attention to:

- Sources of power and influence over others
- How various roles relate to the functions in an organisation to meet its needs.

The role leaders play, in relation to any organisation, highlights the emphasis on not *what they have* but what leaders actually *do*, who they *influence* and how this *relates to the function* a particular leader plays in an organisation. In examining what leaders actually do, Fayol (1925) first identified the main management functions seen as essential at the time as Planning, Organising, Coordination and Control, while Gulick (1937) expanded the scope of these functions to include:

- Planning
- Organising
- Staffing
- Directing
- Coordination
- Reporting and
- Budgeting.

(These functions are denoted by the acronym **POSDCORB**.)

These were, however, set in the context of scientific management and administration, rather than relating to the specific concept of leadership, and were underpinned by the assumption that the 'manager knows best'. Daft et al. (2008: 7) confirm the four functions to managing effectively are still planning, organising, leading and controlling. The functional approach relates the overlapping ideas of appointed leaders and naturally emerging leaders in an attempt to argue that there are some similarities in the two roles as well as some differences. Again this will highlight the nature/nurture debate while being aware of the needs of staff in their developing roles. Kotter (2008) suggests that organisations should 'grow' their own leaders to function effectively within that organisation, that is, current employees should be encouraged to develop their leadership skills in order to advance their careers within that particular organisation or Trust.

▶ Activity

Debate the notion of 'growing' your own leaders vs appointing 'new' blood to enhance organisational and procedural change.

In terms of connecting the functions of the organisation to the people, Adair (2010: 24) uses the idea of 'action-centred leadership' where the group leader, in order to be seen as effective, needed an ability to meet three functions:

- To achieve the required task(s)
- To maintain the team
- To meet the needs of individual team members.

> ◆ **Activity**
>
> How could this model of leadership apply in clinical practice?

It can be seen that clinical practice fits with this simple model. When exploring patient care, the *task needs* are related to specific aspects of care being undertaken at the time and the resources required to undertake those tasks; *individual needs* relates to ensuring staff understand what is expected of them and have an understanding of the purpose of their task, but it is also to do with ensuring that individual needs are addressed. If these elements and group cohesiveness are achieved then the integrity of *team maintenance* to meet *team needs* should follow. His three-sphere model highlights the overlapping areas of functions that the leader must be aware of in order to achieve the desired outcomes (Figure 4.1).

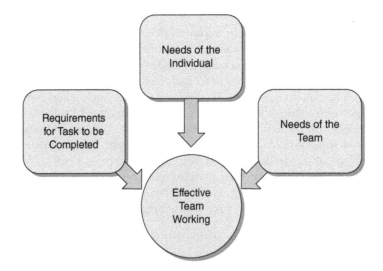

Figure 4.1   Functional needs to be fulfilled for effective team working adapted from Adair, J. (1997) *Decision Making and Problem Solving.* London: Institute of Personnel and Development

TASK NEEDS

An organisation must undertake various activities in order to fulfil its objectives. In health care, there are a number of tasks that are undertaken by various levels of staff. These tasks often involve overlap of input from members of the multidisciplinary team. The tasks, the required resources and the organisation of skill-mix all contribute to the overall task being completed. For instance, a diabetic patient may require blood glucose monitoring. At first sight this may look easy as it appears simply to involve time, the patient and a health care professional to take the blood, but on further analysis it can be seen to be a much more complex process. More specifically, the task may be analysed as set out in Table 4.3.

Table 4.3 Task needs

The individual task	Monitor the blood glucose of patients
The allocation of resources to achieve that task	Calibrated blood glucose monitoring equipment Haematology laboratory facilities/ technology Time
The organisation of skill mix in order to ensure the quality of performance	Trained health care professionals to judge the level of monitoring required Trained health care professionals who can take and test the blood samples Trained health care professionals who can interpret and take action – including advising the patients, referral to other professionals as necessary and documenting the relevant issues

► Activity

Do you think that the 'task' can be easily learnt by an individual within a team?

In health care, the 'task' not only relates to the delivery of effective and efficient physical care for the patient but should also be about addressing the emotional care required by the patient. All patients are individuals; they have very different needs physically, socially and mentally. Individual staff have to know how to deal with all these aspects of care as they are carrying out the tasks for, or with, patients. Teams also vary; some teams are more effective than others and leaders need to understand how each person works within the team, and how their skills and strengths can be best utilised – this relates to the use of Emotional Intelligence (Chapter 10).

Leading out on this complexity is challenging. Leaders in health care have to think about the type of work and jobs that have to be done for the health service to address the needs of patients. For example, there are certain tasks that have to be planned and organised in a surgical unit.

> ◆ **Activity**
>
> Can you think of any examples of tasks required, for instance, around midday?

In relation to the Activity, there are patients who will be hungry and thirsty after returning from their surgery and will want to be offered something to eat and drink. Others may have only just returned from surgery and airway management is required. They or their relatives will expect to see their doctors to discover whether there are any results from the surgery or diagnostic tests, and medical rounds/consultations have to be organised. There may be patients who will need to be prepared for afternoon theatre or other procedures such as X-ray or MRI scans. New patients may be arriving into the area and will need to be 'admitted' and some will be waiting for discharge from hospital. The various patients' needs will have to be addressed in order of priority. In the community there are similar tasks that have to be done, such as the administration of referrals, telephone contacts, visits to book, patient/client visits to make, clinics to run as well as management meetings to attend. Filling the car with petrol is also a task that has to be fitted in!

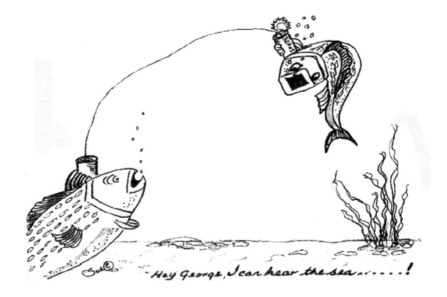

"Hey George, I can hear the sea.......!"

Managing and leading teams will require leaders to think about *how* the following activities will be achieved:

1. Setting and achieving goals and objectives to get the required work done
2. Communicating goals and objectives to the rest of the team
3. Defining the tasks to meet the objectives

4. Planning the work
5. Bargaining for and mobilising resources, for example, beds, linen, people
6. Delegating the work, organising responsibilities and supporting the team
7. Monitoring performance and quality management
8. Reviewing progress.

Leading from the front in order to ensure all eight elements are addressed is an accepted part of effective leadership, whichever style is adopted.

THE NEEDS OF THE TEAM

When we consider the *team*, we must consider training needs, communication systems and team development in order for the multi-professional teams to function. Teams require leaders and followers (Chapter 2) who may not always be the same people, as various roles change and take shape. The people in a team should have the right skills, knowledge and attitudes for the tasks to be completed, if the team is to be a success. All team leaders must consider:

1. Team development and encouraging a team spirit
2. Encouraging a working cohesive team unit
3. Setting standards and professional behaviour
4. Setting up systems of communication within the team
5. Learning and training within the team
6. Delegating and team growth.

These features may be addressed formally within a team meeting as part of the recognised agenda or addressed within an informal situation – say a night out ten-pin bowling, encouraging team growth, team spirit and cohesion. It may be difficult at times to address the needs of the team where there is no single leader identified, for example:

- **Job sharing leaders** When one leader has one way of doing things and the other holds a different view
- **Rotational leaders** Where leaders change on a rotational basis or with specific functions and accountabilities within a specific situation
- **Distant leaders** Where the team members are working throughout the geographical community and only have limited face-to-face contact. (Barr and Dowding, 2008)

Differing philosophies and styles may affect how the team functions but, through open discussion, a central path and philosophy can be devised to satisfy all concerned.

THE NEEDS OF INDIVIDUALS

This area focuses on a leader giving attention to personal needs or individual problems while giving praise and status to those concerned. Again, professional development and training has to be recognised in order to raise the quality of care delivery. Individuals will have personal as well as professional needs. They will come to work for a variety of reasons besides financial gain. They will want to be valued and developed within the working team. Leaders may well need to think about the following:

1. Appraising and listening to the needs of individuals
2. Attending to personal issues
3. Giving praise and status to individuals
4. Reconciling conflicts between team needs and individual needs
5. Training and developing individuals
6. Clinical supervision and reflective practices.

Working within the three spheres of Adair's model (see Figure 4.1) is challenging for any leading individual. The ideal is, of course, to occupy the position in the centre where all three areas are integrated, the needs are adequately met and the team or group is satisfied. Adair (2006) suggested the seven qualities of a strategic leader as being:

- Direction (purpose and aim of the business)
- Strategic thinking (bridging the gap between now and the future)
- Making it happen (details)
- Relating the whole to the parts
- Establishing allies and partners outside the business
- Releasing corporate energy
- Developing leadership in others.

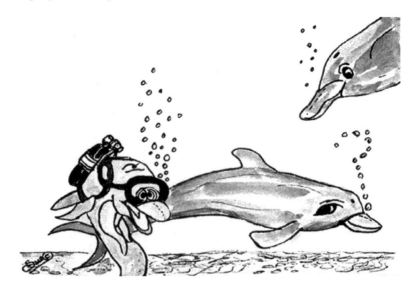

The implications of this focus within the complexity of the Health Service are related to the need to build the capability and capacity within the leadership of the NHS. The Institute for Innovation and Improvement (DH, 2007) recognises this will bring huge benefits for patients, carers and staff as well as increased quality and value. The latest developments – of GP consortia commissioning and the impact of the Health and Social Care Bill (DH, 2011a) overall – have stimulated mounting debate for many stakeholders in the shaping of the future of the NHS.

LEADERSHIP AS AN EFFECT ON GROUP BEHAVIOURS

This category overlaps with 'Leadership as a Function' but has a greater focus on the behavioural aspects of people relationships. The Human Relations Management era greatly influenced the humanistic view of leadership and the importance of people over productivity. The theories that emerged within this category focused initially on how leaders behaved towards their team; but later the importance of the effects of team behaviour *on leadership* was realised. The various *leadership style* and *motivational* theories, which concern how to get the best out of people to get the work done, are seen as wide ranging. The motivational theories of people such as Herzberg (1966), Ouchi (1981), Maslow (1987) or McGregor (1987) 'fit' within this section but will be discussed in greater depth in Chapter 7.

LEADERSHIP STYLES

The way an individual leads, within an organisation or a team, has been seen in terms of their style of behaviour and relates to the underpinning behavioural theories. Lewin (1951) and White and Lippitt (1960) identified various types of leader behaviour that signalled different styles. One way of looking at leadership style is in connection to the *power* that a managerial leader exerts over any subordinates in a team and these were situated on a continuum (Figure 4.2).

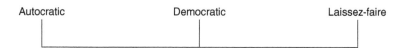

Autocratic   Democratic   Laissez-faire

Figure 4.2 Leadership behaviours

- **The autocratic or authoritarian style** The leader exercises ultimate power in decision making and controls the rewards and punishments for the subordinates in conforming to their decisions
- **The democratic and participative style** The leader encourages all members of the team to interact and to contribute to the decision making process

- **The laissez-faire style** The leader *conscientiously* makes the decision to pass the focus of power on to the subordinate members in genuine laissez-faire style. This is distinct from abdication or 'non leadership' when the 'leader' refuses to make any decisions.

A person's leadership style has a great deal of influence on the work environment. For many years, it was believed that leaders employed a consistently dominant style. It was also felt that autocracy and laissez-faire styles were less acceptable than democratic leadership. Later on, it was felt that there was a continuum of styles between autocratic and laissez-faire behaviours and those leaders moved dynamically between styles in response to new situations. Go back to Chapter 2 and look at the results of your leadership/followership quiz to see where you might 'fit' in Table 4.4. The table highlights how this categorising of styles is influenced by situations and is, therefore, more complex than was first suggested.

Table 4.4　Comparative elements of leading styles

Comparative Criteria	Autocracy Style	Democracy Style	Laissez-faire Style
Situations where valued	Where predictable group action is required to reduce group frustration and develop group security Useful in crisis situations	Where groups are together for long times and cooperation and coordination are necessary	Where problems are poorly defined and all views can be considered to get solutions
Possible negative outcomes	Creativity, self motivation and autonomy are reduced	Time consuming and frustrating when decisions need to be made in a short time Less efficient than autocracy	Group apathy, disinterest leading to frustration
Possible positive outcomes	Well defined group actions reducing frustration and producing security	Promotes autonomy and growth in individual workers Communication flows up and down	Group cohesion when trying to deal with ambiguity
Cultural issues	'You' and 'I' signal the different status Coercion is used to motivate Decision making does not involve others	'We' is emphasised Rewards are used to motivate Decision making involves others	The group is emphasised Motivation by support when requested Decision making is spread within the group

The notion of a continuum model from laissez-faire to autocratic leadership has also been challenged. The work of Tannenbaum and Schmidt (1958) highlighted that the continuum model is too simplistic, that a mixture of autocracy and democracy is needed, and elements such as leadership skills, the situation, and the abilities of the group are needed for effective leadership.

The ideas of Hersey and Blanchard (1977), Blake and Mouton (1985), Blake and McCanse (1991) and Yukl et al. (2002) are also reflected in this section, concerning the multiple dimensions involved in leadership behaviour.

EMERGENCE OF CONTINGENCY THEORIES

Theories that identified the impact of the situation on the behaviour of a leader high-lighted that leadership styles of individuals *could* be changed. From this a range of contingency theories emerged in order to explain the variety of contexts which influenced leadership (Fiedler, 1967; Vroom and Yetton, 1973; Vroom and Jago, 1988). In essence one can think of these theories as being quite fluid and manoeuvrable – an 'if/then' sort of relationship between a number of variables – so that *if* a certain situation arose *then* it would be dealt with in the most appropriate manner. Within the clinical situation we work a good deal within the confines of such theory; we rarely know what is going to happen next, so we have to adapt to each situation as it occurs.

FIEDLER MODEL

The work of Fiedler (1967) concluded that no one particular style of leadership met the needs of every situation so developing the contingency model of leadership. Fiedler came from a background in psychology and used the assumption that personality is relatively stable but that *situations* changed the effectiveness of the leadership style. The relationship between the leader and the group was affected by the leader's own ability, the task to be met and the positional power of the leader. Fiedler's interpretation of his research was that there were leaders who were good in terms of developing interpersonal relationships with the team. Conversely, there were leaders who derived most satisfaction from knowing that a specific task had been completed, rather than considering the implication of relationships within that achievement. However, as a piece of scientific research this has been challenged over the years. Fiedler's work has been subject to much criticism but it is worth recognising the contribution it has made both to gauging leader effectiveness and to stimulating further research.

THE VROOM-JAGO CONTINGENCY MODEL (1988)

This model focused on the degrees of people relationships of the leader and their impact on decision making. The starting point is the idea that a solution is needed to solve a problem and the amount of involvement of others depends on the leadership influence. The model is made up of three main parts:

- Leader participation styles
- Diagnostic questions
- A set of decision making rules.

The seven diagnostic questions that accompany this model relate to:

1. The importance of the decision for the organisation
2. The commitment of the group to implement the solution
3. The level of leadership expertise in the decision
4. Likelihood of group commitment to the decision
5. The group's support for the organisational goals
6. The group's expertise
7. Competence of the group to team problem solving.

This model is complex but interesting in its view of the relationship between the group, the organisation and the leadership. It has since been integrated into a computer-based model to add more complexity. Despite being less than perfect, it is a useful model for learning to make timely, high quality decisions by managers (Daft, 2005).

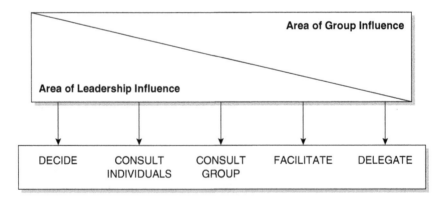

Figure 4.3   Vroom-Jago contingency model (Vroom and Jago, 1988)

LEADERSHIP AS AN INFLUENCE ON FORMING AN ORGANISATIONAL CULTURE

Having examined the last three forms of leadership theory, the latest era concerns the different cultures set within the organisation in which the leadership operates.

Transactional culture and transformational culture have been differentiated as being part of organisational life. The *transactional era* stems from the work of Bass, who stimulated new management thought around transactional leadership between the 1960s and 1980s. This was a time when there was more employment stability in the UK and transactional leadership was based on the notion of a *contract process* between the leader and the group. Bass (1985) noted that transactional leadership concerned:

- rewards and incentives to influence motivation
- the ability for the leader to monitor and correct subordinates in order to work effectively
- an explicit promise of tangible benefits for followers
- an ideological appeal.

The bureaucracy of the National Health Service benefited from the contractual or transactional leadership style in the stable environment at the time. The growth in policies, procedures and employment law started at this time. It was also felt that leaders and groups found mutual satisfaction within these transactional relationships, 'knowing where they stood'.

Marquis and Huston (2006) identified the characteristics of a transactional leader as someone who:

- Focuses on management tasks
- Caretakes
- Uses trade-offs to meet goals
- Does not communicate shared values
- Examines causes
- Uses contingency rewards.

Transactional leadership has been criticised in less stable environments where creativity is needed to deal with today's more complex business worlds.

However, a culture of 'following the rules' has been noted to be effective, especially where planning, organising and budget management are essential – as in the British NHS. When traditional industry in Britain was changing in the 1980s and 1990s there was a shift away from a culture formed through transactional leadership. We began to lose our manufacturing base for employment and the information revolution started to take hold on a global basis. Traditional ways of working, where employees had a job for life and were rewarded for their loyalty to the employer, were starting to dissipate. More creative problem solving was required to look for new markets, new products and services and 'fit' within the emerging global economy. This environment also affected the health services, within the public services, and quasi management modelling, based on the private sector, occurred. *Transformational leadership* theories started to surface, in contrast to transactional leadership theories. Transformational theories of leadership are based on the idea that leaders are people who *motivate* others to perform by encouraging them to see a vision and change their perception of reality. Such leaders are seen as committed individuals with long-term vision and a need to empower others, and who are interested in the consequences. They use:

- Charisma
- Individualised consideration
- Intellectual stimulation to produce greater effort, effectiveness and satisfaction in followers
- Inspiration through symbols. (Bass and Avolio, 1990)

Burns (1978) identified that the transforming process is one in which leaders and followers raise each other to higher levels of morals and motivation. So values such as liberty, peace, equality and humanitarianism are often emphasised rather than values based on individual benefits. However, it has been noted that transformational leaders can have the potential for accruing a good deal of control and power, which can lead to the exploitation of large numbers of followers. Great leaders can be seen as very positive; however, there may be transformational leaders who are portrayed in a negative light (Table 4.5).

Table 4.5   Positive and negative transformational leaders

Positive	Negative
• Pope John Paul II	• Charles Manson
• Mohandas Gandhi	• David Koresh
• Martin Luther King	• Adolf Hitler
• John F. Kennedy	• Saddam Hussein
• Nelson Mandela	

Other criticisms of transformational leaders may be that they tend to focus on the bigger issues of life and, because of their high visibility, are unwilling to spend time facilitating the implementation. Thus, to followers, it may seem that leaders are autocratic and success is about the detail of getting things done. The old adage, 'the devil is in the detail', might be appropriate here.

> ◆ **Activity**
>
> - Have you ever been inspired and motivated by someone else's charisma in practice?
> - Jot down three reasons why you think they made such an impact on you.
> - How do you think these ideas relate to trait theory?

An anaesthetist I worked with was amazing with children; he was so calm that the parents left knowing that their child was in good hands, irrespective of how ill he/she was. I'm not sure why he made such an impact on me but I think it was the calm, quiet way he went about his work. I believe the fact that he was so positive in his outlook, and encouraging to junior colleagues, made him approachable when one didn't quite understand an element of care.

ANTI LEADERSHIP ERA

It is interesting that some management theory from the 1970s recognised the important relationship between leaders and their team workers and, although the focus of the time was on leadership styles, the relevance of the team situation was underplayed. Hersey and Blanchard (1977) highlighted that the characteristics of the team ethic *influenced* their leadership behaviour. The readiness of the work team to take on board the required organisational tasks was reflected in the way their managers/ leaders approached them (Table 4.6).

Table 4.6 Team readiness and leadership approaches

Team Readiness	Leadership Approach
Low	TELLING
Moderate	SELLING
High	PARTICIPATING
Very high	DELEGATING

This is an interesting perspective for health care work teams. More recently there has been a developing perspective of anti leadership theory moving towards the importance of teams of 'followers'. Servant leadership theories are more recent and may combine views from any of the other theories above.

Greenleaf (1977), as a director of the communication company AT&T, first raised the idea of servant leadership. He noted that successful managers led in a different way and put 'serving others' as a priority. He noted they had certain qualities:

- Listened deeply to others to try to understand
- Kept an open mind without judging
- Dealt well with ambiguity and complexity
- Shared critical challenges with all and asked for input to solutions
- Shared clear goals and gave direction
- Served, helped and taught first
- Chose words carefully to avoid damage
- Used insight and intuition
- Had a sense of the whole and relationships/connections with that.

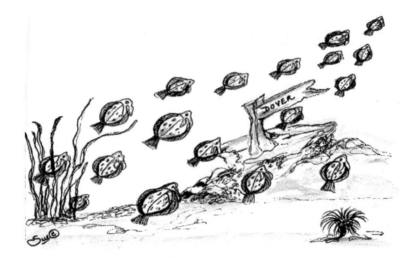

Howatson-Jones (2004) highlights that understanding the followers' perspective in servant leadership offers a valid way to promote health care effectiveness. The style involves mature mutual trust, collegiality and empowerment of multidisciplinary or multi-agency professionals. Greenleaf (1998) noted that, contrary to traditional leadership, the two leadership stages involved in servant leadership are reversed:

1. Serving the needs of followers to empower them to reach their potential
2. Aspiring and maturing into leading.

There seems to be more acceptance of servant leadership in the health industry (Lucas, 1999; Mullaly, 2001) because of the complexity of professional relationships. However, it has been debated whether vision and direction get lost in this type of leadership; as the direction of the NHS is well set within the total goals and governance of quality patient care, this may not be a valid argument here (Snow, 2001). McAlpine (2000), however, challenged the idea of serving in a moral and ethical style and drew an analogy between Machiavelli (1469–1527) and organisational achievement. In highlighting the role of leaders and followers, the principles that are not good indicators for success are that:

- Leaders require the souls of their followers
- Leaders should never fail to express gratitude and appreciation; followers need flattery as recognition of their success
- Leadership loyalty, fairness, trustworthiness in prosperity and adversity are keys to success
- True leaders have a sense of history and awareness of the present position
- Leaders must never blame or penalise followers for their own misjudgement
- Leaders should resist exchanging old friends for new.

Jealousy, competition, skulduggery and treachery keep the power and leadership in place; an interesting idea in politics but, when patient care is the centre of the business, these principles could also work against the quality of service provision. How these ideas may influence an organisational culture will need to be evaluated. Interestingly, one cardiac surgeon in the UK decided to raise concerns about the safety of patients in 2010 when beds were increased in a cardiac unit. He was sacked from his position and despite a tribunal finding he had been unfairly dismissed he was never given back his position (www.theguardian.com/society/2014/apr/17/legal-victory-heart-doctor-whistleblower-hospital-safety-fears accessed 4 June 2014). The question is, who has the right to lead out on clinical excellence and patient safety, who is competing for this power and how can managers and clinicians work together to be accountable to the public purse?

Leadership has thus emerged in the context of changing cultures and dynamics, which is especially important within different health care environments, even within the NHS. Schein (1985) felt that leadership needs to be seen in context and the culture of that context is important: 'Leadership is entwined with culture formation.' The type of leadership required in health care is, therefore, one that fits with the culture of the organisation in which that health care is delivered. Schein (1992: 237) defined organisational culture as:

> The pattern of basic assumptions that a given group has invented, discovered or developed in learning to cope with its problems of external adaptation and internal integration and therefore taught to new members as the correct way to perceive, think and feel in relation to those problems.

These levels of culture (Table 4.7) can be seen within the organisation of a hospital or community placement and also within university life itself.

Table 4.7 Levels of culture (www.12manage.com/methods_schein_three_ levels_ culture.html accessed 28 July 2014)

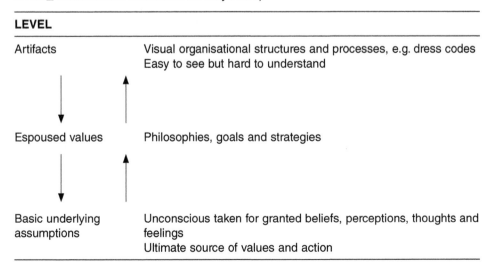

LEVEL	
Artifacts	Visual organisational structures and processes, e.g. dress codes Easy to see but hard to understand
Espoused values	Philosophies, goals and strategies
Basic underlying assumptions	Unconscious taken for granted beliefs, perceptions, thoughts and feelings Ultimate source of values and action

Induction at the start of a new course, meeting up with lecturers, mentors and other students on the course as well as people who have nearly finished their courses integrates us into what is expected in terms of our behaviour within the university. During our induction into new clinical placements we note the way other professionals behave and react to patients/clients and their relatives. This idea will be explored further in Chapter 7.

NEW LEADERSHIP

New roles and expectations are driving health care professionals into a more prominent position. Non medical prescribing, nurse-consultant led clinics, integrated community teams, hospital and community matrons and nurses managing doctors are signs of this challenge for clinicians. Kanter (1991) identifies some specific skills for new leadership:

- Self mastery
- Strategic visioning
- Continual learning
- Creator of partnerships
- Team facilitator.

Multi-agency teams will be a feature of the future and they too will require appropriate leadership. Mintzberg (1998: 588) highlighted vision, shared ideals, creation of organisational pride, developing environments for energies and innovation as essential attributes of leadership. He also identifies that a unique and essential leadership function is to build an organisation's culture and shape its evolution. He goes on to suggest the leadership roles of designer, teacher and steward were required for contributing to leadership in the past but propose that new meanings will be needed for 'learning' organisations of the future.

Through personal mastery, group synergy, learning and sustainable development, a new leadership theory will emerge. Bennis et al. (1994) and Malby (1994) support this view and identify that the time is right for leading in this way within a framework of increased accountability. Scott (1998) points to the value of improving relationships between settings, process-based skills and professional judgement for the future of clinical leadership.

Daft (2006: 682) noted that we are now in a post-heroic leadership era and focuses on the need for leaders to show more humility. He also notes the importance of:

- Servant leadership
- Interactive leadership
- Moral leadership
- E-leadership and
- Level 5 leadership.

These ideas have connected themes within leadership theories. E-leadership concerns the situation found in many industries, where communication is often not on a face-to-face basis and, with increasing amounts of e-communication, there are thus further challenges for leaders. Building trust, maintaining open lines of communication and being open to subtle cues of concern are crucial in what are seen as virtual working environments. Level 5 leadership emerged from a five-year study by Collins (2001), where a model of five hierarchical states to top leadership was proposed. Not everybody can climb to be a level 5 leader but, in line with many of the new leadership theories, the ultimate leader is not seen as someone who is egotistical and overly ambitious, rather as someone who works ethically, humbly and gives credit to others.

Level 5: Level 5 Executive
Builds enduring greatness through a paradoxical blend of personal humility and professional will.

Level 4: Effective Leader
Catalyzes commitment to and vigorous pursuit of a clear and compelling vision, stimulating higher performance standards.

Level 3: Competent Manager
Organizes people and resources toward the effective and efficient pursuit of predetermined objectives.

Level 2: Contributing Team Member
Contributes individual capabilities to the achievement of group objectives and works effectively with others in a group setting.

Level 1: Highly Capable Individual
Makes productive contributions through talent, knowledge, skills and good work habits.

Figure 4.4 The level 5 hierarchy model

Source: Good to Great by Jim Collins © 2001. Used by permission of Curtis Brown, Ltd. All rights reserved.

Kouzes and Posner (2007) focused on leadership as a human relationship and noted the five exemplary practices of leadership:

- Model the way
- Inspire a shared vision
- Challenge the process
- Enable others to act
- Encourage the heart.

Daft (2006) indicates that these newer paradigms of leadership, involving change facilitation, creating a learning environment, sharing vision and shaping cultural values are important in the complexity of working life. Weberg (2012) proposes the value of 'Complexity (adaptive) Leadership' to provide a newly coined framework of continual process that focuses on collaboration, complex systems and innovation mindsets with the promise to improve costs and quality in health care. It has its roots in chaos theory, situational and servant leadership as well as the shared leadership approach of Mintzberg. Leadership professor Jim Clawson noted that a leader is not about status but about a perspective (2013: 1). In his opinion, leadership has three elements:

1. Seeing what needs to be done;
2. Understanding all the underlying forces at play in the situation; *and*
3. Having the courage to initiate action to make things better. (Clawson, 2013: 3)

This fits in well with Radcliffe (2012: 29) who developed his recent model to stress that successful leadership is not about leadership personality or characteristics or even whether leaders are born or made but shaped on what *needs to be done* through three ingredients that focused on the:

• Future
• Engagement
• Delivery.

He noted this FED recipe signified effective leadership:

> Powerful and effective leaders are guided by the future they want. And more than this, the leader is stronger when that future is powerfully connected to what he/she cares about. If you need others then you need to engage with them and encourage and support them to deliver.

The notion of 'big shoes' leadership was coined by Flaum (2009) to convey a sense of power that a new leader may have in crafting a new winning culture in an organization and leaving behind big footprints which will be remembered. One of the most important aspects of all of these ideas is the ability to encompass human skills in order to build a culture of performance based on trust and integrity. These ideas will be discussed in greater detail as we progress through this book.

Will clinicians be able to rise to these demands? Hopefully, they will not accept the traditional followership roles of the past. The following quote is a useful ending for this chapter:

> As for the best leaders, the people do not notice their existence. The next best, the people honour and praise. The next, the people fear, and the next the people hate. When the best leader's work is done, the people say 'we did it ourselves!'.
> Lao-Tsu (604–531 BC), cited in Robertson (1997: 278)

Summary of Key Points

This chapter has briefly looked at various aspects of leadership theory in order to meet the identified learning outcomes. These were:

- **Identify the evolution of leadership theories** There is a direct link to psychology and social sciences in the adopted styles of the leader; however, it is generally felt that – depending on the situation – the role of leadership may change.
- **Compare and contrast the various leadership theories** Trait theory originated prior to the turn of the twentieth century and around the time of the second Industrial Revolution. It was felt that leaders exhibited distinct qualities or traits in order for them to function effectively. Conversely, what leaders do in terms of Action Centred Leadership to meet the needs of an organisation was discussed. However, it is necessary to be aware of the effects different leadership styles have on the overall behaviour of the group in order for that group to become effective.
- **Critically discuss the application of these theories in relation to health care** A wide range of leadership theories has developed over time and these theories have contributed to the drive to make the health service more effective and efficient. However, it has been debated whether these theories have always been scientifically substantiated. The influence of these theories can be seen through the recruitment, work practices and appraisal processes in organisations and these have an impact on the performance of the individual or the team.

FURTHER READING

Kouzes, J.M. and Posner, B.Z. (2007) *The Leadership Challenge* (4th edn). San Fransisco, CA: Jossey-Bass.

Northouse, P.G. (2011) *Introduction to Leadership: Concepts and Practice* (2nd edn). London: Sage.

Prosser, S. (2002) 'Servant leadership', *Professional Nurse*, 18 (4): 238.

Van Seters, D.A. and Field, R.H.G. (1990) 'The evolution of leadership theory', *Journal of Organizational Change Management*, 3: 3.

www.theguardian.com/society/2014/apr/17/legal-victory-heart-doctor-whistleblower-hospital-safety-fears (accessed 4 June 2014).

Visit the companion website at https://study.sagepub.com/barr3e for more resources.

PART 2

THE TEAM

5   TEAM LIFE

Learning Outcomes

By the end of this chapter you will have had the opportunity to:

- Define what is meant by 'group' and 'team'
- Examine the values of team membership
- Discuss the value of group/team unity
- Discuss the importance of group/team formation
- Debate the classification of work groups
- Investigate the application of team leadership
- Evaluate the notion of effective leadership teams and their impact on the learning environment.

INTRODUCTION

Over the last four chapters, you have been investigating yourself as an individual preparing for the role of leader, taking into account the expected behaviours, beliefs and values you may hold. It is now prudent to scrutinize the team from the point of view of group/team formation, team dynamics and how you might expect individuals to react within a given situation. It is important to recognize the dynamics of the team in order to lead effectively for best patient care outcomes. To enable us to do this we must examine group formation and dynamics prior to studying the effects these elements have on leadership skills. Following this, we will attempt to offer suggestions as to the best method or style of leadership within given hypothetical health care situations.

GROUP AND TEAM CHARACTERISTICS

Individuals do not often work in isolation; rather they are members of a group. Indeed, you may well be a member of one or more groups related to both work and leisure activities. Groups are an essential feature of any organisation; their power cannot be underestimated and so the ways in which they work together are fascinating phenomena. It is interesting to study children at play to see how they interact with each other. If you watch what is going on in the playground, crèche, or any group of children you will see different behaviours emerging – from leader to subservient member. The effective leader should consider the impact of diversity such as age, gender and ethnicity (Chapter 3) on group processes and work pressures. These pressures can, in turn, have a great influence over the behaviour of group members; for example, society expects health care workers to dress and act in a particular way. It is useful to think of other areas where expectations in fads and fashions influence the way groups of people dress and act together – 'Mods' 'Rockers', 'Teddy Boys', and today's 'hoodies' or Goths, where group members have to dress in a particular way in order to be accepted into the prevalent teen society.

Activity
What do you think a group is?
Write a definition.
List how many groups you belong to.

Honey (1988: 88) notes that a group is seen as 'a collection of individual people who come together to achieve some purpose'; Sullivan and Garland (2010: 78) concur with this but differentiate between:

- formal groups – existing within the organisational structure to complete a specific task, for example, Task and Finish Groups
- informal groups – evolving naturally from social interactions despite organisational structure, for example, golfing or theatre work societies.

Mullins (2013: 300) offers the suggestion that any number of people who interact with one another are psychologically aware of one another, and those who perceive themselves to be a group are therefore a group. Other authors add to this by highlighting the need for a communication network, complementary goals and a group structure. Buchanan and Huczynski (2004: 283) state that 'it has been estimated that the average person belongs to five or six different groups and about 92% of people are in groups of five people or less'. Whatever groups you may have listed, the identified group members should share a common purpose with shared norms, values and beliefs.

It is often fudged but it is important to explore the difference between groups and teams. Humphries (1998: 11) states:

a group is a collection of individuals each with their own thoughts, ideas, abilities and objectives – the sort of gathering you might encounter on a social occasion, or indeed waiting at a bus stop.

He goes on to say that:

a team is a group of people working together to achieve common objectives and willing to commit all their energies necessary to ensuring that the objectives are achieved.

Honey (1988) distinguishes a group from a team in that the latter evolves from the former and performs at a much higher level of cohesion than a group needs to. Sullivan and Garland (2010: 79) discern that there is a blurred boundary between groups and teams. They note that not all work groups are teams, giving a General Practice (GP) as an example; it may have six General Practitioners (GPs) working alongside each other but they do not necessarily need to work as a team to care manage their patients. The practice management administration does, however, need to work as a team to arrange appointments, maintain records and ensure referrals are managed appropriately. This could be seen as a 'community of practice' which is a concept where individuals work together with a shared practice goal and is further explored in Chapter 6. Whether we concentrate on work or leisure activities, we all have roles to play within a team or a group and we all seem to function better when we work with others rather than working in isolation.

Loyalty within a team or a group is often seen as a requirement. Those who question the actions or decisions of the group may run the risk of being ostracised or subtly made to conform. For instance, within the workplace allied health professionals may work in directorate groups, standard setting groups and workplace audit groups to name a few. There are also the Royal College of Nursing (RCN) Forum groups, supporting different professional groups such as operating theatre, rehabilitation, primary care nursing, emergency care working. If you wish to maintain membership of these groups then you might, at times, feel a need to suppress or restrain your feelings to retain your membership without any loss of face. So it is clear that group and team formation is an important area to understand when endeavouring to lead; it is this knowledge that will help the effective leader to understand better the ways people behave. If leaders or managers are to avoid the negative aspects of a group, it is important for them to understand the dynamics of work groups and the advantages and limitations of using them to accomplish different types of tasks.

Try the self-assessment of your own position in dealing with people in teams provided on the companion website. If you answered mainly yes to these statements, your role is seen as having a *people focus* within the role of dealing with groups and teams. It is important to realise that a work team strongly influences the overall behaviour and performance of individual group members. Belbin (2000) describes teamwork as being a fashionable term and it seems to have replaced the more usual reference to the group; therefore, every activity conducted by a group is referred to as teamwork. Mears and Voehl (1994) are more specific in describing the differences between groups and teams to include skills exhibited by members.

There were many changes in the way people viewed groups during the twentieth century. However, it appears that for universal purposes the word 'group' is taken to have a general sense, whereas 'team' has a more specific context; so in order to 'get the job done', a team needs to be formed. In general, we refer to 'group' or 'team' according to the particular focus of attention and the spirit, style and perception of the group/team. Confusion arises due to the duality and interchangeability of the terms and many writers do not differentiate between the two. The dynamics of the group are about the forces within a group that are ever-changing in order to meet specific situations; it is also about the science investigating the action of these forces relating to the strength of the demands of given situations on individual members. Not only does this affect the way in which we interact at work but also when we are in our homes and within our individual communities.

RELEVANCE FOR PERSON CENTRED CARE

If we now consider the relevance of groups and teams in relation to person centred care it is clear that by considering the patient as a person rather than a condition, care can be devised to meet individual needs. Person-centred care aims to be user focused, promote independence and autonomy, provide choice and control and be based on a collaborative team philosophy. It takes into account service users' needs and views and builds relationships with family members. Considering services from a user's point of view is a fantastic way of helping the professionals involved to take a step back and see their services from a new perspective. This becomes a powerful motivator and driver for change, and can help to increase clinical engagement in the project. When staff hear how patients experience their services, the need for improvement is immediately apparent and the case for change becomes compelling.

The Health Foundation (2013) suggests person-centred care involves:

Compassion, dignity and respect – these are the essential foundation for the greater involvement of people in their own care.

Shared decision making – this requires the involvement of patients as equal partners in their health care. Tools to support shared decision making can include self-management support, access to personal health records, personal health budgets, care planning and shared treatment decisions.

Collective patient and public involvement – this is about involving people in decisions about the design and delivery of services. Examples of collective patient and public involvement include consultation of communities of patients in commissioning decisions and public engagement in reconfiguration decisions.

In England the White Paper *Equity and Excellence: Liberating the NHS* (DH, 2010a) emphasises the importance of giving people more autonomy and control over their health care. The principle of 'No decision about me without me' underpins the NHS reform plans. The intention is that patients will get more choice and control, backed by an information revolution, so that services are more responsive to patients and designed around them, rather than patients having to fit around services. We make many assumptions that we, as clinicians in whatever speciality, know what it is like for patients and carers, but taking the step of actively finding out and involving them is critical not only when designing or changing a service but also when we devise a plan of care for the current need episode.

There is a need to validate and prioritise problems with patients, clients and their families in order to meet with their individual values and life goals. The use of standard care plans is often not agreed on an individual basis; patients with communication difficulties are thus compromised. Hibbert and Peters (2003) highlight the complexity and quantity of information given to patients and that the skill of the professional is in how to present and target that information for patients so that it is actually used in their decision making.

> ### ▶ Activity
>
> How do you think the use of standard care plans might assist/inhibit personalised care planning and taking the patients' individual needs into consideration?

You might have thought about the constraints of using a particular model of assessment as inhibiting choice, but by the same token it could enhance the situation because you will have the basic building blocks on which to discuss how changes in lifestyle, treatment or therapy can help move the person towards their optimum health and activity. An example of personalised care might be thinking of the diabetic patient who is at increased risk of circulatory problems so it is vital that the subject of diet, cessation of smoking and taking effective exercise needs to be raised. The rise of integrated care specialists goes some way to deal with the problem of helping the patient adapt to their new lifestyle, maybe attend combined clinics where diabetes and cardiovascular specialists are present to share expertise; or there may be sessions where guest speakers talk about their experiences in coping positively with the situation. Diabetes care has evolved, and will continue to do so over the years. The introduction of new technical advances and changes in working practices has provided health care professionals with excellent opportunities to deliver best practice, so improving patient outcomes.

VALUE OF GROUP/TEAM MEMBERSHIP

> ### ◆ Activity
>
> Why do you think working in a group is so popular?
> What benefits does it offer to individuals?

There are both positive and negative aspects to the use of work groups or teams. On the positive side you might have thought about the feedback, support and praise you get from others as you attempt to complete a task. There is also the togetherness and friendships formed which may give you a feeling of self-worth. Look at the success of websites like Friends Reunited, where people are able to reach out to members of groups they have lost contact with, in order to see how they are getting on. On the negative side, group membership may apply peer pressure on an individual to perform at a certain level. Similarly, an individual may find the behaviours of the group unacceptable but, due to the power within the group, find it difficult to rail against the 'norm', which is a form of 'groupthink' (Janis, 1982). This concept will be discussed further in Chapter 8.

Humphries (1998) highlighted specific benefits from teamwork where the team can:

- Achieve goals more quickly and efficiently than individuals working alone
- Support each other to improve skills
- Become more confident and develop interpersonal skills
- Be more creative
- Take more risks
- Be more flexible
- Show commitment to the task and each other
- Share information, knowledge and feelings
- Be self-motivated
- Enjoy their work by being with other people
- Be easier to lead.

> ### ◆ Activity
>
> Do you agree with this or does team working seem to take too much time?

The work of West (2002) and West et al. (2002, 2003), highlighting research work, established a relationship between staff working in teams and patient mortality. The leadership team processes and innovation in clinical contexts can be seen to have practical and theoretical implications. Mukamel et al. (2009) suggested that a higher quality of care was linked to better teamwork in nursing homes. Dackert's (2010) quantitative research in Sweden examined the positive importance of team climate and innovation in nursing the elderly.

It is interesting to read how management theory and research relates to the benefits of teamwork. The classical approach to management and organisational behaviour tends to ignore the importance of groups/teams. Indeed, Taylor (1947), commonly thought to be the 'father' of scientific management, described the concept of the 'rabble hypothesis' wherein he made the assumption that people should carry out their work as solitary individuals, unaffected by others and with no interaction. He may also have thought that allowing people time to mix would only lead to trouble and rebellion! This assumption was challenged by the Hawthorne experiments at the Western Electric Company in America (1924–1932). The experiments were designed to demonstrate a positive correlation between the amount of light in the workplace and worker productivity. One of the experiments took a group of 14 men working in a bank wiring room. It was noticed that the men formed their own subgroups and that, despite financial incentive, the group had decided that 6,000 units per day was a fair level of output. The group felt that if they started to produce in excess of the 6,000 units then it would ultimately become the 'norm'. Although 6,000 units was well below the level the group was capable of producing, group pressure not to 'over work' was stronger than the financial incentive, so the actual output was kept to the perceived 'reasonable' limit.

The four general conclusions drawn from the Hawthorne studies were that:

- **The aptitudes of individuals are imperfect predictors of job performance** Although they give some indication of the physical and mental potential of the individual, the amount produced is strongly influenced by social factors.
- **Informal organisation affects productivity** The Hawthorne researchers discovered a group life among the workers, and also showed that the relations that supervisors develop with workers tend to influence the manner in which the workers carry out directives.
- **Work-group norms affect productivity** The Hawthorne researchers were not the first to recognise that work groups tend to arrive at norms of what is 'a fair day's work', however, they provided the best systematic description and interpretation of this phenomenon.
- **The workplace is a social system** The Hawthorne researchers came to view the workplace as a social system made up of interdependent parts.

The notion of the Hawthorne effect also arose from these experiments. The effect can be defined as 'an increase in worker productivity produced by the psychological stimulus of being singled out and made to feel important', hence team or group members experienced a boost to their self-esteem when their work was being valued (www. nwlink.com/~donclark/hrd/history/hawthorne.html accessed on 24 March 2014).

Activity

How do the groups you identify with meet your social needs and enhance your social identity?

Do they stifle your individuality and freedom?

It can be argued that better ideas emerge when a number of people work on a problem separately and come together at a later date than when they work face-to-face in a group. This is possibly because group situations can inhibit the generation of ideas from less vocal members. Which begs the question: why form work groups or teams? Groups will often take greater risks (possibly because responsibility is shared and, therefore, less threatening) and groups make fewer errors because there may be more rescuers – members who see potential problems and set out to rectify them before they become problems. In a group there is also greater total knowledge and information. By discussing the situation, a more thorough review is accomplished and a particular proposal strengthened. Most importantly, problems require decisions that depend on the participation and support of a number of individuals. By forming groups, more members will accept a decision based on the group solving a problem than when one person solves it alone. Furthermore, communications relating to the decision can be speedy in the group process; communication breakdowns are reduced when the individuals have ownership.

GROUP UNITY

Group unity is an important aspect of work group dynamics. When establishing a new work group, it is important to cultivate a feeling of unity among the group members at an early stage. Unities in a group develop slowly as members open up and learn about each other. In the beginning, members are not sure whether they will be accepted and may hold back until they feel more secure. If the group has an unfriendly atmosphere or there is a chance of rejection, unity may not develop at all. As a leader, you can help the group to be more unified by providing a safe environment for all. Today, for the most part, groups are usually composed of people possessing some basic idea upon which they are all agreed and which they are trying to express through the medium of their clashing personalities and, frequently, in obedience to someone in a leadership role. Groups also come together in order to exploit and use methods which are regarded as essential to attaining the prevailing definition of 'successes'. Whatever degree of unity is achieved in such groups is often based on expediency or good manners. Ambition, conflict, hurt feelings and bruised egos can still be the 'normal' in-group experience. A number of factors have been identified which affect the cohesiveness of a group.

Size As the size of a group increases, its cohesiveness tends to decrease.

Achievement of Goals The attainment of goals increases cohesiveness, especially if the group establishes the goals.

Status of the Group Generally, the higher a group ranks in the hierarchy of an organisation, the greater its cohesiveness. A group can achieve status for many reasons, including:

- Achieving a higher level of performance or attaining other measures of success within the organisation
- Achieving recognition because individuals within the group display a high level of skill
- Conducting work that is dangerous or more challenging than other tasks
- Receiving more financial or material rewards than other groups
- Recognition that members of the group are considered for promotion more often or more quickly than those outside of the group. However, it should be noted that a sense of 'eliteness' might cause friction with other groups.

Dependence of Members on the Work Group The greater individual members' dependency upon the group, the stronger will be the bonds of attraction to the group. A group that is able to satisfy a number of an individual's needs will appear attractive to that individual. These needs may include status, recognition, financial rewards, or the ability to do his or her job more easily.

TYPES OF GROUPS

In every organisation, people are assigned to groups to perform tasks that one person could not accomplish alone. Some work groups, such as departmental teams, are formal parts of the organisation's structure, for example, operating department teams and ambulance teams, while some are ad hoc groups established to meet a short-term objective. Other groups may be formed where members operate individually but with equal commitment to achieving a set goal, such as integrated teams/multi-agency teams. An example of this type of group may include nurses, radiographers, physiotherapists, speech and language therapists and doctors working with patients in a stroke care unit. Still others are informal working arrangements that evolve to meet the various needs of the organisation e.g. a pastoral church group who visit the housebound parishioners.

The formal group is one created to accomplish a defined part of the organisa- tion's collective purpose. It has specific tasks allocated to it for which it is officially responsible. On the other hand, the informal group is a collection of individuals who influence one another's behaviour within the formal group. The informal group normally develops spontaneously and the people within the group talk and joke with one another; they have 'in jokes'; they associate with one another outside of the working environment and may be referred to as 'cliques' or be part of the grapevine system of communication within an organisation.

FORMATION OF GROUPS

A discussion related to the formation of groups must start with an examination of the members of the proposed group. They are a collection of people who will meet for the first time and then go on to form a group. Forsyth (2010) notes the work of Tuckman and Jensen (1977) who suggest that groups pass through five clearly defined stages of development that they call Forming; Storming; Norming; Performing; and Adjourning (sometimes listed as Mourning). They admit that not all groups go through all the stages; some find that they are stuck in the middle, and remain inefficient and ineffec- tive. With others, passage through the stages may be slow, but that passage appears to be necessary and inescapable. These stages are explained further below.

Forming

This is the orientation phase where individuals have not yet gelled. Each person is busy finding out about the others' attitudes and backgrounds; from this, ground rules (that is, codes of behaviour) for the group are established. Members often like to establish their personal identities and a leader is chosen. Task-wise they seek clarity/instruction about what they are being asked to do, what the issues are and whether everyone in the group understands the task.

How to Address the Forming Stage

Help team members get to know one another by the use of name badges or by introducing each other to the group. Make sure the purpose and task are clearly defined and share management expectations of the group. Give the team time to get comfortable with one another, but move the team along as well.

Storming

This is a conflict stage in the group/team's life and can be quite an uncomfortable period. Members bargain with each other and try to sort out their position within the group and, occasionally, hostility may result as differences in goals emerge. The key element for the leader here is to manage and resolve the conflict.

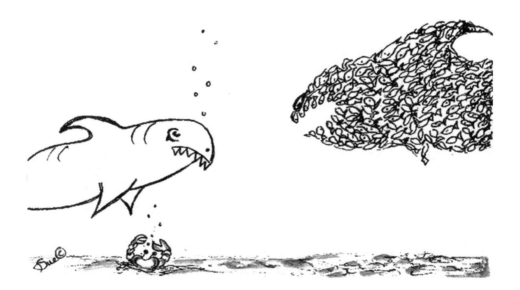

How to Address the Storming Stage

Do not ignore the storming stage. Acknowledge it with the team as a natural developmental step. Facilitators should acknowledge the conflicts and address them. This is a good time to review ground rules, revisit the purpose and related administrative matters of the team.

Norming

In this cohesion stage, members of the group/team develop closer relationships with each other; overall working roles like norms of behaviour and role allocation are established, and group cohesion becomes obvious.

How to Address the Norming Stage

At this stage, the team has established process fairly well. The task will take on new significance, as the team will want to accomplish its purpose. Facilitators should keep this in mind and remind the team of the task. In addition, facilitators should be more diligent in adhering to the road map, providing time for feedback or closure.

Performing

Here the group/team has developed an effective structure and is actually concerned with getting on with the job. Interestingly, not all groups reach this stage, with many becoming 'bogged down' in an earlier and less productive stage. Within the performing stage members are equally happy to work alone, in subgroups or as a single unit.

How to Address the Performing Stage

Teams at the performing level are generally self-regulating. Road maps, processes, decision making, and other matters of team management will be handled independently by the team.

Adjourning/Mourning

In this final stage, the group may disband or shift its dynamics, as its work is complete. The final stage (adjourning) is a more recent addition because it is thought to be a natural performing conclusion as the purpose of the team has been achieved. Tuckman and Jensen (1977) go on to suggest that groups may oscillate between the stages and pass through some stages several times without ever becoming effective.

▶ Activity

Consider the teams you are a member of and think of the following:

- What stage are you at in the formation of your team?
- If you believe you are at the performing stage, did it take you a long time to get there?
- Has there been a change in membership of the team?
- If so, has it affected the performance level of the team?

Humphries (1998) discusses the need to identify team roles, recognising that each team member will have two roles: their professional role and their team role. He then listed seven team roles:

- natural leader
- activator
- thinker
- organiser
- checker
- judge
- supporter.

He suggests that the role undertaken will be related to the personality of the team member but will not be under the control of that person, that is, you would not be able to select the role you think you might wish to undertake. As each role has some advantages, it is useful to have a mix of the attributes within the team so that as the team leader you would be able to develop the positive features and reduce the negatives. In an ideal world, a team would have one member from each category together with several supporters. Belbin (2000) lists eight similar roles but gives slightly different descriptions of each role, the overall intent being for the leader to recognise and utilise these roles effectively. It might be useful to go to Belbin's website (www.belbin.com) in order to compare and contrast the team roles described. Barr and Dowding (2012) reflect on the member roles identified by Belbin (2000); Marquis and Huston (2008: 457) similarly identified that tasks within a team are encompassed within 11 roles but agreed that managers and leaders have to be aware of how teams carry out these specific roles and tasks.

1. **Initiator:** proposes or suggests group goals or redefines the problem in order to make sure all members understand what is to be achieved
2. **Information Seeker:** searches for a factual basis for the group's work
3. **Information Giver:** offers an opinion of what the group's values are
4. **Opinion Seeker:** seeks opinions that clarify or reflect other members' suggestions
5. **Elaborator:** gives examples or extends meanings of suggestions and may indicate how they might work
6. **Coordinator:** clarifies and coordinates ideas and activities of the group
7. **Orienter:** summarises decisions and actions, questions departures from original intention
8. **Evaluator:** questions group accomplishments and compares them to the standard
9. **Energiser:** stimulates and prods group into action
10. **Procedural Technician:** facilitates group by arranging the environment, *and*
11. **Recorder:** records the group's activities and accomplishments.

Together with this, managers and leaders need to examine the importance of team-building. It is necessary to identify supportive roles in order to provide care for the members of the team. They also need to identify roles that negatively affect the team dynamics.

> ◆ **Activity**
>
> Look at the resource on the companion website and see if you can identify any of these roles you or others play in a regular meeting you attend.
>
> How do you think these relate to conflict and conflict management (Chapter 9)?

It could be that the negative behaviour on the right-hand side is not meaningfully destructive but simply indicates that the individual has found no other arena in which to convey their work dissatisfactions; leaders need to confront these dissatisfactions in a one-to-one supportive meeting. These individuals may be seen as helpful in raising creative expressions of the value systems of the team but it must be noted that an individual may feel excluded from the team unless the leader manages this positively. Their behaviour will continue to impact negatively on the team's ability to reach its goals unless the individual feels valued as a member and has their concerns taken seriously.

How to Handle the 'Not Always Helpful' Roles

There are a number of ways team members may appear to be unhelpful ranging from outright hostility towards the change to quiet but grudging acceptance. In order to recognise and address these issues it is vital that the team leader is aware of the non-verbal as well as the verbal manifestations of the members' concerns; by understanding the roles described by Belbin and further discussed by Marquis and Huston many problems can be avoided. Strategies for dealing with these 'not always helpful' roles can include the following:

- Set clear time limits for making decisions and remind people often of the time – jokers are less likely to intrude or delay if they are regularly informed of the time and process.
- Clarify expectations – get team 'buy-in' upfront for the work to be done. Agree by consensus that everyone will accept responsibility for any extra work. If the 'Busier Than Thou' person begins to complain, remind that person of his or her agreement.

In general, individuals disrupt meetings for myriad reasons. Skilled facilitators will acknowledge the fears or anxieties behind the behaviour and then move on.

Remember This ...

Team members must commit to the success of the group and promise to participate. Here is another activity that reflects the interrelationships of individuals within a team.

▶ Activity

The Drawbridge

Go to the resource on the companion website. In the story there are six characters. They are (in alphabetical order): the Baron; the Baroness; the Boatman; the Friend; the Lover; and the Gatekeeper. Put the characters in order of their responsibility for the death of the Baroness.

There should be 100 per cent agreement between all members of the group undertaking the exercise.

The exercise is designed to challenge your attitudes, beliefs and values. In doing so you can see that there is more than one side to an argument with each of the characters feeling that they are correct in what they do to support – or not – the Baron. The exercise may cause a great deal of discussion among your colleagues and it will become extremely difficult to come to the same outcome between different team members – and, indeed, teams.

Clearly, people do not necessarily elect to adopt one of the highlighted roles (see the resource on the companion website) but their individual personality and knowledge will mean that certain people will not be able to avoid working in a particular way. This knowledge can be utilised by an effective leader when allocating tasks but it is also of use to the followers when learning to deal with appointed managers.

◢ Activity

Have you worked with people in the clinical area who fit into the categories mentioned? (Refer to the resource on the companion website.)

I well remember a colleague who clearly functioned within the 'dominator' role. I seemed to spend a great deal of time reassuring new members of staff that it was 'just her way' of achieving objectives and that her attention to detail when delegating work was not personal – she did it to everyone irrespective of role or position within the hierarchy. Once they had realised that it was not personal, members of staff were able to function effectively and not take her comments to heart. In this situation, I could be seen as the 'harmoniser'; the new staff became effective 'followers' until they took on their preferred roles.

Whilst, in the main, diversity within a team may lead to creativity, it can also contribute to a healthy level of conflict. The effective leader must remember that there can be negative effects of teamwork. Sullivan and Garland (2010: 180) highlight the negative aspects of 'groupthink' (Janis, 1982), which is a phenomenon occurring in highly cohesive, isolated groups in which group members start to think alike. In turn, this can interfere with critical thinking and may lead to inappropriate decision making.

You may have found that it took you longer to reach the performance level in one group than it did in another; indeed, you may never have reached high performance in one of your groups and found that you remained at the storming stage for most of the time until the group was disbanded. The problem may have stemmed from the lack of effective leadership, where the leader may have been unaware of the roles of some of the group members. Dynamic leaders will inspire followers towards participative management by how they work and communicate in groups. Effective leaders will need to keep group members on course, draw out the shy, politely cut off the talkative and protect the weak. At all times leaders must be aware of the team but remember that they should not be 'hung up' on the roles but recognise that all roles are valuable. The long-term consequence of this is 'labelling' a person, which may lead to the 'halo' or 'hero' effect (Hartley, 1997).

CLASSIFICATION OF WORK GROUPS

Mullins (2013) discusses the classification of work groups as being either formal or informal. These groups may coalesce in order to accomplish a specific task or may arise naturally in order to meet the needs of a particular group of people working within the organisation. Understanding the functions of these groups is important in becoming an effective leader.

Formal Groups

These include a variety of groups and teams whose roles can be clearly defined. In the main, they are permanent groupings of personnel specified in the organisational chart. Within the NHS these groupings could be speciality based, for example, operating theatres, ambulance trust, ward based, community and NHS Trusts that are concerned with the commissioning of care in the community setting. Subordinates report directly to a designated supervisor and the relationships among personnel have some formal basis. This might take the form of duty rotas where there is a rota chart that relates to who is working with whom on what days, in order to ensure all care is given to the patients/clients within a specific area. Other formal groups may be termed 'task groups' and are formed by a number of personnel assigned to work together to complete a project. There are different levels of task group. Task groups may comprise personnel from two or more departments and are, thus, cross-departmental. A 'committee' is a special-purpose task group. The purpose of committees is to:

- exchange views and information
- recommend action
- generate ideas *and*
- make decisions.

Here the term 'committee' refers to a group of people whose job is to define the parameters of tasks, while a 'work group' is assigned the job of accomplishing tasks.

> ◀ Activity
>
> Go back to the purposes of a committee above where the exchange of views and information, recommending action, generating ideas and making decisions are identified.
>
> What views do you have about the effectiveness of the committees you know?

You might wonder about the outcome or output of many committees. One can think of areas where a committee may be necessary in deciding a long-term strategy or business plan but it sometimes seems out of touch with reality. Indeed, remember that 'a camel looks like a horse that was designed by a committee' (Sir Alec Issigonis 1906–1988, July 1958) (http://en.wikiquote.org/wiki/Alec_Issigonis accessed 24 March 2014). It's an ironic expression, used to show that deciding anything by committee – and therefore taking too many opinions and wish-lists into account – will result in something that's probably vaguely similar to what was originally planned but which won't be anywhere near as effective as was wanted. A camel and a horse are both ungulates, but the point is that the camel is both ugly and slow in comparison to a horse. Strategic decisions do not always translate into operational tasks. Leaders should read and try to understand fully any committee documents produced and appraise them for their effectiveness and workability. Often it feels as though nothing ever comes from a committee; we hear of people/managers 'going to meetings' but then go on to ask, 'What has been achieved?'. The routine of meetings for meetings' sake has to be challenged and there are now more references made to task and finish groups in order to prevent stagnation. However, these may in turn be seen as a 'quick-fix' solution to a problem that requires more sustainable action. Task groups in the form of unilateral or multidisciplinary teams may also be charged with reviewing policies and procedures governing clinical practices. Here we may think of a project such as ensuring all procedures are documented and updating any research that informs practice towards better quality patient care.

Advantages to teamwork include broader experience and wider knowledge, and members may be more committed to implementation if they have the opportunity to share in the decision making process. Disadvantages might include any decisions that come from a group process being open to social pressures, with decisions made for the wrong reasons and weaker members being strongly influenced by stronger ones.

Informal groups

Within a work setting, people may band together informally in order to accomplish an objective. This objective may be related to the work of the organisation; for example, a group of people such as nurses, physiotherapists, pharmacists, and dieticians may join up in order to produce a health education poster. Informal groups are likely to develop when the formal organisational structure does not accommodate their joint needs. Another example is where all the paramedics within a shift might get together informally to compare notes, talk about practice, and socialise in the context of clinical support groups. Workers who want to promote a particular interest or point of view also form interest groups within an organisation; these are the most important non-formal groups for the manager to consider.

'Friendship groups' are informal associations of workers developed as an extension of their interaction and communication in the work environment. They are formed for a variety of reasons, including common characteristics (such as age or ethnic background), political sentiment, or common interests. In this book, we will not explore friendship groups in detail. However, managers should be aware that many actions (such as assignment of tasks and the establishment of other types of working groups) influence the interaction and communication patterns among subordinates, causing individuals to affiliate with each other so that interests and friendship groups inevitably emerge. These groups can have both positive and negative consequences for an organisation, and managers should be alert to ways in which these informal friendship groups affect overall performance.

TEAM LEADERSHIP

Within the management of the NHS workforce, the notion of team and group appear to be interchangeable. Teams emanate from groups. Earlier in this chapter, we were discussing the differences between groups and teams; we highlight the differences and note that it is important to ensure the team is empowered to do what is necessary to achieve the overall goal. The complex process of leadership is highlighted by Barge (1996), who sees leadership as 'mediation' and 'coordination'. Owen (2009: xxi, 383) also discusses the 3½ Ps of leadership where he highlights People Focus, Professionalism and Positive Attitude as being the three main elements of leadership performance. The *performance* element is then the odd one out (Owen, 2009: xxi) as most leaders in his survey saw performance as a symptom rather than a feature of leadership; it therefore achieves only a ½ in the 3½ Ps. He then goes on to discuss what good leadership might look like at each level of the organisation.

These descriptions draw together factors that have been discussed throughout this chapter in terms of group/team formation and the personalities of people in the situation. Moving on from this we can revisit the application of information from the MBTI® (Chapter 2). From the results of the indicator and by learning to know yourself – and how you prefer to work – you can construct your 'style compass' (Figure 5.1).

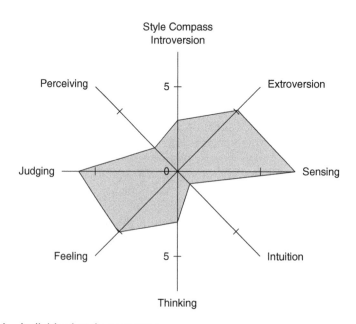

Figure 5.1 Individual style compass

Following this, you can use your judgement of what you know about others to plot their shape over yours (Figure 5.2). Now you will see how alike/different you are and note the degree of overlap. Clearly, it would not be of great benefit for us all to be the same otherwise nothing would be achieved; there needs to be a balance so that decisions can be made, thus making it easier to move forward as a team. The style compass is only a quick way of thinking about any style and can be adapted to highlight interactions among people within a team.

Certainly, while we both appear to be extroverts, I appear to be more judgemental than my colleague is but she has more perception of what is required – hence, we work well together, recognising each other's differences and building on each other's strengths.

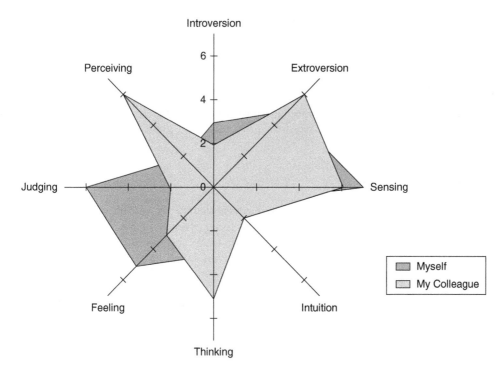

Figure 5.2   An example of a style compass for two people

Activity

Plot your own style compass and that of a colleague. Having completed the Myers-Briggs MBTI type test (discussed in Chapter 2 and the companion website) you can plot the initial totals by constructing a graph in a spreadsheet programme; this is of most use for visual learners.

Highlight where you differ and discuss how these differences may enhance your abilities to lead effectively.

GROUP CONFLICT

Effective team development can help to resolve conflict. Initially the group needs to plan what they are going to do, identify goals and decide, if appropriate, on a mission statement (Marriner Tomey, 2008). There are techniques that can be utilised in order to do this, the best known of which is 'nominal group technique'; alternatives include 'consensus', ' majority rule' and 'independent listing', so that items can be considered in order of importance. This is very similar to nominal group technique, which has the following pattern:

- First, the group members are asked to list, on paper, what the group wants to achieve and how they will behave in order to reach that identified goal.
- Second, each person will read out one item from their list, which will be recorded on paper or whiteboard for all to see, discuss and agree to.
- Third, discussion will take place to prioritise the items prior to them being typed up for all to have a copy.

By having all members of the group agree to the list of objectives and behaviours a feeling of identity is engendered and the group should function well.

LEADERSHIP TEAMS

In general education, the notion of distributed leadership is becoming the 'norm'. It is a notion that has been around for a long time, either as delegated or as shared leadership. It is essentially about sharing out leadership across the organisation. However, we are aware that while there is a strong belief in the idea, there is not a great deal of evidence about how it works in practice. Therefore, we need to explore the idea in some depth. We know that effective leadership makes a difference, so it follows that the caring professions need effective leaders at all levels.

Leadership teams, it is believed, are one way of giving power to everyone. As the caring professions and the NHS in general become more complex to manage and lead, we need many more leaders than ever before, enabling us to create pools of talent from which we can grow tomorrow's leaders. A key to successful planning and implementation is the development of teams. Table 5.1 provides a description of three types of teams and their relative advantages and disadvantages.

When we talk about sharing leadership, we ought to mean sharing learning-centred leadership. We should create and develop many leaders who influence and improve the quality of learning and teaching. Although distributed leadership is not a difficult idea, when put into practice it can take many different forms. For example, you will find that there are assortments of teams within the health service that have powers in a variety of situations (Table 5.2). It is useful to understand how they work in order to function effectively.

Barr and Dowding (2012: 94) highlighted the relative features, advantages and disadvantages of leadership teams that are seen to be necessary to ensure the smooth

Table 5.1 Three types of team and their relative advantages and disadvantages

Model	Features	Advantages	Disadvantages
Functional	A manager and subordinates for a particular function in organisation (e.g. ward nursing team)	There is a whole team focus on implementing continuous nursing care across a 24-hour period for patients on the ward Skills can be learnt within the team and cost effective to use different grades of staff Hierarchical management to ensure policy/procedures are followed	There may be difficulties communicating the needs of patients towards other specialities (medical, physiotherapy, pharmacy, etc.) on a regular basis Cross-sector communication to community teams may also prove difficult Rigidity of change
Cross Functional	Experts of various specialities or functions working together on specific organisational tasks (e.g. Accident and Emergency staff in a Trust)	Uses the skills and knowledge of a breadth of practitioners (for instance-surgical, nursing, radiology, social work functions) for the care management of complex trauma needs of patients	Complexity of functional cultures where poor communication issues may affect care and thus patient outcome
Self-directed	Self-managed teams work without managers to deliver services to internal or external customers (e.g. alternative health therapy centre)	Problem solving and decision making left in the hands of each consultant, practitioner or therapist	Difficulties when specialist is off work to cover their speciality Difficulty in internal monitoring of quality provided by each specialist

Table 5.2 Team and administration responsibilities

Management Team	Governance Team Responsibilities	Administration Responsibilities
Vision (planning)	Creates, reviews and approves	Recommends process, develops and plans (decides what) and implements plans (decides how)
Structure (policy)	Creates, reviews and adopts	Recommends and implements
Advocacy (communication)	Represents public interest, seeks public input	Acts in public interest, seeks and provides public information
Accountability (evaluation)	Monitors progress toward goals, evaluates the board standards and personnel in accordance	Implements evaluation of programmes

running of a business or institution such as the NHS. The Executive teams are normally quite small (3–8) and able to make decisions quite quickly, whilst District teams are often mid-sized (15–20) where key representatives are present to ensure their views are taken into account. However, when teams or committees get bigger than this (Community teams, 25–30) there are often so many individual issues to be satisfied that decisions take longer to be made and opportunities may be missed.

When a unit has leadership in teams, the whole institution can evolve towards becoming a learning organisation. Learning organisations are able to retain staff due to their commitment to those staff. It is, therefore, part of the role of the effective leader to ensure students and staff are supported within their clinical areas, which in turn requires effective mentorship programmes and updating of staff to ensure accurate and professional assessment within that clinical area. The following characteristics may go some way to define the effective learning environment:

- People feel they are doing something that matters – to them personally and to the larger world
- Every individual in the organisation is somehow stretching, growing or enhancing his/her capacity to create a learning, caring environment
- People are more intelligent together than they are apart
- The organisation continually becomes more aware of its underlying knowledge base in the hearts and minds of employees
- Visions of the direction of the enterprise emerge at all levels. The responsibility of the administration is to manage the process whereby new emerging visions become shared visions
- Employees are invited to learn what is going on at every level of the organisation, so they can understand how their actions influence others
- People feel free to enquire about each other's assumptions and biases
- People treat each other as colleagues
- There is a mutual respect and trust in the way they talk to each other, no matter what their position is.

All this is led by the effective leader and done within the framework of the team. Staff retention and team morale will be supported and maintained; together with this, students will feel that there is a place for them within the organisation and as they complete their individual courses they will apply for a permanent post.

Summary of Key Points

This chapter has briefly looked at various aspects of team life in order to meet the identified learning outcomes. These were:

- **Define what is meant by 'group' and 'team'** The various definitions, and interchangeability, of the two labels were discussed. Ultimately, it seems from the literature, there is ongoing debate related to whether or not there is a need to differentiate between the two.

- **Examine the values of team membership** Teams are valued because they can achieve cohesiveness and effectiveness within our working environments. The Hawthorne Experiment demonstrated the ability to enhance worker productivity through boosting self-esteem due to work being valued.
- **Discuss the value of group/team unity** This is an important aspect of work group dynamics. As a leader, you need a unified team in order for the workplace to become effective.
- **Discuss the importance of group/team formation** It is important to remember that groups and teams form for specific purposes. The stages of formation are important if the effective leader is to encourage the team to meet their final objectives.
- **Debate the classification of work groups** Here we note that there are two main classifications of groups: formal and informal. Each has its own role and responsibility but working effectively relies on all types of groups/teams.
- **Investigate the application of team leadership** Effective team leadership is vital. In order to achieve this, a number of tools have been developed to identify personal strengths and weaknesses to enable team leadership to work effectively.
- **Evaluate the notion of effective leadership teams and their impact on the learning environment** Learning from general education we can see that employee retention is affected by staff perception of involvement with the decision making process. The knock-on effect of this may be to enhance the learning environment.

FURTHER READING

Department of Health (2001) *A Health Service of all Talents: Developing the NHS Workforce.* London: DH.

Donaldson, L. (1995) 'Management for doctors: conflict, power, negotiation', *British Medical Journal*, 310: 104–7.

Ellis, P. and Abbott, J. (2011) 'What new leaders need to understand about their teams', *British Journal of Cardiac Nursing*, 6 (3): 144–6.

Health Foundation (2013) *Inspiring Improvement.* Available at: www.health.org.uk/areas-of-work/topics/person-centred-care/person-centred-care/ (accessed 11 May 2015).

Kay, L. (2010) 'Leading other midwives: experience of midwife team leaders', *British Journal of Midwifery*, 18 (12): 764–9.

Pattison, S. (2001) 'User involvement and participation in the NHS: a personal perspective', in T. Heller, R. Muston, M. Sidell and C. Lloyd (eds), *Working for Health*. London: Sage/Open University Press.

Rashid, C. (2010) 'Benefits and limitations of nurses taking on aspects of the clinical role of doctors in primary care: integrative literature review', *Journal of Advanced Nursing*, 66 (8): 1658–70.

Salvage, J. and Smith, R. (2000) 'Doctors and nurses: doing it differently', *British Medical Journal*, 320: 1019–20.

Visit the companion website at https://study.sagepub.com/barr3e for more resources.

6   INTERDISCIPLINARY AND INTERPROFESSIONAL WORKING

Learning Outcomes

By the end of this chapter you should be able to:

- Critically discuss the importance of interdisciplinary and interprofessional working in health for effective patient care and safety
- Critically explore the opportunities and challenges of interprofessional working in the contemporary context
- Identify issues of practice communities, tribalism and professional identities and the importance of interprofessional education.

INTRODUCTION

In Chapter 5 we explored the nature of team life and the importance of leadership in relation to team behaviour and management of difficult situations. We also explored the importance of team working in relation to improving patient/client outcomes. This chapter aims to explore another facet of the notion of teams within the context of working across boundaries with people from different backgrounds. The importance of effective interdisciplinary and interprofessional team working for quality health care has long been underpinned by research, inquiries and policy (Firth-Cozens, 1998; Reeves et al., 2010; DH, 2002; HM Government, 2013). Interdisciplinary and interprofessional working does need leadership for success.

Failings in the NHS have become more evident in the last few years especially concerning quality of patient care. There is particular emphasis on interprofessional team working across a number of NHS agencies and partnerships. The Kennedy Report into the child heart surgery in Bristol in 2001 identified a number of poor interdisciplinary practices (DH, 2002). More recently Francis (2013) in his independent inquiry into care provided by a Midland NHS Foundation Trust noted that 'patients were seen intermittently by various members of the multidisciplinary team but there was little evidence that there was a planned multidisciplinary approach to their care'. Bender et al. (2013: 165) noted the challenge of formal collaborative processes and resulting fragmentation of care that exists throughout the healthcare system today.

Ineffective interdisciplinary and interprofessional leadership is seen as a cause of concern. With the need for more effective and efficient health services – and with the finances of public health services being under government scrutiny – working with different disciplines and professions will be essential. The Keogh review of care quality in July 2013 also signalled the importance of health care leadership and proposed the following improvement issues:

Patient experience – understanding how the views of patients and related patient experience data is used and acted upon (such as how effectively complaints are dealt with and the 'visibility' of feedback themes reviewed at board level);

Safety – understanding issues around the Trust's safety record and ability to manage these (such as compliance with safety procedures or Trust policies that enhance trust, training to improve safety performance, the effectiveness of reporting issues of safety compliance or use of equipment that enhances safety);

Workforce – understanding issues around the Trust's workforce and its strategy to deal with issues within the workforce (for instance staffing ratios, sickness rates, use of agency staff, appraisal rates and current vacancies) as well as listening to the views of staff;

Clinical and operational effectiveness – understanding issues around the Trust's clinical and operational performance (such as the management of capacity and the quality – or presence — of trust-wide policies, how the Trust addresses clinical and operational performance) and in particular how Trusts use mortality data to analyse and improve quality of care;

Governance and leadership – understanding the Trust's leadership and governance of quality (such as how the board is assured of the performance of the Trust to ensure that it is safe and how it uses information to drive quality improvements).

NNRU (2013) identifies that research shows there is a close correlation between staff experience and patient care. Patients receive better care by staff working in teams that are well led, have clear objectives and have the time and resources to provide that care.

◆ Activity

Jot down what you understand by the terms interdisciplinary, interprofessional and multidisciplinary working.

There are a number of similar terms – such as interdisciplinary and interprofessional – which are often used interchangeably.

The term **interdisciplinary**, as an adjective, relates to two or more disciplines collaborating together towards a shared goal. In health care, this may be seen as care activity which involves the various disciplines within one profession. So one example may be that of the disciplines of a children's nurse and a senior adult nurse working in accident and emergency collaborating on addressing the needs of children requiring emergency care in that hospital. Another example may be a locality district nurse and a general practice nurse collaborating to work on tissue viability treatments offered in the home and at the surgery for consistency. Interdisciplinary communication will also be required when patients cross boundaries from the community into hospital or on discharge from hospital to home. A breadth of international, national and regional interdisciplinary networks and forums are set up around certain conditions or concerns such as cardiac/coronary care, child health, learning disabilities or mental health.

Interprofessional as a term relates to two or more professionals collaborating together towards a shared goal. In health care this could involve nurses, doctors, allied health professions (such as occupational, speech, podiatrists or physiotherapist), therapists and social workers collaborating in working out a management plan to discharge an older person with complex needs following a cerebral haemorrhage.

The term **multidisciplinary** infers that health care providers from different professions work together to provide diagnoses, assessments and treatment, within their scope of practice and areas of competence. However, this term is somewhat less used as it is now felt that it does not demonstrate an interactive relationship but is probably how health care practice usually manifests itself.

The term **collaboration** has also been defined by Goldman and Kahnweiller (2000: 435) as a 'mutually beneficial and well defined relationship entered into by two or more organizations to achieve common goals'.

HISTORICAL AND CONTEMPORARY CONTEXT OF INTERPROFESSIONAL WORKING

Historically, different health care professionals have tended to work alongside each other. From the 1500s the development from craft guilds to professions has been documented by Reeves et al. (2010). They note the separate development of professions rather than an integrated development and thus health care tension arose. From a sociological perspective, linked to Freidson's (1970) theory of professional closure, different health and social care workers developed their own 'closed' organisation through professional training and indeed cultural values. The early professionalisation of medicine hence resulted in a hierarchical dominance over these other disciplines.

It was only in the mid-1970s that the UK started to collect data on child abuse and set up interdisciplinary child protection management systems. A number of child deaths such as that of 7-year-old Maria Colwell who died in 1973 led to the Fisher review which concluded there was a lack of communication between the agencies that were aware of her vulnerable situation. Eventually child abuse registers were set up in the 1980s; since the late 1980s, health policy has advocated effective inter-agency collaboration. This is in the context of a number of serious child deaths where reviews note the breakdown of interprofessional communication influencing effective child protection. The death of 4-year-old Jasmine Beckford in 1984 also triggered changes in child protection services; and as other children continued to be abused and die, the services and the government attempted to address policy and interagency practice. The rise in recognition of this social problem influenced another high profile case, the 1988 'Cleveland child abuse' scandal which emerged with what the media felt were overzealous medical and social professions removing over a hundred children from their families, most of whom were found to be wrongly diagnosed as abused. However, this posed issues of tension for interagency protection working to focus on the needs of children and the needs of families.

Ongoing policy documentation has presented as a prequel to the Children Acts in 1989 and more recently 2004 (DH 1999a). Following the Laming Inquiry and more child deaths such as Victoria Climbiè and Baby P, more interagency policy has developed. *Working Together* (HM Government, 2013a) now replaces:

- *Working Together to Safeguard Children* (2010)
- *The Framework for the Assessment of Children in Need and their Families* (2000)
- Statutory guidance on making arrangements to safeguard and promote the welfare of children under section 11 of the Children Act 2004 (2007)

It is the most recent statutory guidance for:

- local authority chief executives
- directors of children's services
- local safeguarding children board chairs and senior managers within organisations who commission and provide services for children and families

- social workers and professionals from health services
- adult services
- the police
- academy trusts
- education
- the voluntary and community sector who have contact with children and families.

This reflects the breadth of interagency working at all levels which need to address the social problem in order to safeguard children. All relevant professionals should read and follow the guidance, so that they can respond to individual children's needs appropriately. Policies in themselves do not prevent abuse, it is the commitment and best safeguarding practice of all those who work with children that do this. In 2013 another child, 4-year-old Daniel Pelka, suffered at the hands of his parents and the lack of poor interagency working together.

Activity

Discuss with a colleague the role you both play in safeguarding children.

As a member of the public or as a health care professional it is important to recognise that we all have a role to play in safeguarding children. Vigilance is imperative in society today whether you come into contact with children in your care or within your home or holiday community.

It is not only with children that effective interdisciplinary safeguarding working is essential. Interprofessional care is now an important model for rehabilitation care for older patients with complex needs. Virani (2013: 3) noted five broad primary care categories of models of patient care

- Interprofessional team models
- Nurse-led models
- Case management models
- Patient navigation models
- Shared care models.

These illustrate the variety of care models available to address the diversity of care needs. The population is living longer; relatives are more often faced with caring for older and more dependent parents and family members. Historically the extended family or interprofessional community care provision was more accessible and available. Domestic challenges prove to be a social issue as more people look after their relatives in their own home and the cost of professional care becomes too high. Along with this, the growth of the independent sector in care and nursing homes has meant that often older people without families become more vulnerable in institutional care. The white paper (DH, 2015) *No Secrets: Guidance on Protecting Vulnerable Adults in Care* sets out a code of practice for the protection of vulnerable adults with strong recommendations for an inter-agency framework and policy to manage potential and actual elder abuse. This has been repealed by The Care Act in April 2015.

It explains how commissioners and providers of health and social care services should work together to produce and implement local policies and procedures. They should collaborate with the public, voluntary and private sectors and they should also consult service users, their carers and representative groups. Local authority social services departments should coordinate the development of policies and proce-dures. The importance of protection of vulnerable adults (POVA) is set out in the DH (2010e) *Protection of Vulnerable Adults Scheme Record: Retention and Disposal.*

Domestic abuse is not only an issue for older people as many people also suffer both physical, mental and sexual abuse from their partners, family or carers. Hague et al. (1996) undertook a two-year research study into multi-agency work which was supported by the Joseph Rowntree Foundation. They noted the variation of domes-tic abuse services across the country. There was concern whether the interagency collaborative approach was seen as pioneering work or just a 'smoke screen'. They concluded that there was a need for a national commitment to resourcing intera-gency work in a structured, co-ordinated way. There is now more political pressure for health visitors and other health and social care professionals to screen families for domestic violence (Early Intervention Foundation, 2014). They link domestic abuse to what is termed as the 'toxic trio' of domestic abuse, mental health issues and substance misuse.

Activity

- Have you considered domestic violence as another possible risk factor when you have cared for a patient with a mental health issue and or substance abuse?
- Check out whether you are aware of any domestic violence screening assessment tools.
- Has this section raised your awareness of the health issues related to child abuse, elder abuse and domestic violence?

Screening for domestic violence has been developed in America but at the moment the NICE guidelines do not recommend this in this country. On 13 May 2014, the BMJ online identified that there is no evidence to support domestic abuse screening (www.bristol.ac.uk/news/2014/may/domestic-violence-screening.html). You may think these issues are not related to your role but you may feel you want to raise awareness of this social problem in your own working team or the wider multidisciplinary team if seen as relevant. Population screening is not advocated but raising awareness of services is important.

EXPERIENCE OF INTERPROFESSIONAL WORKING

A simple reflective model influenced by Bloom (1956), Eyler and Giles (1999) and Rolfe et al. (2001) is a useful tool for exploring interprofessional working events and their impact. The basis of this eclectic reflective model can be seen in Table 6.1.

Table 6.1   Reflective model

What?	Report the facts and events of an experience objectively
So What?	Analyse the experience
Now What?	Consider the future impact of the experience on you and the wider community.

> ## Activity
>
> Using the eclectic model in Table 6.2, reflect on a recent interprofessional experience.

The activity shown in Table 6.2 may be useful for realising the complexity of working in an interdisciplinary way while caring for patients and clients, and does link to improving your health care leadership skills.

Table 6.2   Your reflection

Features	Underpinning Ideas	Your Practice Reflections
What? *What happened?* *Knowledge and comprehension*	**Describe event** Describe the situation: achievements, consequences, responses, feelings and problems.	
So What? *Analysis/ Evaluation*	Debate, compare and contrast Discuss what has been learnt: learning about self, relationships, models, attitudes, cultures, actions, thoughts, understanding and improvements.	

Features	Underpinning Ideas	Your Practice Reflections
Now What? *Application and synthesis*	Demonstrate, construct, predict Identify what needs to be done in order to: improve future outcomes and develop learning What did you learn professionally and what skills do you need to learn about for the future?	
Can you now write three personal action points relating to improving your interprofessional working skills?		1. 2. 3.

CONTEMPORARY HEALTH CARE PRACTICE ACROSS ACUTE AND COMMUNITY SECTORS

The NHS as an organisation is an important and governmentally scrutinised public service element of what is known as the health industry in the UK. However, there are a great many health and social care industries that organisationally impact on the health of the nation – or even on global health.

Generally the local arrangements for health care in the UK have a three-part structure:

- Primary Care (community care/walk-in centres)
- Secondary Care (acute/hospital care)
- Tertiary Care (residential nursing/care facilities).

Primary care usually involves the services that patients and clients can access directly from their home locality and does not require referral to specialist services. However, there are many views about what it exactly involves and a specific definition is hard to pin down. It may be seen as a number of services accessed via the local general practice or health centre but 'walk-in' centres or even accident and emergency provision are seen as primary care, although they may be located in both acute and community centres. The World Health Organization (WHO) is also now less specific about a definition, but notes that the ultimate goal of primary health care is better health for all. There are five key elements identified to achieving that goal:

- reducing exclusion and social disparities in health (universal coverage reforms)
- organising health services around people's needs and expectations (service delivery reforms)

- integrating health into all sectors (public policy reforms)
- pursuing collaborative models of policy dialogue (leadership reforms)
- increasing stakeholder participation.

The WHO Report (WHO, 2008b) notes the importance of primary health care in global terms, now more than ever, in economically challenged health industries. Secondary care usually requires referral from a primary care service for more specialist services in an outpatient service or more directly via the hospital inpatient system. Interestingly, district nurses were formerly perceived as a primary care service but, in today's context, an external referral is usually required and patients cannot always self-refer. Tertiary care usually means a service referred from secondary or even primary care, for example, a specialised rehabilitation service, a nursing home or a hospice. The notion of quaternary health care is also emerging as a concept of highly specialised or even experimental treatment, but this is not yet clearly defined. The boundaries between these care services are sometimes very blurred for patients as well as professionals.

Professional groups have in the past either seen themselves as working in community services or within institutionalised acute hospitals or specialist treatment centres. This has sometimes caused challenges for patient care when the patient moves from the community to hospital or when being discharged from hospital to the community services. Learner (2010) explored a quality-based programme which has resulted in improvements in an acute trust. The programme competitively ranked different wards on their standards of care, which included effective discharge planning.

There have been a number of other models that aim to ensure that the patient journey from primary and community care into secondary or tertiary care, or secondary care back to primary care, is well planned and seamless. Services set up as 'inreach' community provision bring staff from community across into hospital services, a residential home or even prison services. Nelson et al. (2009) conducted evaluative research into an innovative inreach nursing and physiotherapy service in a residential home. They noted the challenges of cultural differences between the different services but concluded there was successful up-skilling by the staff in the home. Outreach specialised services are about bringing the hospital specialised services out into the home territory. There are also differences between skills, even within the same discipline. In community nursing there is a tendency for nurses to develop generalist skills covering a wide range of skills around medical conditions, in a similar way to the practice of general practitioners. In contrast, those nurses who work in the acute sector tend to specialise in certain conditions in line with the medical direction of the clinical area. Generalist skills and specialisms in midwifery, mental health and learning disability are also evident. Interdisciplinary conflict may manifest itself when either a generalist or a specialist professional feels threatened. However, the generalist and specialist model of care offers the best of both worlds for patient journeys.

POLICY, LEADERSHIP AND WORKING TOGETHER

The Coalition Government's structural framework for the National Health Service – with an emphasis around commissioning focused on GP consortia and new arrangements for public health which cross over from local authority and the NHS – continues to stress the importance of interprofessional working for the needs of patients and children (DH, 2010a, 2010b, 2010c). Clinical Commissioning Groups (CCGs) were created following the Health and Social Care Act in 2012, and replaced Primary Care Trusts on 1 April 2013. CCGs are clinically led statutory NHS bodies responsible for the planning and commissioning of health care services for their local area. There are now 211 CCGs in England (www.nhscc.org/ccgs/).

Team working, with various professions involved, requires skills and competencies in this area. All professional-based pre-registration education identifies multidisciplinary team working skills. Leadership in collaborative practice for patient care is recognised as an advancement competency. The NHS Leadership Academy (2011) highlights the new NHS Healthcare Leadership Framework which was introduced November 2013, as a development from the original seven dimensions of the NHS leadership framework.

The nine dimensions of the Healthcare Leadership Model are:

- Inspiring shared purpose
- Leading with care
- Evaluating information
- Connecting our service
- Sharing the vision
- Engaging the team
- Holding to account
- Developing capability
- Influencing for results.

You will find the framework a useful improvement tool to review your own SWOT analysis.

> **Activity**
>
> Having thought about the Health Care Leadership Model it is appropriate to read the Kings Fund improving leadership paper *How Can Improving Leadership Help Transform the NHS?*

RATIONALE FOR COLLABORATIVE WORKING PRACTICES

It is generally seen as important that we work together across the disciplines and professions in order to address the following:

- Population health needs and demographical changes which reflect complex issues that cannot be addressed by a unilateral approach
- Public protection where health care staff support each other but also are charged with public protection in their codes of conduct and standards of practice

- Consumerism/public confidence
- Governmental targets
- Resource management
- Budget control
- Complexity of work
- Role expansion/extension
- Specialism vs generalist skills (escalators).

However, from some patient/public perspectives, the notion of interprofessional working has presented challenges. The public often have a much simpler perspective on the NHS and perceive it as made up of doctors and nurses. Depending on their experience of their care/treatment, however, patients/the public come to realise a number of other professional groups are involved – though they do not always understand the differing expertise or skills. The patient experience does not always receive consideration by interprofessional services and patients do not always feel at the centre of the activity (Howarth and Haigh, 2007).

In terms of the perspectives of the patient, interprofessional working has therefore provided some challenges. Some older people have found the complexity of various personnel roles, uniforms and badges they have met during a hospital stay some-what confusing. If they need a home service, they may be confused by the number of professions who ask to assess their needs. A patient once stated that she had just experienced a 'circus' of visits from health care professionals which was traumatic, troublesome and extremely tiring – particularly as they often asked the same questions, sometimes within an hour of each other.

Activity

Can you identify the discipline/professional groups which could be involved in the scenarios in Table 6.3?

Table 6.3   Interprofessional scenarios

Health Event	Professionals and Support Staff Involved
Having a baby	
Bringing up a child until age 18	
Screening events:	
• Cervical	
• Breast	
• CVD	
• Prostate	
• Bowel	
Mental health episode	

Health Event	Professionals and Support Staff Involved
Surgical intervention	
Eye issue	
Foot issue	
Stroke	
Problems with getting pregnant	
Children with a diagnosed learning difficulty or developmental delay	
A challenge where an older person in a family is told they are terminally ill	

EFFECTIVE COLLABORATIVE TEAMS

Activity

What do you think makes a good interdisciplinary or interprofessional team?

You may have had experience of interprofessional team working that provided satisfaction for you on a number of personal and professional levels. The factors you may have thought about relate to any kind of team effectiveness:

- patient-centred goals
- openness
- collaborative decision making
- clear communication channels
- good conflict management
- good leadership.

One aspect of effective interdisciplinary or interprofessional teams is how well the members of the team collaborate with each other. McCrae (2011) notes that the multidisciplinary context of care has provided challenges for nursing models and thus the nursing-based theory which was taught in the 1970s and 1980s tended to be unilateral in focus. This issue has some resonance with Sommerfeldt (2013: 519) who believes that in practice, assumptions, stereotypes, power differentials and miscommunication can complicate the interactions of health care professions where there is lack of clarity of knowledge, skills and roles in nursing.

Professional power is a complex concept especially in its relationship to patient empowerment. Gilbert (1995) suggests that you need to understand power to realise the real meaning of empowerment. Bradbury-Jones et al. (2007) note that power is a contested concept:

- It has a diversity of interpretation
- Everyone has an opinion of what it means
- Power has a value (nebulous)
- Power is perception
- The concept of power is interwoven with empowerment.

◆ Activity

Jot down four ideas linked to the notion of power in health care practice.

You may have thought about the various power issues linked to different professions such as doctor, social worker and pharmacist. You may have thought about the types of knowledge they use or their skills in health and social care. Wilkinson and Miers (1999) highlight the work of Freidson, a medical sociologist who saw a profession as an occupation that has succeeded in controlling its own work and has been granted legitimate autonomy, usually through the state. This in itself is a form of hierarchical occupational power in society. Some occupations are considered professions and others semi-professions. Social work and nursing may have been consigned to the category of 'semi-profession' on account of the perceived limitations of their knowledge base, training and autonomy (Etzioni, 1969). Democratic accountability and bureaucratic hierarchies are presumed to imply a degree of lay interference in professional activity which does not correspond with the traditional ideal of professionalism.

Orchard (2010) notes the importance of interprofessional patient-centred collaborative practice. The relative importance of the health care team and the patient/family and their choices, however, are often seen as being in competing spheres. Patients may 'move' into the sick role and don't realise or even desire a role in major decisions about their care within the context of the interprofessional team. The patient needs to be helped to retain control over their own care within the context of having access to the knowledge and skills of the interprofessional team. For instance, patients often feel confused when facing complex symptoms relating to the involvement of more than one medical specialty and dealing with various hospital and GP appointments. Bergman (2014) highlights that the health care world has a good deal of conflict among caregivers, patients and their families. He notes that medicine's scientific, psychological, and language complexities, high stakes, fragmentation of care, multiplicity of players, time constraints, institutional politics, cultural differences, competing philosophies and economic dimensions can hinder patient/family understanding. For those requiring acute secondary care, hospital life in itself also compounds the situation. Public involvement in shaping health care is fraught with difficulties in engaging with ill patients or the multi interest factors but as the health service moves away from a paternalistic culture, public involvement is now a key principle for policy, research, delivery and medical education (Coulter, 2011). Pollard et al. (2010: 186) identify that policy has helped in the shifting of power though they note the ongoing challenges of the role of 'lead professional' and that of information sharing. Snape et al. (2014) identify the various values involved with public engagement and question whether this agenda addresses the power imbalance.

McDaniel and Stumpf (1993) did identify that when there were good interprofessional relationships in the health care team there was a positive link to patient outcomes. Laverack (2005) argues, however, that in professional practice someone can only possess a certain amount of power if another person loses an equivalent amount of the same. Do you think this is really true?

Foucault (1995) noted in his work on the deconstruction of power, that:

- It is 'exercised rather than possessed'
- It is not a thing, it cannot be relinquished
- It is embedded in everyday practice and interaction.

In exercising power this can be seen in:

- Control
- Politics
- Wealth
- Hierarchy
- Reaffirmation of social order.

Cooke (2006) noted that those 'without power' are marginalised. Disempowerment, then, can then reaffirm one's own identity with others in the same issues, leading to a solidarity movement embracing loyalty and conformity for those within the marginalised group. The issues of power present within each professional group are an interdisciplinary challenge as well as an interprofessional one. Some groups of nurses feel less powerful and marginalised than other groups of nurses. Similarly, this is true for allied health professionals, social workers and doctors.

OTHER CHALLENGES TO EFFECTIVE INTERPROFESSIONAL WORKING

The issues of power obviously pose a challenge in working with different teams but there are specific issues relating to interprofessional working.

> ### ◆ Activity
>
> What do you think are the main barriers to good interprofessional team working?

You may have thought of the following challenges or barriers:

- Differing professional philosophies, priorities, funding and status rewards
- Differing professional education and training
- Different professional uncertainties
- Gender/class differences
- Staff vacancies
- Agendas – personal
- Structural barriers within health care.

Stereotyping how we perceive different professions and even disciplines can hinder how well we communicate with each other. If we perceive the doctor as the top of the hierarchy, then upward communication may be more of a challenge. Nurses may either be seen as angels, battleaxes, handmaidens or sex objects. Doctors are an admired group in society but often perceived as male. Physiotherapists are linked with fitness and activity. Social workers have been described as wearing sandals and tank tops and health visitors linked with twinsets and pearls. Of course these are all inaccuracies but it's a way of identifying the pigeon-holing and stereotyping of the range of professions. Rushmer (2005) in her research identified blurred boundaries between professional groups. She noted that informally staff are encouraged to blur the boundaries, in order to reduce protectionist and rigid demarcations which adversely affect service provision. Pollard et al. (2010) highlight the difference between the 'old' models of professionalism stressing autonomy and specialist expertise which may inhibit health care transformation and 'new' models of professionalism that emphasise the importance of teamwork and reflective practice.

There is therefore seen to be a need for professionals to be more flexible in their approach to working with other professional groups. They question what blurring of the boundaries may actually involve and whether it offers a way forward in resolving the difficulties experienced by differing health professionals in working together. Some of the challenges here concern what is termed 'professional tribalism', which is discussed in the following section.

COMMUNITIES OF PRACTICE, TRIBALISM, POWER AND PROFESSIONAL IDENTITIES

Lave and Wenger (1991, in Walmsley et al., 1997) argue that many professional groups behave in similar ways to tribes and suggest the notion of communities of practice:

Communities of practice are formed by people who engage in a process of collective learning in a shared domain of human endeavour: a tribe learning to survive, a band of artists seeking new forms of expression, a group of engineers working on similar problems, a clique of pupils defining their identity in the school, a network of surgeons exploring novel techniques, a gathering of first-time managers helping each other cope. In a nutshell: Communities of practice are groups of people who share a concern or a passion for something they do and learn how to do it better as they interact regularly.

(http://wenger-trayner.com/introduction-to-communities-of-practice/ accessed 9 April 2015)

Walmsley et al. (1997) suggest that individuals belonging to the same professional group exhibit many attitudes in common, especially at the ideological level. Individuals working in common circumstances, in similar positions, hold certain views in common; this has implications for professional boundaries.

Activity

Can you suggest a variety of attitudes concerning care delivery in your present practice?

As a paediatric link health visitor in an outpatient clinic I was mainly concerned with child development progress, nutrition and growth as well as home support via the health visiting service across the city. The liaison social worker was mainly concerned with supporting parents – with benefit and charity advice as well as social work and housing support in their district – but also focused on child protection social work liaison across the city. The paediatrician had requested the liaison roles in the clinic but her main role concerned the medical condition of each child and their medical treatment. Interestingly, as a team, this was seen as a holistic approach to care. The downside was that these morning clinics often overran into the afternoon as the needs of each child/family were considered from our triple perspectives.

Child protection issues are the main political challenge to interprofessional working, in the media limelight with respect to the dilemma of safeguarding vulnerable children and supporting parents. Errors of judgement have been seen in too many cases over the years but as the health and social care context of our society becomes more complex – with the mobility of families, complex family structures and the diversity of health and social care services – it is envisaged that safeguarding children will now pose a major future societal challenge. However, it must be recognised that although children are a vulnerable group, there are many other vulnerable groups such as older people, those with learning disabilities or severe mental health difficulties, victims of domestic violence and more recently the slavery of women involved in human trafficking. It is a sad indictment that safeguarding vulnerable adults has not got the same political emphasis. Many older people, the mentally ill or those with a learning disability are abused by families, carers and even staff in the caring services. These are often seen as the forgotten groups, overlooked by the political strategists.

> ### ▶ Activity
>
> Do you agree that poor interprofessional working in adult care has not been addressed with the same importance as child care?
>
> Why is this?

You probably work with a wide range of patients and clients but you will obviously see individuals and families who appear more vulnerable than others. Adults often find difficulty getting health and social care support particularly if they have some mental or learning disability challenges. There are limited safeguarding laws to protect these groups and often the individuals involved do not have the capacity to understand fully the risks to them. It is, therefore, important that interprofessional care encompasses a more interprofessional learning model for the future.

LEARNING AND WORKING TOGETHER

Interprofessional education (also known as IPE) refers to students from two or more professions learning together during all or part of their professional programme with the objective of cultivating collaborative practice (CAIPE, 1997) for providing client- and/or patient-centred care. Laurenson and Brockelhurst (2011), using a triangulated method of research into interprofessional care in long-term conditions, concluded that educational providers and professional awarding bodies need to enshrine interprofessionalism into curricula and qualification accreditation, thereby instilling collaboration intrinsically into care provision.

Barr (2002) earlier conducted a systematic review of the literature concerning interprofessional education (IPE) in health care and from the literature it is noted that successful IPE needed to demonstrate/include the following:

- Service users at the centre of the programme
- Promotion of collaboration
- Reconciliation of competing objectives
- Reinforcing collaborative competence
- Clear rationale of IPE in learning and practice
- Incorporation of interprofessional values
- Common and comparative learning
- Utilising a range of interactive learning methods
- Can be used towards self-assessment and qualifications
- Evaluation programmes
- Disseminating findings.

> ### ▶ Activity
>
> - What are your experiences of IPE?
> - Can you say whether they have been positive or negative?
> - Did they fit with the recommendations of Barr (2002)?

Horsburgh et al. (2001) undertook research with a multi-professional group of health care students in New Zealand and found that the majority of students reported positive attitudes towards shared learning. The benefits of shared learning, including the acquisition of team working skills, were seen to be beneficial to patient care and likely to enhance professional working relationships. However, professional groups differed: nursing and pharmacy students indicated more strongly that an outcome of learning together would be more effective team working. However, medical students were the least sure of their professional role, and considered that they required the acquisition of more knowledge and skills than nursing or pharmacy students. The research concluded that developing effective team working skills is an appropriate focus for first-year health professional students. The timing of learning about the roles of different professionals may yet need to be resolved though.

CONFIDENTIALITY AND ETHICAL ISSUES

One of the challenges for interprofessional working relates to the ethical issue of patient confidentiality. The Nursing and Midwifery Council (2015) identify confidentiality as a fundamental part of professional practice that protects human rights. This is identified in Article 8 (Right to respect for private and family life) of the European Convention of Human Rights which states:

- Everyone has the right to respect for his private and family life, his home and his correspondence.
- There shall be no interference by a public authority with the exercise of this right except such as is in accordance with the law and is necessary in a democratic society in the interests of national security, public safety or the economic well-being of the country, for the prevention of disorder or crime, for the protection of health or morals, or for the protection of the rights and freedoms of others.

They also note that it is not acceptable for nurses and midwives to:

- discuss matters related to the people in their care outside the clinical setting
- discuss a case with colleagues in public where they may be overheard *and*
- leave records unattended where they may be read by unauthorised persons.

Discussing the care of patients across the boundaries of a single care delivery setting is less clear. Sharing of information between medical teams in the NHS and social work teams in the Local Authority has been a long-term challenge. The important ethical consideration is about patient choice and consent when information sharing would benefit patient outcomes. Safeguarding children is a specific area where the rights of the child are more important than those of the adults involved.

INTERPROFESSIONAL WORKING AND GLOBAL HEALTH

On an international level, the importance of interprofessional collaboration has been more recently highlighted in trying to deal with global health inequalities. As the economic downturn across the world impacts on the health industry, the need for more effective use of the skills and knowledge across the professions globally will be even more imperative.

The World Health Organization (WHO) convened a WHO Study Group on Interprofessional Education and Collaborative Practice in 2007 to review the inequality issues, to tackle the challenges within a global health workforce and to maximise human resourcing. A framework for world health interprofessional education and collaborative practice was produced in March 2010: *Framework for Action on Interprofessional Education and Collaborative Practice*. It highlights the current status of interprofessional collaboration around the world, identifies the mechanisms that shape successful collaborative teamwork, and outlines a series of action items that policymakers can apply within their local health system. It also provides strategies and ideas that can help health policymakers implement the elements of interprofessional education and collaborative practice that will be most beneficial in their own jurisdiction.

Summary of Key Points

This chapter has briefly looked at various aspects of team life in order to meet the identified learning outcomes. These were:

- **The importance of interdisciplinary and interprofessional working in health for effective patient care and safety** This was seen in the context of inquiries into poor health care standards but more positively in terms of working to improve patient care outcomes nationally and globally.
- **Critically explore the opportunities and challenges of interprofessional working in the contemporary context** The issues of policy attempting to address the economic recession, stereotyping and the diversity of cultural differences between professional groups were explored. The opportunities for leadership and effective team working were highlighted.
- **Identify issues of practice communities, tribalism, professional identities and the importance of interprofessional education** These issues were explored to raise awareness and support the need for improved interprofessional education.

FURTHER READING

Day, J. and Wiggens, L. (2006) *Expanding Nursing and Health Care Practice: Interprofessional Working*. London: Nelson Thornes.

Freeth, D., Hammick, M., Koppel, I. and Barr, H. (2002) *A Critical Review of Evaluations of Interprofessional Education*. York: The Higher Education Academy.

See also:

- ✓ http://safeguardingchildrenea.co.uk/wp-content/themes/vc_org_1/ChildProtection TimeLine/childprotectiontimeline.html
- ✓ www.nuffieldtrust.org.uk/talks/videos/clare-gerada-commissioning-impact-patient-care?gclid=Cj0KEQjwopOeBRC1ndXgnuvx8JYBEiQAq4RPt3cVo90D mJXX8aLFWPNCgXDH2ESPWksfHFYRasLDMPAaArlC8P8HAQ
- ✓ www.leadershipacademy.nhs.uk/wp-content/uploads/2013/11/Mapping-Leadership-Framework-to-Healthcare-Leadership-Model.pdf
- ✓ www.health.heacademy.ac.uk/projects/miniprojects/completeproj.htm
- ✓ www.nice.org.uk/guidance/PH50/chapter/introduction
- ✓ www.bristol.ac.uk/news/2014/may/domestic-violence-screening.html
- ✓ http://domesticabuse.stanford.edu/screening/how.html
- ✓ http://psychcentral.com/dvquiz.htm Deritaecest omnihil evel inciis volupis cillaut hit qui dolut occusandae sum, aut eaquo eium ad qui qui dolecuptam, sit ea dolupta dolupid quatur, in renda consequ idempos excea con nis voluptata vendit explaccabo. Repelessim ea doluptas que as con eum as ium quundist, is maximagnisit ut dolor ad que estionem qui apis aliqui tem quiandit ommolup tinihit, con re, ut pra dicipsundis dolest fugit, solupta eratiam rem nieniet volecea vel ento tem imus.
- ✓ Uptis natecat atibus sapernam hilis dipidus ut velecus.
- ✓ Pudi tem fugit quaeper spicaernam solore sum quid quis con proritate latis dionemposae vollabor accae nestia saeceribusae pellatem nis int qui asperunt aut eaque sitatquidi dollab ium expero beruptas dolore veriae num nos aut laceped mil magnaturi que quodis sae quam viti ide eosapit asperat emoditat.
- ✓ Solutem demolum velita dolore desciet odias aliquunt ut est, to omnis am cus sanis sunt dolor milit volorep eruptatust volenda epeless imaiorem. Nam ex es molorer ibusciae velentius pori dolum quid quam quam, nesequo dicturio od mo conserum invel maio corestio. Itat quat officae ped esequo occum reseque sae voluptaspero dis dipsapit, tessus modioris et des alit aspis sum etur, occum aut omni sunt.
- ✓ Puditat qui opta doluptaquas aut ad mil ipient, od es aute omnis aut ex expelen dissuntempor re odit utet inctur? Qui soluptur aut im volore comnihit atenet aut quibusam facercidel ma necerum faccull oreprovit venias peribus est, ulparchil experum harum quidel modictia que aspis velestia intiore reiunt quaepudandis estia verem sanders pitias as evelleniet volo illaut volores sitiscil ma nam num qui aut dent laut etur, cone susda discil es si dit ut fugitat uriandiae et as dolu

Visit the companion website at https://study.sagepub.com/barr3e for more resources.

7 COMMUNICATION AND LEADERSHIP

Learning Outcomes

By the end of this chapter you will have had the opportunity to:

- Discuss the application of the 6Cs
- Describe various forms of communication
- Describe a variety of communication networks and their effects on clinical practice
- Discuss the importance of effective communication
- Debate motivational theory and its place in the clinical area
- Discuss the benefits of written and electronically stored information
- Identify the benefits of audit in clinical practice
- Consider the benefits of active listening
- Consider the benefits of Neuro-Linguistic Programming
- Discuss the legal and ethical issues related to effective communication.

INTRODUCTION

> Leadership is primarily trust and communication. When you communicate well with people and treat them with respect, they will go through brick walls for you. (Hackman, 2006)

Effective leadership means communicating with others in such a way that they are influenced and motivated to perform actions that achieve common goals and lead toward desired outcomes (Daft, 2010); so in order to be an effective leader it is vital to be a good communicator. This chapter will examine various forms of communication to enable you to understand how knowledge and ideas are shared. If you can't get your message across clearly, then whatever the message is won't matter and nothing will happen. Maxwell (1999: 23) stated: 'Educators take something simple and make it complicated. Communicators take something complicated and make it simple.' This alludes to the fact that things can be made to sound more complicated than they really are by poor or ineffective communication. So effective communication can be seen to influence the ways in which a team will function by motivating through planning and effective delegation. It must be remembered that leadership and communication are always affected by the overall structure of the organisation. Where there are many layers of line-management, information passed either down or upwards may become distorted.

Within any organisation there are pre-defined communication pathways, but within these pathways there are also sub-divisions e.g. night and day staff within a department; the pre-defined pathways may be circumscribed i.e. the grapevine. Many definitions of communication are used in order to conceptualise the processes by which people navigate and assign meaning.

THE 6CS

Within health care it is recognised that there are a number of elements that contribute to effective care which are known as the 6Cs (NHS England 2012).

1. Care
    Care is our core business and that of our organisations and the care we deliver helps the individual person and improves the health of the whole community. Caring defines us and our work. People receiving care expect it to be right for them consistently throughout every stage of their life.

2. Compassion
    Compassion is how care is given through relationships based on empathy, respect and dignity. It can also be described as intelligent kindness and is central to how people perceive their care.

3. Competence
    Competence means all those in caring roles must have the ability to understand an individual's health and social needs. It is also about having the expertise, clinical and technical knowledge to deliver effective care and treatments based on research and evidence.

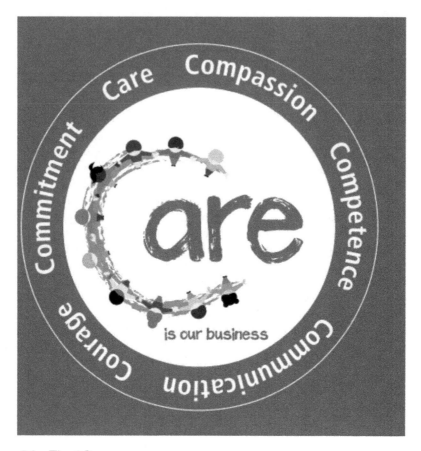

Figure 7.1   The 6Cs

(*Source*: www.england.nhs.uk/nursingvision)

4. Communication
    Communication is central to successful caring relationships and to effective team working. Listening is as important as what we say and do. It is essential for 'no decision about me without me'. Communication is the key to a good workplace with benefits for those in our care and staff alike.

5. Courage
    Courage enables us to do the right thing for the people we care for, to speak up when we have concerns. It means we have the personal strength and vision to innovate and to embrace new ways of working.

6. Commitment
    A commitment to our patients and populations is a cornerstone of what we do. We need to build on our commitment to improve the care and experience of our patients. We need to take action to make this vision and strategy a reality for all and meet the health and social care challenges ahead.

◆ **Activity**

How have you used the 6Cs in your last week of practice?

Discuss these with your colleagues.

FORMS OF COMMUNICATION

It is important that the effective leader is able to adapt their communication style to each situation depending on the needs of the audience. That is not to say that this is always a conscious decision. Communication styles, like leadership styles, are often intuitive. It is useful, however, to understand how communication can be made more effective in order to reduce the risks of misunderstanding and unplanned confusion.

A model, as a representation of reality, may help to describe the communication process and consecutive stages through which someone or something has to pass in order to achieve a specified aim (Weightman, 1999: see Figure 7.1). The model also acts as a checklist to ensure each stage has been negotiated successfully i.e. preparation for communication; delivery of the message; receipt of the message; analysis of how effectively you deliver the message and take corrective measures where necessary. However, exponents of models recognise that, as with many theories, the effective communicator is often unaware of using a model as they are doing 'what comes naturally' to them.

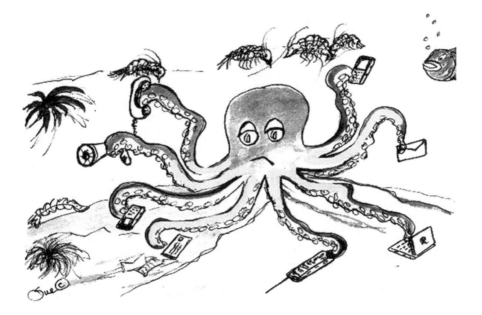

	PROCESS	**CHECK POINTS**
Encoding	Formulating the message. Selecting the right words or symbols. Understanding the person.	Clarify your objectives; is the message clear to the other person? What will be the emotional impact of the message?
Transmitting	Selecting the right method. Sending the message. Giving non-verbal signals.	Make sure there are no more than approximately seven ideas to transmit. Are verbal and non-verbal signals consistent? Is the language suitable?
Environment	Coping with distractions. Dealing with distortions.	Avoid noise and interruptions. Is the seating right?
Receiving	Understanding the message. Active listening.	What phrases, facts and inferences am I looking for? How can I test my understanding of the message?
Decoding	Making sense of the message. Understanding the other person.	What do they mean? What is the hidden agenda? How will I handle it?
Feedback	Encoding the response. Starting the message.	Nod, smile and agree to continue. Look interested, stop eye contact to end.

Figure 7.2   The basic communications model

Source: adapted from Weightman, 1999, with permission

Problems may occur at any of the points of the model so it is worth sitting down and working out where the potential problems might originate so that they can be addressed. This is applicable within all individual or group interactions. The over-all purpose of communication is to ensure that messages are received and understood in order to make life easier, both in working and in home environ-ments. Of course the system goes pear-shaped at times and communication is not as effective as it could be, but if we understand what is happening then we can do something about it.

An example of another model is one described by Shannon and Weaver (1954) and depicted in Figure 7.3. However the cycle is depicted, it can be seen that there is a purpose and direction for messages to travel in order for effective communication to take place. It assumes the communicator wishes to influence the receiver and therefore sees communication as a persuasive process. It also assumes that messages always have effects and thus can exaggerate the effects of mass communication. However you think of them, models are a simplified description of a complex entity or process that allows you to understand the process and so make it work for you.

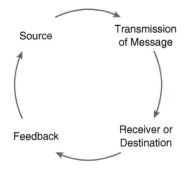

Figure 7.3 Communication feedback loop

Source: adapted from Shannon and Weaver, 1954

Activity

Consider the stages of effective communication and attempt to formulate a message for a patient within your sphere of practice.

- Ask whether the patient can move their right arm up and down.
- Apply this same messaging task to a patient who is deaf, then for one who is blind, then for one who does not speak English.

You might have discussed the need for written material, Braille, or an interpreter; you might also have thought of the type of environment you were in to see if it helped or hindered conversation/communication. I am sure we have all tried to carry on a conversation in a night club or where there is a loud TV, where it is difficult to hear yourself think let alone understand what is being said. Following anaesthesia there may be distortions in understanding due to the drugs. It is important to check that the receiver understands the matter being communicated by considering their response or by asking further relevant questions following the transmission of a message.

COMMUNICATION NETWORKS

A variety of networks can be depicted to demonstrate how messages get passed from one person to another. As children many of us have played 'Chinese Whispers' and have noted that in a linear chain, messages may become distorted or altered. But the majority of organisations use this model to communicate with and listen to their workforce i.e. downward communication (Figure 7.4) where directives are passed down to the workforce from above. However, bottom-up or upward communication (Figure 7.5) is encouraged within the realms of humanistic management techniques whereby the workforce are encouraged to share ideas with their managers and will be involved in the decision making process. Both types have their place within an organisation but the effective leader *must* recognise which will be the most effective within any given situation.

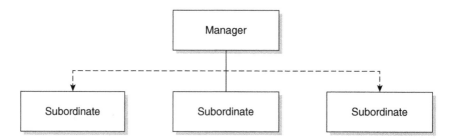

Figure 7.4   Downward communication

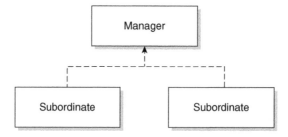

Figure 7.5   Upward communication

EFFECTIVE COMMUNICATION

Hargie and Tourish (2009: xv) state '.... a highly educated, articulate and assertive workforce no longer wishes to be consulted and listened to – Generation Y demand and expect that this will be the case. One result of this is that the workforce wants communication like modern food – instant and always available when they need it'.

Innovation communications may be seen in policies for new initiatives. Team meetings and 'away days' may help to encourage and achieve integration among a small group. Information may emerge as emails or memoranda. Dowding and Barr (2002) suggested a few reasons why you may actually communicate with others in the team as a leader:

- To ensure that everyone gets the same message (**Regulation**)
- To change someone's behaviour (**Innovation**)
- To sort out a problem and raise motivation (**Integration**)
- To give factual information that people need to proceed efficiently with their work (**Information**).

Activity

- Think back over the last 24 hours.
- Make a note of how much time was spent in communication with someone else.
- What form did that communication take?
- What purpose did the communication serve?

You might have identified any of the vast number of communication forms that can be used, for example, speaking/verbal (v), writing (w) and non-verbal (nv). Some of these are formal (f) and some informal (if), for example, department meetings (f); team briefings (f); saying hello (if); coffee break conversations (if); shift changeover (f); memos (f); eye contact in the corridor (if); and so the list goes on. Effective communication should ensure that messages are received and understood by relevant parties, especially in health care environments – whether in an institution, an ambulance or in a patient's home. It is important we are clear what our message is.

More recently the communication skill base of therapeutic communication techniques has developed in the context of treatment, behaviour change and health promotion. Solution-focused therapy and cognitive behaviour therapy (CBT) are relatively well known. Other examples, which are less well known, are motivational and promotional interviewing techniques. Motivational interviewing originated from the early work of Miller and Rollnick where they defined it as a client-centred, directed method for enhancing intrinsic motivation to change by exploring and resolving ambivalence (Miller and Rollnick, 2002). The five key principles are:

1. Expressing empathy by use of reflective listening.
2. Exploring discrepancy between client goals and current problem behaviour.
3. Avoiding arguments by assuming the client is responsible for the decision to change.
4. Avoiding resistance and confrontation.
5. Supporting self-efficacy and optimism for change.

MOTIVATION AND COMMUNICATION

There are numerous theories related to motivation, some of the most well-known being those of Herzberg (1966), Ouchi (1981), McClelland (1984), Maslow (1987), McGregor (1987) and Adair (2003). They all believe that the job of the leader/manager is to get the work done. In order to do this they must motivate their team members. Laschinger (2010) argues that staff who feel they are empowered are more likely to empower patients which results in better patient outcomes. In line with this Rank et al.'s (2009) work in Germany and Apekay et al. (2011) in their research using postal questionnaires note that leadership is an essential element of quality and innovation culture.

Theory X, Theory Y and Theory Z form part of the motivational theories. McGregor in the 1980s proposed various assumptions about how individuals are motivated. He highlighted that Theory X assumes that individuals are lazy and self-centred in nature, lack ambition and will avoid work activity. Managers who have a preference for Theory X assumptions utilise a more authoritarian style and one-way communication. The use of threats and disciplinary action is more common. He compared this to a more positive set of beliefs, Theory Y, which assumes individuals prefer to be involved in the work they do, seeking responsibility and need for creativity and engagement in their work. Managers who have a preference for Theory Y assumptions utilise a more participative style of management and prefer multiple communication. There is a more developmental and liberating culture where performance management is favoured. Theory Z relates to Ouchi's (1981) work as well as Maslow (1987) and Reddin (1970) and is seen in the nature of Japanese cultures which reflects a culture of lifelong employment. It assumes that people enjoy interaction, interdependence and use of reasoning and thus managers' behaviours need to play to these aspects of work life.

Motivational theory is still not clearly understood but McClelland (1984) pioneered workplace motivational thinking, developing achievement-based motivational theory and models. He also promoted improvements in employee assessment methods, advocating competency-based assessments and tests, arguing that they were better than traditional IQ and personality-based tests. His ideas have since been widely adopted in many organisations, and relate closely to the theory of Herzberg (1966). McClelland (1984) is most noted for describing three types of motivational need:

- Achievement motivation (n-ach)
- Authority/power motivation (n-pow)
- Affiliation motivation (n-affil).

The needs-based motivational models are found to varying degrees in all workers and managers, and this mix of motivational needs characterises a person's or manager's style and behaviour, both in terms of being motivated, and in the management and motivation of others.

- The *need for achievement* (n-ach) person is 'achievement motivated' and seeks realistic but challenging goals and advancement in the job. There is a strong need for feedback as to achievement and progress, and a need for a sense of accomplishment.
- The *need for authority and power* (n-pow) person is 'authority motivated'. This driver produces a need to be influential and effective and to make an impact. There is a strong desire to lead and for their ideas to prevail. They also seek increasing personal status and prestige.
- The *need for affiliation* (n-affil) is 'affiliation motivated' and is motivated by friendly relationships and interaction with other people. The affiliation driver promotes motivation and a need to be liked and held in popular regard. These people are team players.

McClelland said that most people possess and exhibit a combination of these characteristics. Some people exhibit a strong bias to a particular motivational need and this motivational or needs 'mix' consequently affects their behaviour and working/managing style. He goes on to suggest that a strong affiliation motivation undermines a manager's objectivity, because of their need to be liked, and that this affects a manager's decision making capability. A strong authority motivation will produce a determined work ethic and commitment to the organisation, and while people motivated by authority and power are attracted to the leadership role, they may not possess the required flexibility and people-centred skills. He also argues that people with strong achievement motivation make the best leaders, although they can demonstrate a tendency to demand too much of their staff in the belief that they are all similarly and highly achievement-focused and results driven, which of course most people are not.

McClelland's particular fascination was for achievement motivation, and through a laboratory experiment he illustrated one aspect of his theory about the effect of achievement on people's motivation. He asserted, via this experiment, that while most people do not possess a strong achievement-based motivation, those who do display a consistent behaviour in setting goals: for instance, volunteers were asked to throw rings over pegs rather like the fairground game; no distance was stipulated, and most people seemed to throw from arbitrary, random distances – sometimes close, sometimes farther away. However, a small group of volunteers, whom McClelland suggested were strongly achievement-motivated, took some care to measure and test distances to produce an ideal challenge – not too easy and not impossible. Interestingly, a parallel exists in biology, known as the 'overload principle', which is commonly applied to fitness and exercising, that is, in order to develop fitness and/or strength the exercise must be sufficiently demanding to increase existing levels but not so demanding as to cause damage or strain. McClelland identified the same need for a 'balanced challenge' in the approach of achievement-motivated people.

McClelland contrasted achievement-motivated people with gamblers, and dispelled a common preconception that achievement-motivated people are big risk takers. On the contrary, typically, achievement-motivated individuals set goals which they can influence with their effort and ability and, as such, the goal is considered to be achievable. This determined, results-driven approach is almost invariably present in the character make-up of all successful business people and entrepreneurs. McClelland suggested other characteristics and attitudes of achievement-motivated people:

- Achievement is more important than material or financial reward
- Achieving the aim or task gives greater personal satisfaction than receiving praise or recognition
- Financial reward is regarded as a measurement of success, not an end in itself
- Security is not a prime motivator, nor is status
- Feedback is essential, because it enables measurement of success, not for reasons of praise or recognition (the implication here is that feedback must be reliable, quantifiable and factual)
- Achievement-motivated people constantly seek improvements and ways of doing things better
- Achievement-motivated people will logically favour jobs and responsibilities that naturally satisfy their needs, that is, offer flexibility and the opportunity to set and achieve goals, for example, sales/business management and entrepreneurial roles.

McClelland firmly believed that achievement-motivated people are generally the ones who make things happen and get results, and that this extends to getting results through the organisation of other people and resources although, as stated earlier, they often demand too much of their staff because they prioritise achieving the goal above the many varied interests and needs of their people. There are interesting comparisons and relationships to be drawn between McClelland's (1984) motivation types and the characteristics defined in other behavioural models (Table 7.1).

More recently, motivational theory has been linked to a 'VICTORY Model' which reflects the relationship between self-motivation, motivation of others, Neuro-Linguistic Programming (NLP) and the mastery of motivation (Landsberg, 2003). The model encompasses the following themes:

- Vision
- Impetus (money, power, respect)
- Confidence
- Taking the plunge
- Observing outcomes
- Responding to feedback *and*
- You.

This motivational model clearly supports the newer focus of the leadership activity of coaching and mentoring staff in the workplace. Malloch and Porter-O'Grady (2005) raise the importance of coaching, mentoring and emotional intelligence (EI) for the twenty-first century and recognise these as advancing leadership skills and

Table 7.1 Comparative features of McClelland's leadership types

McClelland Motivational Type	Achievement-motivated Leaders (n-ach)	Authority-motivated Leaders (n-pow)	Affiliation-motivated Leaders (n-affil)
Focus	Task	Individual self	Team and individual
Favoured style of behaviour	1. Telling	3. Delegating	4. Participating
Hersey and Blanchard (1977)	2. Selling		
McGregor (1987) style typology	X theory	X theory	Y theory

behaviours (see Chapter 10 for further discussion). Within the health industry this is particularly important in supporting non-hierarchical multidisciplinary teams and in the context of clinical supervision.

Together with the need for effective oral communication we must ensure that all paper and electronic records are maintained correctly in order to validate the care given in whatever setting. Audit is a process that aims to promote quality and ensures that all care facilities are meeting the standards of the Care Quality Commission.

ACTIVE LISTENING

Active listening is a way of listening and responding to another person which improves mutual understanding. Klagsbrun (2011) suggests the importance of active listening in the therapeutic context; professional active listening helps patients clarify their inner thoughts and concerns. She explores the situation of patients, many of whom often feel isolated and invisible in a hospital setting; it is the skill of active listening which can help the patient rebuild their sense of self.

In more general terms, when people talk to each other, they don't listen attentively. They are often distracted; half listening, half thinking about something else. When people are engaged in a conflict, they are often busy formulating a response to what is being said. They assume that they have heard what their opponent is saying many times before so, rather than paying attention, they focus on how they can respond to win the argument. In order to become more active in the process the listener must take a structured approach to listening and responding that focuses the attention on the speaker. The listener must take care to attend to the speaker fully and then repeat, in the listener's own words, what he or she thinks the speaker has said. The listener does not have to agree with the speaker; he or she must simply state what they think the speaker said. This enables the speaker to find out whether the listener really understood. If the listener did not, the speaker can explain some more. Elements that tell the speaker that you are listening can be seen in eye contact, posture and gesture.

We can all tell if someone is listening. How many times have you been involved in a conversation and the listener is looking all around the room rather than at you, or they are sitting with their arms folded and leaning away from you. One gets the feeling that they are just not interested in what you have to say and this can make you angry enough that the point of the conversation is lost.

Active listening has several benefits. First, it forces people to listen attentively to others. Second, it avoids misunderstandings, as people have to confirm that they do really understand what another person has said. Third, it tends to open people up, to get them to say more. When people are in conflict, they often contradict each other, denying the opponent's description of a situation. This tends to make people defensive, and they will either lash out or withdraw and say nothing more. However, if they feel that their opponent is really attuned to their concerns and wants to listen, they are likely to explain in detail what they feel and why. If both parties in a conflict do this, the chances of being able to develop a solution to their mutual problem become much greater.

The skills associated with active listening are normally denoted by the mnemonic SOLER, proposed by Egan (2013), which stands for:

Squarely face the person

Open your posture

Lean towards the sender

Eye contact maintained

Relax while attending.

Active listening is used in many ways by health care professionals e.g. counselling; advocacy; restating/interpreting what other professionals have said to the patient in order to aid understanding and ensure the patient knows what their treatment options are. There are a number of tactics that can be employed in order to effectively listen and understand the other persons' point of view, including:

Paraphrasing is a useful tool. By restating a message, but often with fewer words, the listener is encouraged to interpret the speaker's words in terms of feelings. So, instead of just repeating what happened, the active listener might add 'I gather that you felt angry or frustrated or confused when … [a particular event happened]'. Then the speaker can go beyond confirming that the listener understood what happened by indicating that he or she also understood the speaker's psychological response to it. It tests your understanding of what you heard and communicates that you are trying to understand what is being said. If you're successful, paraphrasing indicates that you are following the speaker's verbal explorations and that you're beginning to understand the basic message.

Clarifying helps you to understand exactly what is being said. It brings vague material into sharper focus so that unclear or wrong listener interpretation is disentangled, more information is given, the speaker sees other points of view, and it identifies what was said: for example, 'I'm confused, let me try to repeat what I think you were trying to say', or 'You've said so much, let me see if I've got it all'.

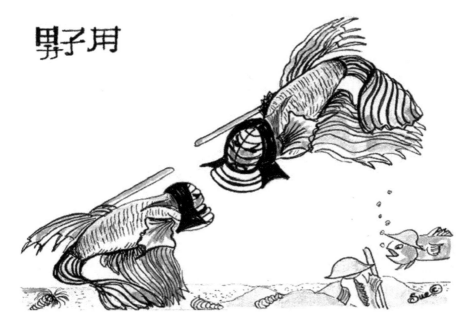

Perception checking again helps you to understand by giving and receiving feedback and checking out your assumptions: for example, 'Let me see if I've got it straight. You said that you love your children and that they are very important to you. At the same time you can't stand being with them. Is that what you are saying?'

Summarising is about pulling together, organising and integrating the major aspects of your dialogue, paying attention to various themes and emotional over-tones, putting key ideas and feelings into broad statements but *not* adding new ideas. By doing this there is a sense of movement and accomplishment in the exchange. It may also establish a basis for further discussion and pull together major ideas, facts and feelings: for example, 'A number of good points have been made about rules for the classroom. Let's take a few minutes to go over them and write them on the board.'

Primary empathy is a reflection of content and feelings in order to show that you understand the speaker's experience; and that allows the speaker to evaluate his/her feelings after hearing them expressed by someone else. The basic formula for this is: 'You feel [state feeling] because [state content]', for example, 'It's upsetting when someone doesn't let you tell your side of the story.'

Advanced empathy, by contrast, is a deeper reflection of content and feeling to achieve greater understanding: for example, 'I get the sense that you are really angry about what was said, but I am wondering if you also feel a little hurt by it?'

Active listening intentionally focuses on who you are listening to, whether in a group or one-on-one, in order to understand what he or she is saying. As the listener, you should be able to repeat – in your own words – what they have said, to their satisfaction. This does not mean you agree with, but rather that you understand, what they are saying.

NEURO-LINGUISTIC PROGRAMMING

Linking to the ability to actively listen is the notion of being able to understand and 'read' how people are reacting to any form of communication or situation. Interestingly, the notion of Neuro-Linguistic Programming (NLP) may help with the ability to 'read' how people are reacting within a given situation and, thus, what course to follow to achieve the best outcome. NLP was advocated in the mid-1970s by a linguist (Grinder) and a mathematician (Bandler) (Bandler and Grindler, 1990) who had strong interests in:

- Successful people
- Psychology
- Language *and*
- Computer programming.

It is difficult to define NLP because those who started it and who are involved in it use such vague and ambiguous language that it means different things to different people. While it is difficult to find a consistent description of NLP among those who claim to be experts at it, one metaphor keeps recurring. Neuro-linguistic programming claims to help people change by teaching them to programme their brains. Furthermore, consciously or unconsciously, it relies heavily upon:

1. The notion of the unconscious mind as constantly influencing conscious thought and action
2. Metaphorical behaviour and speech, especially building upon the methods used in Freud's *Interpretation of Dreams* (1911)
3. Hypnotherapy as developed by Milton Erickson (2002).

A common thread in neuro-linguistic programming is the emphasis on teaching a variety of communication and persuasion skills, and using self-hypnosis to motivate and change oneself. NLP is said to be the study of the structure of *subjective* experience, but a great deal of attention seems to be paid to observing *behaviour* and teaching people how to read 'body language'. I am not aware of signalling my feelings because the message is coming from my subconscious mind, so how might we test these kinds of claims? Probably the answer is that we can't test them with any degree of reliability and there is no empirical evidence to back up the claim. Sitting cross-armed at a meeting might not mean that someone is 'blocking you out' or 'getting defensive'. He or she may just be cold or have a backache, or simply feel comfortable sitting that way. It is dangerous to read too much into non-verbal behaviour. Finally, NLP claims that each of us has a Primary Representational System (PRS) – a tendency to think in specific modes: visual, auditory, kinaesthetic, olfactory or gustatory. A person's PRS can be determined by words the person tends to use or by the direction of one's eye movements. Supposedly, a therapist will have a better rapport with a client if they have a matching PRS. None of this has been supported by the scientific literature.

The BAGEL Model (Dilts, 2006) specifies the five elements (in mnemonic form) purportedly comprising the behavioural cues that indicate an individual's internal processes. The BAGEL Model is predicated on the notion that internal processes are subjectively represented in sensory terms: visual, auditory, kinaesthetic and, least likely, olfactory and gustatory.

- Body posture (e.g. leaning back, head upwards and shallow breathing indicates visual representation)
- Accessing cues (e.g. fluctuating voice tone and tempo indicates auditory representation)
- Gestures (e.g. gesturing below the neck indicates kinaesthetic representation)
- Eye movements (see eye accessing cues and the representational systems below)
- Language patterns (specifically sensory-based, e.g. 'I see!', 'Sounds right!' or 'I feel that ...').

Most of the cues we already know about and use within a meeting situation. A leader can tell when members of the meeting have started to lose interest because they fidget or fiddle with their pen – the worst case scenario would be that the person goes to sleep. However, the eye accessing cues of NLP, normally out-lined for the naturally right-handed person, are interesting and mainly unused. They are the core for NLP training exercises and involve learning to calibrate eye movement patterns with internal representations. According to NLP developers, this core tenet loosely relates to the VAK guidelines below:

- Visual: eyes up to left or right according to dominant hemisphere access; high or shallow breathing; muscle tension in neck; high pitched/nasal voice tone; phrases such as 'I can imagine the big picture'
- Auditory: eyes left or right; even breathing from diaphragm; even or rhythmic muscle tension; clear mid-range voice tone, sometimes tapping or whistling; phrases such as 'Let's tone down the discussion'
- Kinaesthetic: eyes down left or right; belly breathing and sighing; relaxed muscu-lature; slow voice tone with long pauses; phrases such as 'I can grasp a hold of it'; 'I feel that ...'.

NLP theory explains this breathing and mental processing according to the varying levels of chemical composition in the blood that affects the brain. 'Visual' people tend to be fast visual thinkers and can seem untrustworthy to 'kinaesthetic' thinkers because thinking by feeling is inherently slow. So by using judgements from your style compass together with observing others you can become effective leaders, although most effective leaders will say that they continue to learn as leaders and are open to new situations and new opportunities. Some authors use internal verbal/auditory/kinaesthetic strategies in order to categorise people within a thinking strategies or learning styles framework, for example, that there exist visual, kinaesthetic or auditory types of manager. Certainly it is worth being aware of this but without empirical evidence it is difficult to say, with any degree of certainty, that it is an effective practice.

These communication techniques offer valuable insight into advancing your leadership skills when dealing with patients, relatives and staff in your team or outside agencies.

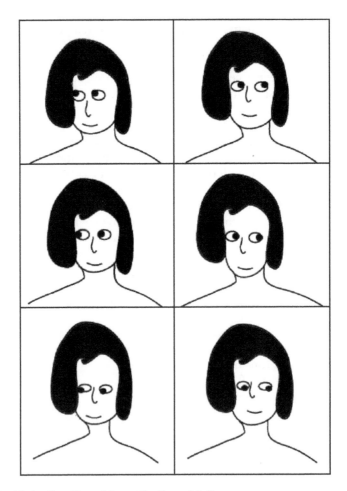

Figure 7.6 Verbal/auditory/kinaesthetic guidelines

LEGAL AND ETHICAL ISSUES

Another important aspect of leadership is the legal and ethical issues that can be seen in the context of professional standards of practice and within the legal framework of health care. Beauchamp and Childress (2001) consider four ethical principles in health care:

- Respect for autonomy
- Non-maleficence
- Justice
- Beneficence.

These relate to health care leadership and are linked to the ethical leadership model. Zydziunaite et al. (2010) identify, through a systematic literature review in Scandinavia, that there were three levels of ethical decision making within health care leadership:

- **Institutional:** related to the organisation
- **Political:** related to the organisation's management
- **Local:** professional expertise.

It is also recognised that record keeping in any of the above decision making levels is seen in the context of professional and ethical standards of practice and within a legal framework. The ethical issues concern:

- **Integrity:** The quality of possessing and steadfastly adhering to high moral principles or professional standards
- **Truth:** Something that corresponds to fact or reality
- **Respect:** Consideration or thoughtfulness
- **Confidentiality:** Being entrusted with somebody's personal or private matters
- **Consent:** To give permission or approval for something to happen
- **Informed decision making:** Based on proper knowledge and understanding of a situation or subject.

The importance of documentation will grow in the future as the culture of litigation increases and health care expectations rise. Paper records are beginning to be overtaken by computerised records so that, while previously there was a need to retain records of care delivered for some time before they are destroyed, this will become a thing of the past as giant computer mainframes store information electronically. This then brings into the discussion the continued vigilance required to maintain confidentiality. Similarly, the notion of explicit (if someone signs a consent form) and implicit (if someone arrives for a blood test) consent has to be dealt with in keeping records safe, which allows them to be shared only with the people who need to know about the medical history, treatment and any other factors regarding health care.

Accountability within the health service is influenced by employment, criminal, civil and professional action. Legal and ethical issues are therefore important professional considerations. Ethics is the study of what our conduct and actions *ought to be* (rather than what they actually are) with respect to others, the environment and ourselves. It is sometimes difficult to separate out ethics and legal issues.

It is interesting to note that health care professionals, once held in high esteem, are now less trusted and are held to account more than before, as cases where individuals who have abused their autonomy for personal satisfaction and criminal activities have become more visible. The health care industry is also facing the ethical problem of trying to meet infinite demand with finite resources. Financial, physical and human resources are being allocated on a priority basis. This had been the case previously but there is now more openness. The implications for these points are that ethical considerations form an important component of health care management. Ethical dilemmas also face clinical staff daily. Haddad (1992: 46) defines an ethical dilemma as a novel, complex and ambiguous problem that does not lend itself to programmed or routine problem solving for which a precedent has been set. In other words, ethical dilemmas are forms of 'messy' problems.

◆ Activity

Can you make a note of any recent clinical problems where you felt ethics played a part?

It may be that you have thought about resuscitation decisions made in your area or maybe decisions about withholding medical treatment for certain groups of people such as the elderly, those with a disability or those who have problems considered to be self-inflicted. You may have identified that screening for certain abnormalities may also pose ethical decisions.

The utilisation of *ethical principles* is useful in examining the issues within any ethical dilemma. Marquis and Huston (2006: 79) identify the following:

1. **Autonomy:** This infers freedom of choice or accepting the responsibility for one's choice. Legal items around the right to self-determination support this moral principle.
2. **Beneficence:** This refers to the point that actions and decisions should be taken in order to promote good.
3. **Non-maleficence:** This goes further and states that if one cannot do good, then at least one should make every effort to avoid harm.

4. **Paternalism:** This principle is related to the positive good that could occur when one individual makes decisions on behalf of another individual. This has to be balanced with the issue that paternalism may limit the freedom of choice for another as one individual makes judgements and decisions for that person. Paternalism is possibly only justified to prevent harm to others.
5. **Utility:** This principle reflects a belief in utilitarianism, where common good outweighs what is good for an individual. This justifies paternalism in also restricting the choice of the individual.
6. **Justice:** This principle is based on the point that equals should be treated equally and 'unequals' should be treated according to their differences.
7. **Veracity:** There is an obligation to tell the truth.
8. **Fidelity:** There is a need to keep promises.
9. **Confidentiality:** Privileged information must be kept private.

Legal issues stem from the statutes and the law of the land. As a health care professional, you should be aware of the legal controls surrounding your practice. Professional negligence in health care concerns any form of malpractice. Malpractice is the failure of a professional with a body of knowledge to act in what is considered a reasonable and prudent manner. This would imply a manner expected of the average health care professional in that discipline, based on expected judgements, foresight, intelligence and skill. Health care professionals hold their own personal liability concerning practice. Fletcher and Buka (1999: 53) identify that it is a professional code of conduct that will enable a judge to decide whether a practitioner was acting within the expectations of their particular profession. This point is known as the Bolam Test from a notable legal test case (Bolam *v* Friern Hospital Management Committee, 1957). Issues such as the position of trust afforded to the professional and the action taken to protect patients' or clients' best interests will be of particular interest in the eyes of the law.

Employers have no legal right, within a contract of employment, to ask you to account for your professional action. They could, however, bring a disciplinary case against you if you failed to account for care, which was deemed poor, and this could thus lead to unemployment. It is only when there is a legal enquiry (criminal or civil) that a health professional may need to go to a court of law – for example, child protection, murder or assault/harm cases – and account for their action. In legal enquiries, the health profession may have to account for any breach in their 'duty to care'.

The NMC or HCPC may also ask professionals to account for their actions but they have no statutory right to force an account. They can, however, through their disciplinary procedures make certain decisions concerning registration; it is obviously important that accurate records of care are kept if one is to maintain registration and practise safely. As role models, leaders should be exemplary in their conduct and accurate in their communication and record keeping.

Summary of Key Points

- **Discuss the application of the 6Cs** NHS England postulated the notion of six elements of compassion in clinical practice and it can be seen that effective communication is one of the main components; together with this we have seen that the model can also be adapted to be used within decision making.
- **Describe various forms of communication** Here we examined the notion of chain, wheel and all channel communication, recognising that these are models that depict the phenomena of effective communication.
- **Describe a variety of communication networks and their effects on clinical practice** By recognising the available networks and understanding their potential shortfalls one is better placed to communicate effectively with the team.
- **Discuss the importance of effective communication** Without effective communication it has been shown that nobody would know what they were supposed to do within a given situation.
- **Debate motivational theory and its place in the clinical area** Motivational theory must be recognised in the clinical area, because without motivation people will not work to achieve the common aims of clinical care.
- **Discuss the benefits of written and electronically stored information** All professions need documented evidence of care delivered and its effect on the patient in order to prove that 'best practice' was always in the forefront of the carer's mind.
- **Identify the benefits of audit in clinical practice** Audit is not a whip to ensure 'best practice' is being delivered; it can also have positive effects e.g. ensuring adequate staffing levels.
- **Consider the benefits of active listening** This is an essential tool of caring, as without it we may not really hear what our patients/clients are telling us. On occasion we know that even though someone is telling us that everything is OK there is something about the way they say it that indicates that it isn't really the case.
- **Consider the benefits of Neuro-Linguistic Programming** This is debatable. On occasion NLP has been shown to work. It is used within the court systems of some countries but it is still necessary to be sceptical.
- **Discuss the legal and ethical issues related to effective communication** It is vital that legal and ethical issues are understood and adhered to. Being an exemplary role model, and using all elements of legal and ethical perspectives, helps one to become an effective health care professional.

FURTHER READING

Bach, S. and Grant, A. (2009) *Communication and Interpersonal Skills for Nurses (Transforming Nursing Practice Series)*. Exeter: Learning Matters.

Bavister, S. and Vickers, A. (2004) *Teach Yourself NLP*. London: Teach Yourself.

Burton, K. and Ready, R. (2010) *Neuro-Linguistic Programming (NLP) for Dummies* (2nd edn). Oxford: John Wiley.

Cassedy, P. (2010) *First Steps in Clinical Supervision: A Guide for Healthcare Professionals*. Maidenhead: McGraw Hill/Open University Press.

Fiske, J. (2010) *Introduction to Communication Studies* (3rd edn). London: Routledge.

Northouse, P. (2012) *Introduction to Leadership: Concepts and Practice*. London: Sage. Chapter 3.

Pierce, J.R. (2010) *An Introduction to Information Theory, Symbols, Signals and Noise* (2nd edn). New York: Dover Publications Inc.

Visit the companion website at https://study.sagepub.com/barr3e for more resources.

8   PROBLEM SOLVING

Learning Outcomes

By the end of this chapter you will have had the opportunity to:

- Discuss the concept of problem solving
- Critically review the models of problem solving
- Critically examine the theory and skills associated with decision making
- Examine the relevance of ethical decision making in practice
- Critically explore the importance of clinical decision making within the context of problem solving for health care practice.

INTRODUCTION

Health care practitioners spend a good proportion of their clinical and management time involved in dealing with patient needs and problems as well as dealing with professional decision making. Leadership therefore involves the need to have experience and skills in problem solving and effective decision making. Having examined the team, it is prudent to now focus on some of the relevant theoretical perspectives associated with problem solving and decision making both for the health care professional and from a patient perspective. The chapter will offer possible solutions and explore the clinical decision making process. Muir (2004) notes the importance of clinical decision making, its effect on patient health care and also the impact on the health care professional. Due to the complexity of health care, and the constant need to keep up to date, the professional is faced with a multitude of problems that require their attention. Professional accountability in the context of clinical governance and evidence-based care (Chapter 12) has also made health care professionals aware of the need to understand the nature of problems and the need to recognise the rationale for the professional judgements they make (DH, 1997b; Muir Gray, 1997, 2007; NMC, 2015).

Goodwin (2014: 46) suggests that as the culture of managerialism has risen in the NHS, accountability is laced throughout professional practice and linked to autonomous practice and decision making. This is at its clearest in the codes of practice produced by professional bodies such as the General Medical Council (GMC), the Health and Care Professionals Council (HCPC) and the Nursing and Midwifery Council (NMC). These regulatory bodies dictate the standards to which each practitioner should conform and against which their performance may be evaluated.

WHAT IS PROBLEM SOLVING?

Problem solving is a key management skill that involves complex cognitive processes. It was VanGundy (1988: 3) who noted that a problem could be defined as 'any situation in which a gap is perceived to exist between what is and what should be'. On the other hand, Armstrong (1990) noted ambitiously that there were no real problems – only opportunities.

 Activity

What do you think?

Think about a recent problem you have faced and decide which of the above ideas fits the situation in your view.

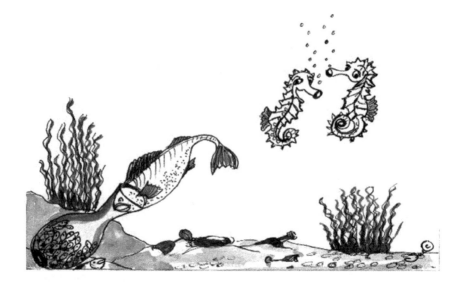

Although Armstrong offered a useful 'glass half-full' perspective it is not always true for certain life events, for instance when the King family took their child out of hospital in 2014 to Spain for treatment which UK doctors thought inappropriate. They were hounded by Hampshire police and the father was taken into custody when the family was found. The media reversed their perspective of a criminal event to one where the family were pursuing the opportunities for treatment they thought was in the best interests of their child.

From a health visiting, teaching and personal perspective, the Government's Health Visitor Implementation Plan 2011–15 has challenged Trusts and universities alike to increase the number of health visiting students to meet the government targets to over 4,000 more health visitors. Ultimately it is seen that this will be an opportunity which will be better for children's health and the success of the 'Healthy Child Programme'.

Problem solving and decision making are often seen as the same activity. Problem solving assumes a fuller analysis of issues than pure decision making issues because it relies on trying to discover the root cause of the problem. Decision making, however, may not address these issues in-depth and this can mean that the process will not take the same amount of time and energy (Tappen et al., 2004; Whitehead et al., 2009).

In some of the literature you may find that decision making involves problem solving while in others decision making is seen as part of problem solving. For the purposes of this chapter, we will assume the latter model. Neither is wrong but is simply a different perception of the link between the two concepts. Huber (2014) identifies a tripartite relationship between problem solving, decision making and critical analysis. The reality of focusing in on problems may present a negative aspect of our professional work so care is needed to balance this leadership activity with a proactive stance seeking solutions to potential problems. Problem redefinition is often helpful in seeing a particular issue from a number of perspectives.

PROBLEM MANAGEMENT

Problem management can be considered using the main four-fold organisational management approaches:

- Classical Management
- Human Relations
- Systems
- Contingency.

The scientific (Classical Management) approach, where the need for optimum productivity is sought in an organisation, will relate to how problem management influences the goal. The Human Relations approach focuses on the impact and implications of work-based problems on people and the importance of their human values. A Systems approach highlights the impact and implications of problem management on the interdependency of relationships within an organisation. Finally, a combination of these ideas is seen in the Contingency approach (Barr and Dowding, 2012: 58–62). It was VanGundy (1988) who suggested that success in problem management relied on two elements: the approaches used and the nature of the problem.

The notion of successful problem solving relates to how organisations or individuals address the following issues:

- Recognition of the nature of the problem
- Assessing the intelligence, implications and impact concerning the problem
- Identifying success criteria in problem solving
- Decision making for solution generation
- Communicating solutions.

Simon (1977) identified decision making as 'management itself'. He was also concerned with how decisions are made and how problem solving could be improved. This has real relevance for the health care industry if leaders are to learn how to do things better and smarter. The novice practitioner often looks for the 'quick fix' idea in order to solve a problem, using a 'blueprint' approach, whereas the effective leader uses a reflective approach, considering the wider perspectives or implications. Robotham and Frost (2005) highlight the work of Benner (1984) and describe the proficient practitioner as someone who perceives situations as wholes rather than in terms of specific aspects.

TRADITIONAL AND CONTEMPORARY APPROACHES TO PROBLEM SOLVING

Traditionally, problem solving and decision making used a rational model as a basis. One perspective, known as the 'Economic Man' approach, has underpinning assumptions that rely on two notions:

- That individuals are all working towards the same organisational goals
- Rationally, they use the best methods to achieve these goals.

This model has been criticised because of the unrealistic nature of its assumptions. There is another approach to compare with the 'Economic Man', which is based on the real or actual behaviour of the problem solvers/decision makers (Cyert and March, 1963; Simon, 1994). Linstead et al. (2004) highlight the differences between 'Economic Man' and the more realistic 'Administrative Man' (Table 8.1).

In recent years feminist writings have rejected this patriarchal approach as being politically incorrect and 'man' would be replaced with 'person'. Either way, leaders of both sexes need to understand the nature of problem solving.

Table 8.1   Economic vs Administrative Man

Economic Man	Administrative Man Simon (1960); Cyert and March (1963)
Rational approach	Solves problems that are 'good enough'
Complete knowledge of the problem	Complete knowledge not possible,
Complete list of possible choices	knowledge is always fragmented
Decisions based on maximising effect	Impossible to predict accurate consequences due to their futuristic nature
	Choice is usually from few alternatives
	Choice is based mainly on satisfying.

THE TYPES OF PROBLEMS

In straightforward terms, there are two types of problems. First, there are the *simple* or *bounded* problems that face us every day, and are fairly easy to solve in terms of time and energy spent on them. Second, there are more *complex* problems that need a good deal of our time and often create internal and external tensions. There are many ways in which health care professionals manage the problems they face. It is often much easier to try and position a problem in the 'simple' category, particularly when we face a new situation where we think a quick solution is desirable and valued by others. It is, therefore, easy to jump to conclusions about the type of complexity of some problems.

Ackoff (1981) and Ackoff and Greenburg (2008) described simple or bounded problems as difficulties or hard problems with clear boundaries (Figure 8.1). The more complex ones were referred to as 'soft, messy problems'. These messy problems are seen as unbounded (Figure 8.2), connected to mess or chaos theory. There is uncertainty and there are no straightforward answers to these problems (Table 8.2). It is all too easy to try and solve messy problems quickly, like simple problems, without really thinking what the real problem is all about and who the problem concerns. The real trick is to recognise the type of problem, the stages of solving it, and how to make the process look and feel simple. Leaders unconsciously select an approach in managing problems most closely related to their personal leadership style. There is a

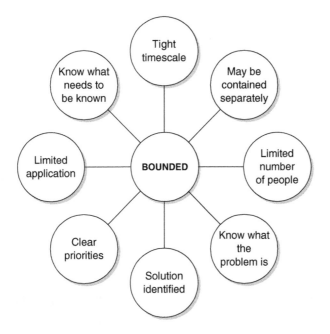

Figure 8.1 Bounded problems

Source: The Open University, 1996 © The Open University. Reproduced with kind permission

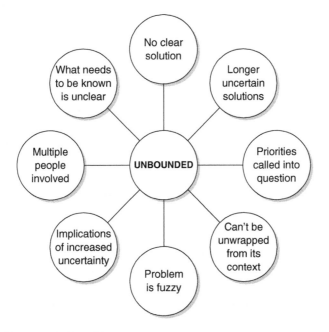

Figure 8.2 Unbounded problems

Source: The Open University, 1996 © The Open University. Reproduced with kind permission

continuum of approaches related to problem solving from a rational approach to a more creative approach. Both approaches have their place depending on the situation being dealt with.

SCIENTIFIC RATIONAL APPROACH

It has generally been accepted in the *rational approach* that there are several stages to problem solving that may help us to understand the concept. Marquis and Huston (2006: 71) illustrate a more traditional Problem Solving Seven Step Model. This can be compared to the handy Six I's model depicted by Stott (1992) (Table 8.3), which emphasises the need to involve relevant people when making decisions.

Table 8.2 Hard and soft problems

Hard Problems or Difficulties	'Soft, Messy' Problems
• One clear problem	• Complex problem
• One clear solution	• No one clear solution
• Know what needs to be done	• Answer can be one of many
• Clear methods for working out solution	• Uncertainty about the problem
• Problem is structured	• No obvious way of working it out
	• Problem is unstructured

Source: Ackoff (1981)

These stages seem like a useful way of logically looking at problems, but it must be said again that human minds do not always work in such a rational, sequential and logical fashion. We do not always work out solutions in a one-to-seven step process. We may look at any of these steps and move through various stages at the same time when dealing with complex problems. However, this traditional problem solving approach is useful to see some of the elements involved and to have some memorable structure to work with. Indeed, this type of problem solving approach has been modified to a four-stage process and utilised as the Nursing or Health Visiting Process in addressing the needs and problems of our patients/clients. Midwifery does not have a named midwifery management process because most of their women/clients are not generally seen as having problems, but are undergoing normal physiological changes during pregnancy and childbirth. There are also some three-stage models that offer the simplest way of approaching problem solving (Table 8.4).

Table 8.3   Traditional v Six I's framework

Traditional Problem Solving Process	Six I's: A Framework for a Staged Problem Solving
1 Identify the problem	1 Identify: Try to understand the problem and its causes
2 Gather data to identify cause and consequences	2 Isolate: Separate the details of the problem and further define the criteria for successful solution
3 Explore range of alternative solutions	3 Involve: Involve necessary and helpful people
4 Review range of alternative solutions against evaluation criteria	4 Investigate: A range of possible solutions and evaluate their application to the problem
5 Select solution	5 Implement: Make a decision, action and communicate decision
6 Implement	
7 Review success	6 Inquire: Ask into effectiveness of decision and reflect on process for future learning

Adapted from Stott (1992: 206)

Table 8.4   Simon (1977) v VanGundy (1988)

Simon (1977)	VanGundy (1988)
• Intelligence	• Problem analysis and redefinition
• Design	• Idea generation
• Choice	• Idea evaluation and selection

INTELLIGENCE OR PROBLEM ANALYSIS

As stated earlier, there are a variety of problems – from simple to more complex ones. There are lots of problems facing health care professionals on an hourly basis which are dealt with quickly and intuitively because the solutions are clear. For more complex problems a number of problem solving frameworks may be useful. The six sigma problem solving and decision making statistical model is another scientific approach (Pyzdek and Keller, 2014). It was developed by Motorola in the 1980s and is a quality model similar to TQM (Chapter 12). Huber (2014: 76) notes that the model is 'error-free' and one decision making application may be in the activity of hospital discharge planning. It is a complex model, in some respects, but Ackoff (1981) indeed felt that there was a need to look for different approaches when dealing with messy problems.

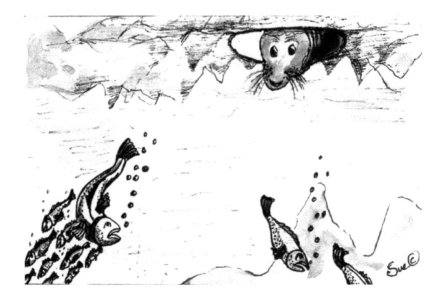

From these rational frameworks, there is more emphasis on analysing the type of problem presented, rather than reaching a quick solution. It is also important to look at who should be involved with the problem analysis as there may be many stakeholders in the context of the problem and the impact of the solutions (Stott, 1992). Stakeholders may be those who have an interest in the problem and possible solutions due to two factors: relevance and expertise.

The problem/solutions may have relevant implications for stakeholders. Other stakeholders may have expertise in supporting the decision making. For example, a team of health professionals are aware of an isolated group of new mothers and their babies in a rural area who have difficulty accessing the health centre/ GP provision in the city. The team leader wants to explore the problem with relevant stakeholders such as the new mothers, the GP, midwifery and health visiting team, social workers and the voluntary sector. It may not be possible to get all these people physically together but if they can set up a communication network they will be able to explore the issues and reach a range of choices for a solution. The team leader may well engage with other stakeholders who can help because of their expertise, for example, a financial expert, charity organiser or legal representative.

In some instances stakeholders may be very few. For example, there may be time to work through health care goals and therapies with just you and your patient/client. Other cases may involve working through the problems with a variety of other professionals and the required quality of the solutions may arise out of a period of reflection and collaboration with others. It is useful, therefore, to identify who might own or be affected by the problem, or even be affected by any solution proposed: these are the problem owners. Remember, then, that the *problem itself* needs to be analysed, redefined and separated from the *symptoms*.

A staged approach to problem solving may offer guidance for complex issues and help you to resist coming up with a *quick fix* solution that has no value in the long term. However, this notion of a staged progress to finding successful solutions is still not without difficulties – or debate – as the approach remains based on the notion of several assumptions, that:

- the problem solving process is a rational one
- there are no conflicting objectives within the process
- there is perfect knowledge which can be shared
- all possible solutions and consequences will be acknowledged.

ROLE OF THE CREATIVE/INTUITIVE APPROACH IN PROBLEM SOLVING

Against the backcloth of the debate concerning the scientific approach is the value put on the creative or intuitive approach. Benner and Tanner (1987) signalled that intuition relates to being able to understand phenomena without any rationale. McCutcheon and Pincombe (2001) used grounded theory to collect data from 262 Registered Nurses, to explore their perceptions of intuition and its impact on practice; they concluded that it is not some mystical power that appears from nowhere but is a product of the synergy that occurs as a result of several factors. It could, therefore, be said that intuition is a linear deductive process (Agor, 1986) and 'The act or faculty of knowing or sensing without the use of rational processes; immediate cognition'. More recently, Green (2012), using contemporary neurophysiology research and the philosophy of Jacques Maritain and Yves R. Simon, claimed that intuition, particularly nursing intuition, is a valid form of knowledge today.

> ### ▶ Activity
>
> Can you recall any decisions you made in the last month where you were not aware of why you made the decision?

I can think of many instances where intuition has played a major part in caring. One example was when working in the recovery unit of an operating theatre and a patient was ready to go back to the ward, but there was just something about her condition that I didn't like. I didn't know what it was but when she was seen by the anaesthetist he said she was developing heart block. On another occasion I remember dealing with a daughter whose father was terminally ill. When she asked whether it was advisable if she went home for a short rest, I made a decision to encourage her to stay a while longer. She was present when her father died about an hour and a half later and was pleased she had stayed with him. Intuition has been linked with personal experiences influenced by prior patterns of knowledge. Having experience in dealing with many people who have died in your care, there are physiological and psychological patterns of events that are not always easily internalised or communicated to others.

Another view on intuition is one of heuristics, or rules of thumb, whereby large amounts of stored knowledge are bypassed using procedural shortcuts.

Intuition is often used to solve problems at a subconscious rather than a conscious level (Buckingham and Adams, 2000). Indeed, the work of de Bono (1990) and others has enabled more creative problem solving approaches to become accepted and allows for fresh idea generation, lateral thinking and innovation, especially where the complexity of the problem may be overwhelming to the team. Creative approaches are often used in leadership courses for health care professionals.

IDEA GENERATION OR DESIGN

There are a huge number of management tools that can help in unpicking a complex problem in more detail. These tools can be shared among any of the problem stakeholders at any part of the process. VanGundy (1988) provides a wealth of ideas for problem solving techniques:

- **PEST/STEP:** (Political, Economic, Societal and Technological context) analysis of problem
- **Six honest serving men:** Kipling (1902) *The Elephant's Child:*

  I keep six honest serving-men:

  (They taught me all I knew)

  Their names are **What** and **Where** and **When**

  And **How** and **Why** and **Who.**

  I send them over land and sea,

  I send them east and west;

  But after they have worked for me,

  I give them all a rest.

  I let them rest from nine till five.

  For I am busy then,

As well as breakfast, lunch, and tea,

For they are hungry men:

But different folk have different views:

I know a person small–

She keeps ten million serving-men,

Who get no rest at all!

She sends 'em abroad on her own affairs,

From the second she opens her eyes–

One million Hows, two million Wheres,

And seven million Whys!

- **Why** method
  - o The problem statement is written down and the team is asked to keep asking 'Why?' to the responses in order to get to the root of the problem.

- Input and output framework
  - o The input and output factors are uncovered to review the contributing elements and results on a situation.

- Cause and effect or Fishbone (Ishikawa, 1985)
  - o The cause and effect factors are uncovered to review a situation. An Ishikawa analysis can use brainstorming to identify possible causes or effects of an issue. The fishbone may involve looking at elements such as man, materials, 'mother nature', machines, measurements and methods related to a problem (www.mindtools.com/pages/article/newTMC_03.htm accessed 24 August 2014).

- **Thought-showering** or **thought-writing**, which can use a verbal or written word method
- **Checklists**
- **Six Thinking Hats** (de Bono, 1990), where six coloured hats (with specific characteristics) can be used for individuals in a group to allow them to abandon their own personalities
- **Six Action Shoes** (de Bono, 1990) This is a similar approach to the above, but allows people to have two personalities/roles
- **Metaphors** or **analogies** These can allow you to see the problem in another context, such as a game, an animal, event or a journey
- **Visualisation** This may help in providing a reflective internal environment in thinking through a problem

- **Reversals** This is where problem statements are made and the wording is reversed. For example:

  o How to deal with relatives of patients parking, when there are limited spaces, can become how to provide relatives of patients with available parking spaces. This could lead to more provision of park and ride facilities where there is ample parking provision.

- **Superheroes and heroines** This is where a hero or heroine is seen as the problem solver and you are asked to identify how they might see the situation.

◆ Activity

Some of these ideas may be useful within your work teams and others may be useful in helping patients to work through their own problems.

Which of these do you think lends itself to patient support?

You may have thought of a superhero type person, the one you can always go to when you have a problem at work, the one who will offer suggestions while not making you feel small for asking for help. There may also be a person who looks on the good side all the time, looking for positives. I remember being on placement with a Sister who was always on my back, to the extent that I used to look at the duty rota to see if I was on with her. If I was, I would consider throwing a 'sicky'. I didn't and a colleague pointed out that although I had another six weeks on placement it could be broken down into 30 days, and as I only worked with her once or twice every five days, that was only another six to ten shifts I had to do with her. That made it all far more acceptable to me, so I survived! Clearly reflection on the situation made sure that I would not inflict a similar experience on students when I became a Sister.

'GROUPTHINK'

Caution must be taken when involving groups of people in identifying problems and solutions. Janis (1982) identified that when groups of people come together to make decisions they are more likely to conform to the majority decision because they do not feel comfortable being an outsider; this means less creative solutions may be offered up. This 'groupthink' is the result of group pressure which prevents members testing the reality and using individual judgement to decide whether something is good or not. The outward signs of 'groupthink' present themselves in different ways; members of the group may be less likely to challenge the judgement of the majority as they don't want to be seen to be rocking the boat. Also, when suggestions within the group are asked for, there is reluctance to voice ideas. Janis further suggests that the following are key characteristics of 'groupthink':

- Illusion of invulnerability
- Belief in integrity of the group
- Negative views of competitors
- Sanctity of agreement
- Erecting a protective shield.

The consequences that flow from 'groupthink' are synonymous with those of poor decision making processes and ultimately could affect patient care. Snell (2009) undertook a quantitative correlation study using a survey method to identify how job stress, conflict and ambiguity affected 'groupthink' in nursing in two acute hospitals. His research showed that the low to moderate incidence of these factors helped explain the low incidence of 'groupthink' in the organizations. As leaders need to bring out a diversity of ideas to address problem solving, they should perhaps work towards counterbalancing the possibility of 'groupthink' within their team.

CHOICE AND DECISION MAKING

The skill of decision making, within the context of health care, alludes to the presence of natural cognitive and learnt abilities. We learn to make decisions in our early childhood days through identifying how to connect with the environment; we learn to deal with more complex decisions as we develop through to adulthood and even into the role of the health care professional.

> ### ◆ Activity
>
> Have you ever had an experience where you felt something was wrong with a patient during your training but didn't actually know what decision to make about that feeling?

I well remember a time when I was a very junior nurse on my first surgical placement during my first week. I had completed a task and noticed that the last patient in the ward didn't look very well. I didn't feel I had enough knowledge of what could be wrong to make a decision about his care. I was unsure what I should do but when the staff nurse told me to go on my break a few minutes later I made the decision to mention my concerns to her. The decision making process took place but I have little recollection of the formality of recognising the various stages in a conscious manner. The staff nurse responded by going to see him and when I returned from my break she told me that he had unfortunately passed away (this episode took place prior to the introduction of Cardio Pulmonary Resuscitation in the 1960s).

Interestingly McCallum et al. (2013) reviewed the awareness of nurses to deteriorating patient conditions in order to refer on for medical support. The evidence base in relation to student nurses' skills in managing patients whose condition is deteriorating may be limited, however the findings from Cooper et al.'s (2010) study are consistent with research undertaken with qualified nurses. It was noted that learning and using 'Early Warning Signs (EWS)' scoring systems are not helpful in developing student nurses' decision making skills. One possible reason for this may be the dissonance between early warning scoring systems and decision making theory involving information processing, professional judgment and intuition. McCallum et al. (2013) indicated that EWS tools can deskill the student experience and development of their own problem solving and decision making skills which involves getting to know the patient and their changing condition.

DEFINITIONS OF DECISION MAKING AND RESEARCH

There are many definitions associated with decision making. Linstead et al. (2004: 489) note that it could be regarded as a commitment to a course of action, rather than the action itself. An example of making a decision could be when a nurse decides to administer a specific dose of a drug from the range that has been prescribed, for example, if one or two tablets are ordered then the nurse must decide how many to give. It is not necessarily their visible action that constitutes the first stage of the decision making process but the cognitive activity prior to this. A Google search (www.google.co.uk) reflects these inconsistencies and uncovers the link with dealing with finite human and other resources, psychology, law and sporting events (Table 8.5).

Table 8.5 Definitions of decision making

- The act of making your mind up about something (wordreference.com/definition/decision).
- A decision is the commitment to irrevocably allocate valuable resources. A decision is a commitment to act. Action is therefore the irrevocable allocation of valuable resources (en.wikipedia.org/wiki/Decision).
- A formal, written judgement or verdict (www.nfa.futures.org/basicnet/glossary.aspx).

Decision making may be seen as a systematic and sequential process of making choices from a number of alternatives and putting that choice into action (Lancaster, 1999). Malloch and Porter-O'Grady (2005: 145) identified that good decisions require insight, creativity and methodology where there is uncertainty and a number of alternative choices are available. Bach and Ellis (2011: 24) however distinguish between effective and ineffective health care team decision making where the former is featured by

Consensus

General agreement

Acceptability

Toleration of dissenters

Acceptance of diverse views

The importance of decision making is thus critical to everyday health care work. It is about giving patients/clients the best care to meet their needs. Bucknall (2000) undertook an observational study of decision making among critical care nurses in Australia and found that they made, on average, patient care decisions every 30 seconds and the three main decision making areas were:

- Intervening – to modify the patient situation
- Communicative – to give or receive information
- Evaluative – to review patient data to evaluate their status.

This shows how critical decision making is within the sphere of everyday health care, and often relates to critical episodes and patient outcomes. Table 8.6 gives you a comparison of how some management theorists have classified problem and decision types.

Table 8.6 Problem/decision types

Drucker (1989)	Simon (1980)	Stott and Walker (1995)
• Simple or generic decisions – decisions are based on using principles	• Programmed	• Standard
		• Crisis
• Unique or complex	• Non-programmed (novel, unstructured, consequential)	• Deep (involving generation of alternatives)

There are similarities between all these ideas sets but Stott and Walker (1995) appear to offer a little more relevance in the real world of health care with their inclusion of crisis decisions. It was Stott (1992: 203) who highlighted that not all decisions are of equal importance and thus will involve greater or lesser time commitment, differing skills needed, who might be involved and what resources you may need.

- **Standard decisions** are those we make on an everyday basis and tend to be repetitive. Solutions are usually found by rules of thumb, procedures or policy, for example, deciding to offer patients or relatives tea when you encounter them in stages of emotional upset.

- **Crisis decisions** arise from unexpected situations and need an immediate response with little or no time to negotiate and plan with others. A quick, precise response is required, for example, in the case of severe haemorrhage or other life-threatening situations.
- **Deep decisions** require more intense planning, reflection and consideration. They may concern forward planning as part of change management and often incur debate, disagreement and conflict. They require a substantial amount of time and networking with a range of people; for example, you may encounter a patient with complex needs who requires a greater understanding of their lifestyle and attitudes to health. At other times a case conference will need to be called to make decisions with a number of health care professionals as well as the patient and carers.

There is an activity on the companion website you might like to undertake in relation to decision making.

ETHICAL DECISION MAKING

Professional leadership involves deeper decision making guided by ethical principles which have been highlighted in Chapter 7. There are a variety of ethical theories that might help you in your decision making:

- Feminist theories which emphasise compassion, kindness, self-esteem and justice
- Care ethics which emphasise the uniqueness of the individual, patient/client or situation
- Virtue ethics which emphasise the behaviour of the professional
- Teleological/utilitarian theories which focus on the perceived end result or outcome
- Deontological theories which emphasise the means/ process of actions planned.

There are a number of ethical decision making frameworks from simple to complex. The IDEA Ethical Decision-Making process is one which is fairly simple in its approach:

- Identify the issues
- Determine the relevant ethical principles
- Explore the options
- Act

STYLES OF DECISION MAKING

There may be a need to use a variety of skills to solve problems – logical thinking, intuition or trial and error – depending on the type or the context of the specific problem. The kind of management skills and styles you have may affect the outcome of the solution and decisions made. Vroom and Yetton (1976) identified different styles of problem solvers depending on their position on a management style continuum. The style of problem solving will depend on who and how other people are involved in the problem solving process (Table 8.7).

Table 8.7   Types of decision makers (Vroom and Yetton, 1973)

A1	Solve problems and make decisions using available information
A11	Get information from subordinates and solve problems themselves
C1	Share problems with individual subordinates, generate solutions, then make their own decisions
C11	Share problems with subordinate groups, generate suggestions then make their own decisions
G11	Share problems with subordinate groups, generate ideas and come to a consensus on a solution.

The quality of decision making may depend upon a variety of factors. Vroom and Yetton (1976) noted the following:

- Values and personal beliefs
- Life experience
- Individual preference
- Willingness to take risks
- 'Our' way of thinking
- Critical, collegial culture.

Buchanan and Badham (2008) concurred with these ideas but noted important principles for being considered a successful political decision maker. These were to be able to develop liaisons, appear conservative, clear the air, ally with power, use trade-offs effectively, strike when the iron is hot, ape the chameleon, limit communication, involve research, and know when to withdraw.

Activity

What do you make of these principles?

How could you apply them in your everyday work?

At first sight the principles appear to be interesting, but they may in part represent a double-edged sword. They imply networking is essential but there is a need to be careful and wary of the power within the environment and keep on the right side of it. Good decision making is therefore seen to be about awareness of the environment, learning from past experiences, wanting and forcing things to happen, and looking for new ways to solve problems while possibly taking risks.

APPLICATION OF RESEARCH

Doherty and Doherty (2005) looked at patients' preference for involvement in clinical decision making using an interpretative phenomenology/triangulated approach. They noted the continuum scale from full patient decision making to health care professional with full decision making rights. The researchers conducted semi-structured interviews of 20 patients in one British Acute Trust; there were equal numbers of medical and post-surgical patients, and nine men and 11 women. Seventeen of the group were over 60 and the youngest was 18. The researchers categorised the patients into active, collaborative and passive, based on their responses (Table 8.8).

Table 8.8   Active vs collaborative vs passive role of the patient

Active Role of Patient	Collaborative Role of Patient	Passive Role of Patient
• Active decision making role 15% (three) medical and 5% (one) surgical; 10% (two) noted the importance of personal autonomy, for example, requesting GP to prescribe steroids. However, they did not know about their discharge plans. • Patient knowledge The surgical patient felt he disagreed with his surgeon's opinion that he needed more surgery but he consented based on the fact that he wasn't asked for his opinion. • Communication issues Concern noted regarding the need for better communication.	• Share decision making 40% (eight) believed they could make their own opinion but still required professional knowledge to help in decision making. • Specific barriers: one noted pain was a barrier to taking an active role; one noted Doctor interpersonal skills; two noted limited opportunity to being involved; one noted there were 'too many on ward round'. 'Sometimes I find the doctors talk to the nurse and they don't consult you. You're the last one to know.'	• Passive role 40% (8) – mainly because they felt 'Doctors had greater knowledge of illness' than they did. Some felt they were powerless.

These are interesting, patient-focused results as most of our research has related to health care professionals dealing with their own problems and decisions. However, more research may be needed concerning patients' roles in this activity. From these results it is suggested that most of the research participants experienced a paternalistic health service and never thought to challenge it.

Activity

How will this research change your practice?

You may have considered becoming a better patient advocate. You need to think about the perceived powerlessness of your patients and how you can help to avoid their passive role developing. This could be achieved by ensuring that the patient is made fully cognisant of the facts about their treatment, and any alternatives there might be, in order that the patient has an involvement in the clinical decision making process. It is important that, whatever your discipline, your patients/clients are able to use informed consent for any treatment or intervention offered.

Summary of Key Points

This chapter has briefly looked at various aspects of problem solving and decision making theory in order to meet the identified learning outcomes. These were to:

- **Discuss the concept of problem solving** Only a small number of the many theories have been explored, but it is noted that problem solving is a key leadership skill that involves cognitive processes.
- **Critically review the models of problem solving** Traditional and contemporary approaches to problem solving were addressed, highlighting the notion that there is more than one way to solve problems.
- **Critically examine the theory and skills associated with decision making** Here we examined two models of problem solving, the traditional and the 'Six I's', together with comparing the three stage models offered by Simon (1977) and VanGundy (1988).
- **Examine the relevance of ethical decision making in practice** Here the use of ethical decision making frameworks was explored in the context of vulnerability and professional practice.
- **Critically explore the importance of clinical decision making within the context of problem solving for health care practice** Clinical decision making was explored by the examination of research to support the need for patient involvement in the process.

FURTHER READING

Dowding, D. and Thompson, C. (2004) 'Using decision trees to aid decision-making in nursing', *Nursing Times*, 100 (21): 36–9 (accessed 5 June 2011).

Dowding, D. and Thompson, C. (2004) 'Using judgement to improve accuracy in decision making', *Nursing Times*, 100 (22): 42 (accessed 8 May 2011).

Higgins, J. (2006) *Creative Problem Solving Techniques: The Handbook of New Ideas for Business* (rev. edn). Florida: New Management Publishing Company.

Thompson, C. and Dowding, D. (2002) 'Decision analysis', in C. Thompson and D. Dowding (eds) *Clinical Decision-making and Judgment in Nursing*. Edinburgh: Churchill Livingstone.

Visit the companion website at https://study.sagepub.com/barr3e for more resources.

9   MANAGING CONFLICT

Learning Outcomes

By the end of this chapter, you will have had the opportunity to:

- Discuss the concept of conflict
- Critically review a range of models associated with conflict management
- Critically explore the importance of conflict management within the context of problem solving
- Recognise the importance of cultural diversity on leadership during conflict.

INTRODUCTION

This chapter explores the notion of conflict management within the context of health care. Forsyth (2010) identifies that conflict involves discord and friction

brought about by differences in ideas, values or feelings between two or more people; however, internal conflict can also occur *within* the individual. Conflict is not
necessarily a bad thing; if you think back to the discussion related to group formation (Chapter 5) the second stage, '*storming*', is all about conflict as the group settles
to become effective (or not) as they begin to work together and as such is an inescapable part of team working. Where there are huge numbers of people with
differing backgrounds interacting with each other daily conflict is an expected
occurrence. With infinite demands being put on the health service, conflict can also
be seen as a result of competitiveness of different groups for scarce health resources.
Results of conflict may be poor team behaviour, time wasting, poor productivity,
absenteeism, stress and ill health. Leadership, therefore, has to be interested in managing conflict; leaders have to try to foresee as well as make sense of conflict
situations, and plan solutions before patient care is compromised. McElhaney
(1996, cited in Valentine, 2001) identified that probably about 20 per cent (about
one day a week) of managerial time is spent dealing with conflict. Marquis and
Huston (2008: 492) suggest that if the manager decides to handle a conflict crisis
when it occurs but does not attempt to identify the real problem then only decision
making rather than problem solving skills are being utilised. However, later they
may decide to address the problem by identifying the root cause of the conflict
before deciding whether or not to do anything about it. They go on to describe five
stages of conflict as being:

- **Latent Conflict** – implying the existence of antecedent conditions e.g. short of
  staff, rapid change
- **Perceived Conflict** – usually involves issues and roles. If addressed the problem
  could be resolved at this stage
- **Felt Conflict** – when emotionalised e.g. hostility, fear, anger
- **Manifest Conflict** – sometimes called Overt Conflict, where action is taken and
  the reaction may be withdrawal from the situation or to seek conflict resolution
- **Conflict Resolution** – this is often influenced by culture, gender, age, power, position and upbringing.

Interestingly the notion of the 6Cs (Figure 9.1) may also be used for decision making
where the 6Cs become:

- Construct a clear picture
- Compile a list of things to do
- Collect information
- Compare all alternatives
- Consider what could go wrong
- Commit to the decision. (www.fgbt.org)

In this way you can be assured that all 'angles' of the problem have been considered
before any action is taken thereby ensuring that time and resources are not wasted
during the actual execution of the task.

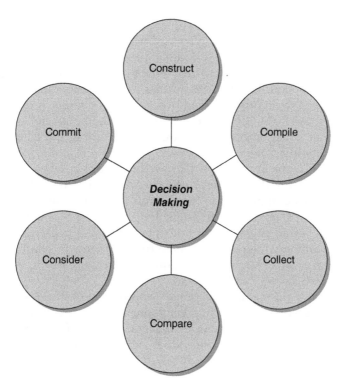

Figure 9.1   The 6Cs of decision making

(*Source*: Full Gospel Businessman's Training, 2014)

THE CONCEPT OF CONFLICT

In the twentieth century, conflict was considered in a negative light. In terms of organisational life it was even seen as a result of poor leadership and as being dysfunctional to the objectives of an organisation. Everything was meant to run smoothly and harmoniously and so conflict was pushed underground or accepted passively. Buchanan and Huczynski (2010) suggested that conflict was a state of mind perceived by the parties involved. Rahim (2011: 1) noted that conflict in organisations is a natural outcome of human interaction when two or more social entities come in contact with one another in attaining their objectives. A variety of organisational behaviours, which are influenced by differing goals and relationships of individuals, could be seen as a result of conflict.

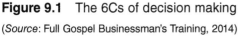 Activity

Think about a recent episode where you experienced a conflict situation. Write down ten words that come to mind when you think about this situation.

Look back on your ten words. Would you say they are negative or positive words? Conflict is now seen as neither bad nor good so you may have written both negative and the odd positive-sounding word. Good conflict management can bring about organisational growth whereas poor conflict management can bring about destruction. Handy (1993) notes the two disparate views regarding conflict. The negative unitary and traditional view of conflict is that it gives rise to deviant, dysfunctional behaviour resulting in emotional and physical stress where a win–lose situation occurs. The outcome is seen as the dominance of the one party over another.

The other side of the argument is that 'well managed conflict' can be energising and vitalise forces that produce constructive group life, which is more of a positive, pluralistic approach and can result in a win–win situation (Handy, 1985; Covey, 2004; Cemi et al., 2012). Figure 9.2 reflects how conflict can affect the performance of an organisation both positively and negatively. On a more positive note, Chan et al. (2014: 943) note that constructive conflict can inspire innovations and creative strategies to address challenging issues, improve teamwork, patient care delivery and outcomes.

A concept analysis using an evolutionary approach was undertaken by Almost (2006) concerning conflict in nursing environments. She found that conflict was a multidimensional notion with both detrimental and beneficial effects. The antecedents to the concept related to individual and organisational issues as well as interpersonal relationships.

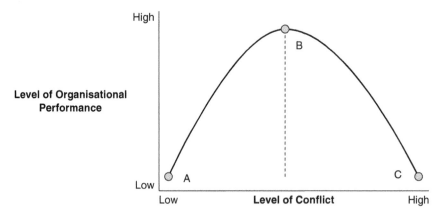

Figure 9.2   Conflict and organisational performance

LEVELS OF CONFLICT

It is useful to understand the three levels of conflict when leading teams in health care. These levels are *intrapersonal*, *interpersonal* and *intergroup* conflict. A good leader should recognise these as different but also recognise how to attempt to manage conflict competently.

Intrapersonal conflict

This takes place *within* an individual who may have difficulty in managing their contradictory felt needs or wants. It may involve role conflict or confusion or it may be about balancing work and home life. Discord and unhappiness might occur before the situation is resolved. It is valuable to turn these internalised felt needs and wants into expressed needs. This can be achieved through self-awareness, peer and leadership support.

Interpersonal conflict

This takes place between two or more people with different values and beliefs. It is becoming a significant issue in health care where the conflict may bring about bullying and harassment, causing discontent, stress and grievance. Farrell (2001) identifies the phenomena of 'horizontal violence' in nursing where some nurses are left squashed and deflated by more powerful members of their own profession. This situation has been widely documented in other countries (Thomas, 2003; Marquis and Huston, 2008: 490).

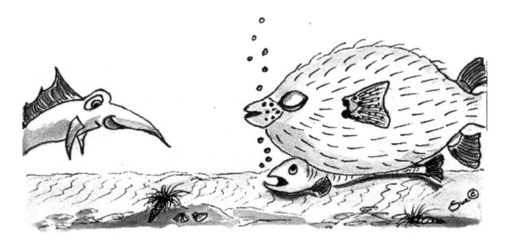

Intergroup conflict

This takes place between two or more groups, departments or organisations. This kind of conflict may be the result of jealousies of others getting more resources, recognition or favourable rewards.

▶ Activity

Jot down any examples of these three types of conflict you have experienced as a health care professional.

From a personal perspective, my own intrapersonal conflict example relates to the dislike of driving to work and back along the motorway with lots of roadworks. I try and leave home very early or later in order to avoid the rush hours. Recent interpersonal conflict related to confronting staff workload in a team, when one member was not happy helping another member of the team, because they felt they had enough to do. Last week, I experienced intergroup conflict when the teachers on the post-registration programmes felt the teachers on the pre-registration programmes got the first choice of classrooms in the university building. It sounds as though I have had a very difficult time but really I see it as everyday working life; however, it can cause stress and disruption if not dealt with.

STAGES OF GROUP LIFE AND CONFLICT

How conflict emerges is important, because if a leader can identify the early stages they can deal with them appropriately. Indeed, in terms of developing a team (Chapter 5), the principles of leadership are related to two main ideas:

1. Diagnosis of the group stage
2. Intervening in order to help 'move the group on'.

It is interesting to relate the stages of group development and where these fit with emerging conflict. As discussed in Chapter 5, Tuckman's (1965) notion of a natural sequence for small groups offers a simple way of identifying with group life.

Forming This is where there is a period of uncertainty

Storming This is where a period of conflict and hostility between members may arise

Norming This is a settling down period and the group starts to pull together

Performing This is where performance is at an optimum.

Tuckman, on reviewing this, later added a fifth stage, **adjourning**, where the group breaks up as a natural activity. Hartley (1997) compared a number of other models about stages of group life which have been proposed through research over the years. Bennis and Shepherd's (1956) work suggested another conflict stage between Norming and Performing, and Bales and Strodtbeck's (1951) three-stage model of orientation, evaluation and control was closely linked to a problem solving model. Hartley (1997), however, paid regard to the more recent research-based model of Wheelan (1994), characterised by fluctuating stages where some groups may get stuck at one stage, resulting in conflict and self destruction (Figure 9.3).

Dependency and Inclusion	Reliance on leader; polite, tentative communication; group members are anxious and shy away from tasks.
Counter-dependency and Flight	Conflict may occur between leader and members or just between members; there may still be a shying away from tasks as individuals try to work out their roles.
Trust and Structure	Conflict resolution. Norms and roles are agreed; more open communication; members feel more secure.
Work	Group works effectively.
Termination	The group disbands having completed the task.

Figure 9.3   Fluctuating stages resulting in conflict (adapted from Wheelan, 1994)

Activity

Can you see any problems with these models of group life?

One of the difficulties in working with staged models is that in reality it can be very difficult to identify the transition from one stage to another. Hartley (1997) hints that chaos and disharmony is more prevalent in reality than some of these models suggest. Do you agree? When conflict arises, it can also be seen in terms of another four-staged model (Pondy, 1992):

- Perceived (latent) conflict is where there is a feeling of unease
- Felt conflict is where the unease is internalised and agreed as a real conflict of interests
- Manifest conflict is where the conflict is externalised and expressed
- Conflict aftermath is where the outcome of the conflict episode affects the individual(s) and group(s) concerned.

While there are many different models it is important to remember that they are just a simple representation of a complex situation. You may find yourself preferring one model to another or use an eclectic approach to leadership during conflict.

CAUSES OF CONFLICT

The causes of conflict may have nothing to do with the work situation but may be associated, as briefly suggested above, with individual differences and may relate more specifically to differences in ideology and personal objectives. Some of the common causes of conflict in the workplace may relate to the following:

- Differences in perception at various levels of the organisation
- Concealed objectives
- Limited resources
- Departmentalisation and specialisation
- Nature of work processes and design
- Role conflict
- Inequitable treatment.

Do these sound familiar? Some of the following situations may be familiar to you.

Differences in perception at various levels of the organisation

The senior manager believes staff should change their practice in Accident and Emergency to get work done quickly in order to get patients transferred home, to the right department, or to another provision. This is set within the context of the government's required target time so staff need to work in a more efficient manner. The A&E staff are trying to effectively care for and treat patients within a given time frame, recognising that there may be fluctuating patient numbers and varying dependency needs. These situational differences are challenging for the staff already working in a pressurised environment. Even though there is a valid reason for moving patients on as soon as possible other departments may have their own pressures that influence the continuity of patient care.

Another example may be that a new unit manager in a residential care setting recognised that the current care staff have been allowed to become less than professional in their dress and attitudes to residents. The staff are reminded that they should wear uniform properly as provided by the employer, that their hair should be clean and tied back; correct footwear worn at all times when on duty and they should speak to residents and colleagues in a civil and respectful manner. Of course the staff rebelled at the thought of this change in their current practices; when they realised that the changes would make them feel more professional their attitude to work changed. They had positive feedback from patients and relatives concerning their appearance and behaviour on duty; suddenly they could see a point in it all.

Another example was in the same setting where a manager was concerned about the correct completion of fluid balance charts. She raised awareness with staff and the discord did not last long when she explained the importance of the charts for some of the residents. Presently standards of care are rising and of course the residents are also benefiting. Chan et al. (2014) in their research related the notion of emotional intelligence links to better outcomes with the use of a compromising style rather than an avoiding style.

Conflict can arise from a variety of reasons. They can generally be grouped under the following headings:

- Hidden Agendas
- Finite Resources
- Departmentalisation and Specialisation
- Work Design
- Role Overlap
- Unfair Situations.

Hidden Agendas

The ward sister was told in July that her rehabilitation ward would close in October and the staff would be relocated to another ward area. She has been told that she must not discuss this with the staff as they will be duly informed at the beginning of September, when plans are in place. Staff become concerned that the ward sister is reluctant to discuss any staffing issues. Rumours, from an unknown source, start to emerge that the ward will be closed.

Finite Resources

A medical ward and a medical admissions unit (MAU) would like to send a number of staff on a clinical update. Due to the turnover of patients in the MAU, staff numbers have been curtailed.

Departmentalisation and Specialisation

A renal ward is introducing a new outreach service into the community. Selected staff will be supporting patients and district nurses in keeping patients at home as much as possible. Some of the senior staff will continue with their inpatient work but those chosen will be given new titles of renal specialists.

Work Design

The general surgical theatre nursing staff have been divided into two teams and their theatre coverage has been allocated between the two theatres. One team, however, appears to complete their elective work by 4:30 p.m. while the other team are faced with elective work until 5:30 p.m.

Role Overlap

The District Nurse has been sent a referral from the hospital to visit a patient. When she gets to the patient's house, the rapid response team is there already and she is told that she will not be required. Here there is confusion about the complexity of community roles and an overlap of role expectations.

Unfair Situations

The night staff in a particular clinical area cannot get access to educational updates while on duty. They have to try and 'fit their professional development' sessions in and around their working hours, which often means they get to the sessions after only a couple of hours' sleep or in the middle of their annual leave. The day staff can get to their updates for these sessions during their working time.

> ### ▶ Activity
>
> How would you manage any of these situations?
>
> Can you identify similar examples from your own clinical experience?

SYMPTOMS OF CONFLICT OR COLLISION

From the above examples it can be seen that conflict can be a result of the multiple competing demands we have in health care. Leadership is required to help deal with past, present and even anticipated conflict situations. There are underpinning symptoms of conflict; these can help us to identify situations before the conflict becomes too oppressive.

These symptoms can be seen as:

- Territorial issues
- Poor communication – laterally or vertically
- Intergroup jealousy
- Interpersonal friction (personalities)
- Escalation of arbitration
- Increasing rules, norms and myths
- Evidence of low morale.

> ### ▶ Activity
>
> Make some notes of these symptoms related to the following:
>
> - Your past work life experience
> - Your current work life situation
> - Possible future work life issues.

You will probably recognise that these symptoms are a feature in all work life experiences. These symptoms may culminate in increasing sickness/absence and ultimately clinical staff retention. When pursuing new positions you may need to critically question why a vacancy has occurred and why the position looks so glamorous. Being aware of 'staff turnover' in that clinical area may influence how you see your application. This should form part of your SWOT analysis. You must also understand how the organisational culture deals with symptoms of conflict when people are joining or leaving a workplace. You need to get a sense of the quality of leadership, past and present, together with histories of conflict so that you are fully aware of the environment you are applying to work in.

CONSEQUENCES OF CONFLICT

Almost (2006) noted that the consequences of conflict related to those highlighted in Figure 9.4. From these ideas you can identify both positive and negative outcomes but, unless it is managed effectively, negativity can dominate the situation.

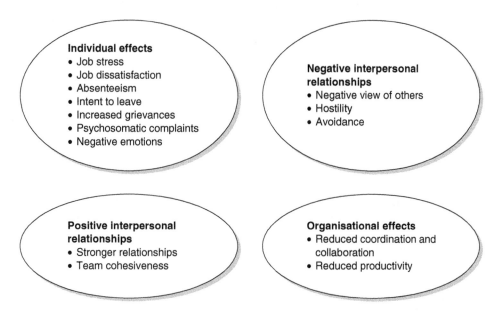

Figure 9.4   Consequences of conflict (Almost, 2006)

Unresolved conflict in the workplace has been linked to miscommunication or lack of communication by leaders and managers which can then result in confusion of role expectations, refusal to cooperate, poor quality output, missed deadlines, increased stress, decreased collaboration and lack of willingness for the team to problem solve. I am sure you can think of many other effects as the list can go on at some length.

MANAGEMENT OF CONFLICT

The Royal College of Nursing (RCN) (2005) highlighted that most people experience negative and positive colleague relationships. They note the importance of good working relationships and support within teams, and have produced an excellent tool to explore relationships on an individual and team basis through observable behaviours. You might like to try the first exercise on the companion website, which is based on a self-awareness exercise.

The resource on the companion website focuses on five aspects of leadership:

- Creating a friendly atmosphere (Qs 1 and 3)
- Helping everyone to feel part of the team (Qs 4 and 6)
- Looking after colleagues (Qs 5, 7 and 9)
- Showing appreciation of the work that people do (Qs 1, 2, 10, 13, 14 and 15)
- Demonstrating respect and consideration (Qs 8, 11, 12, 14, 15 and 16).

Obviously, you have all scored well as we always have a better perception of ourselves than maybe others do! Now try to think about negative behaviours in the workplace and tick whether you have had any experience of these (see the resource on the companion website).

> ◆ **Activity**
>
> Go through the issues in the resource on the companion website and discuss with a colleague the bullying or harassment examples.

Bullying normally involves overt or covert behaviour to another individual who cannot defend themselves effectively and involves an imbalance of power (RCN, 2005). This power may involve status, information, knowledge, skill, access to resources and social position.

Three types of bullying behaviours are identified:

- Downward bullying (superior to subordinate)
- Horizontal bullying (between peers)
- Upward bullying (subordinate to superior).

CONFLICT MANAGEMENT STYLES

There are thought to be a number of styles of conflict management which people use in organisations. Blake and Mouton's (1985) grid for differentiating conflict management styles along two axes stems from their 1960s model and relates to people's motivation in two dimensions:

- Concern for production
- Concern for people.

Thomas (1976) reshaped this model and focused on:

- Desire to satisfy one's own concern
- Desire to satisfy others' concern.

While Rahim (2011) relabelled the dimensions more simply:

- Concern for self
- Concern for others.

Five styles of conflict management have been identified that reflect a degree of how well conflict can be managed.

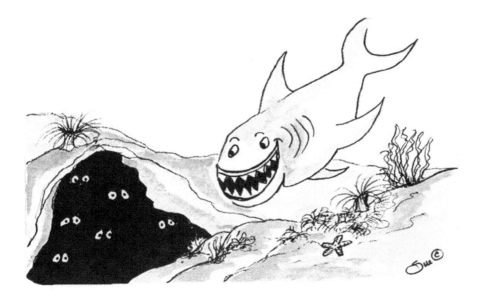

Avoidance

Seen as a passive activity where there is a withdrawal from a difficult situation. Complaints are ignored and there is a closure put on open discussion. This reflects a lack of concern for a healthy team life.

Competing

Seen where power is used to dominate the situation for self-interest and ignores the needs of the team. This is generally a win–lose situation and the style reflects a high concern for self but low concern for others in the team.

Accommodating

Seen as a style to minimise differences as an obliging act and there is surrender to the stronger party. This reflects a low concern for one's self but high concern for others in the team.

Compromising

Seen where there is negotiation and an attempt to meet on middle ground so that all sides win. This reflects a moderate degree of concern for one's self and team life.

Collaborating

Involves exploring and examining each of the differences in order to find a solution that is acceptable and of benefit to all involved. Openness and exchanges of information with good communication and problem solving are evident. This style reflects a high concern for one's self and those of the team.

The model which depicts these styles along the two axes is depicted in Figure 9.5.

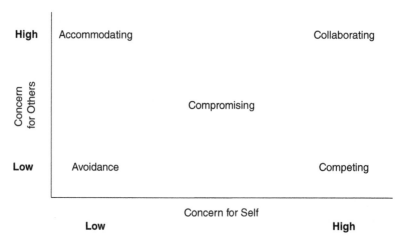

Figure 9.5   Conflict styles

A two-dimensional model of conflict management styles (adapted from Thomas, 1976 and Rahim, 1983)

It appears that the research points to both positive and negative conflict management styles. However, Thomas (1977) indicated that there were occasions when each of the conflict management styles were required and may be active (see the resource on the companion website). Barzey (2005: 62) notes the importance of being aware of behaviour that causes problems and suggests that difficult people elicit negative behaviours to gain control over situations. She suggests there are the following difficult behaviour types:

- **Complainers:** they are quick to find problems but offer no solutions
- **Negatives:** refuse to involve themselves in change
- **Insecure:** they throw tantrums and are critical of others
- **Bull in a china shop:** they are always right and must win, stamping all over others
- **Know it alls:** they are usually valuable to the team but give off a superior attitude and override others
- **Timidly pleasant:** they are quiet and pleasant but are often unresponsive to requests for help
- **Passive aggressive:** they are indecisive in not wanting to disappoint others
- **Oblivious:** they have little regard for the way they come across.

Activity

Do you think we categorise people into these typologies?

Are these behaviours difficult to cope with?

It is important that these behaviours are seen as real but care should be taken not to stereotype individuals. These behaviours happen because of circumstances and indeed may have developed to protect individuals from their external world because of past experience. It is very difficult to change these behaviours over-night. A philosophy for overcoming future conflict in a team may relate to the following points:

- Participative and supportive leadership for a trusting and respecting climate
- Clarifying higher order goals, objectives, roles and standards
- Knowing when to confront, how to diffuse aggression and reduce risk of aggression
- Careful attention to Human Resources policies and procedures
- Focus on problematical systems and processes (rather than individuals)
- Attempt to use initiative/innovation to overcome resource limitations and use of non-monetary rewards
- Attention to factors affecting group dynamics.

In terms of effective strategies to handle conflict, Barzey (2005) suggests that to prevent escalation of any conflict situation, the following actions may prove useful:

- Keep calm
- Remain positive
- Protect privacy
- Be direct and objective

- Address the problem not the person
- Maintain eye contact and be aware of body language
- Be aware of the tone of your voice
- Know when to involve a third party such as your line manager or Human Resources.

Hartman and Crume (2014), using a survey methodology with student nurses concerning team conflict, recommended the importance of designing a framework for conflict competency in nursing programmes. Enhancing conflict competency could be considered a key skill related to EI and leadership development (Waite and McKinney, 2014).

CULTURAL INFLUENCES

The method of conflict management by individual leaders may be influenced by their own cultural background. Hofsted (1980) used a cross-cultural study to identify cultural similarities and differences between 116,000 employees in a large multinational company. He identified four cultural dimensions that could affect conflict management and mapped out 40 cultures into eight categories according to the following dimensions:

- Power distance (PD)
- Uncertainty avoidance (UA)
- Individualism–collectivism (IC)
- Masculinity–femininity (MF).

Power distance (PD)

This related to the degree to which inequality of power was accepted by the culture. Argentina and Spain ranked as high power cultures where leaders were expected to use their full power over subordinates, resulting in low mutual trust and preference for leaders to be more directive in order to avoid disharmony. Australia and Canada ranked as low power cultures, where a more collegial relationship existed with mutual trust being demonstrated.

Uncertainty avoidance (UA)

This dimension related to the extent to which each culture encouraged or discouraged risk taking. Japan, Iran and Turkey were high on uncertainty avoidance and disliked ambiguity and risk taking. Hong Kong and Taiwan were seen as low uncertainty avoidance cultures.

Individualism–collectivism (IC)

Britain and the USA were seen as individualistic cultures as opposed to collectivist cultures such as the Philippines and Singapore, which required loyalty to the family and wider social structures.

Masculinity–femininity (MF)

Some cultures, such as Italy and South Africa, were considered masculine, with an emphasis on material possessions such as money, status and ambition. In contrast, in feminine countries such as Scandinavia and Holland, emphasis was placed on the environment, quality of life and caring with greater equality between the sexes. The eight cultures and their typologies were defined as outlined in Table 9.4.

Table 9.4 Cultural typologies

1 More developed Latin e.g. Belgium, France, Argentina, Brazil, Spain	↑ PD, UA and individualism Medium masculinity
2 Less developed Latin e.g. Columbia, Mexico, Chile, Yugoslavia, Portugal	↑ PD and UA Individualism Mostly masculine
3 More developed Asian e.g. Japan	Medium PD and individualism ↑ UA High masculinity
4 Less developed Asian e.g. Pakistan, Taiwan, Thailand, Hong Kong, India, Philippines, Singapore	↑ PD UA, individualism Medium masculinity
5 Near Eastern e.g. Greece, Iran and Turkey	↑ PD and UA ↑ individualism Medium masculinity
6 Germanic e.g. Austria, Israel, Germany, Switzerland, South Africa, Italy	↑ PD ↑ UA medium individualism High masculinity
7 Anglo e.g. Australia, Canada, Britain, Ireland, New Zealand, USA	↑ PD and low to medium UA High individualism High masculinity
8 Nordic e.g. Denmark, Finland, Netherlands, Norway, Sweden	↑ PD and low to medium UA Medium individualism Low masculinity

What are your thoughts on this research 30 years or so on? Do you think each culture based on a country can be simplistically broken down like this or do you think that gender, age, or social class of individuals as well as the growth of multiculturalism negates these ideas when we think about dealing with conflict?

Despite the question, it appears that the way leaders manage conflict has probably been influenced by the nurturing culture in which they have been socialised, and the work by Hofsted offers some explanation of the diversity in the way people manage and lead their teams.

Summary of Key Points

This chapter has examined various aspects of managing conflict in order to meet the identified learning outcomes. These were to:

- **Discuss the concept of conflict** Here we explored the negative and positive perceptions of conflict and its importance to organisational performance.
- **Critically review a range of models associated with conflict management** Models that underpin conflict levels, conflict causes and conflict management were offered in the context of the leadership role in developing positive collegial relationships and recognising negative behaviours in the team.
- **Critically explore importance of conflict management within the context of problem solving** Conflict management styles were positioned against concern for self and others in dealing with problems faced by leaders in health care.
- **Recognise the importance of cultural diversity on leadership during conflict** Here four cultural dimensions that could affect conflict management were discussed.

FURTHER READING

Almost, J., Doran, D. and Hall, L. (2010) 'Antecedents and consequences of intra-group conflict amongst nurses', *Journal of Nursing Management*, 18 (8): 981–92.

Barton, A. (1991) 'Conflict resolution by nurse managers', *Nursing Management*, 22 (5): 83–6.

Brinkert, R. (2010) 'A literature review of conflict causes, costs, benefits, and interventions in nursing', *Journal of Nursing Management*, 18: 145–56.

Cavanagh, S. (1991) 'Conflict management style of staff nurses and nurse managers', *Journal of Advanced Nursing*, 16: 1254–60.

Cox, K.B. (2001) 'The effects of unit morale and interpersonal relations on conflict in the nursing unit', *Journal of Advanced Nursing*, 35 (1): 17–25.

O'Grady, T.P. (2003) 'Conflict management special, part 2', *Nursing Management*, 34 (10): 34–40.

 Visit the companion website at https://study.sagepub.com/barr3e for more resources.

10 EMOTIONAL INTELLIGENCE

Learning Outcomes

By the end of this chapter you will have had the opportunity to:

- Discuss the notion of emotional intelligence
- List a variety of preferred learning styles
- Identify your preferred learning style
- Critique the value of emotional intelligence in complex team working situations
- Define the emergence and value of positive psychology in leadership
- Discuss the notion of neuro-leadership in the workplace.

INTRODUCTION

An estimated 40 per cent of all managers in general fail in the first 18 months on the job (Carnes et al., 2004) with costs both to the organisation and to individuals being significant. There is, therefore, a need for new approaches that will improve the success rate of clinical leaders in the health industry and have better outcomes for quality patient care. Shanta and Connolly (2013: 174) noted the importance for nurses to understand their own emotions and those of others within a complex health service but this rightly applies to all those who care for others. Indeed Rankin (2013: 2719) notes that 'being compassionate involves a significant degree of emotional expression'. Most leaders develop their personal essence on the basis of education, experience, mental intelligence, emotional intelligence (EI) and the ability to form meaningful relationships. When I first heard of the concept of emotional intelligence I thought it was a 'fad' but, after reading about it further, I realized that it has been around for at least the last two decades and is gaining in popularity.

As long ago as the 1920s Thorndike was discussing social intelligence which, he said, was the ability to act wisely in human relations and, in doing so, he popularised the notion of Intelligence Quotient (IQ) being an important factor in the ability to learn (Thorndike, 1932). Current theory indicates that one should not only take on the idea of IQ but also recognise EI as being a significant part of the effective leader's toolkit. Many of the skills grouped together under the heading of EI appear to be innate. Interestingly some scholars argue that the causal significance of EI has been overstated due to the lack of evidence supporting the relationship between EI and workplace success (Vitello-Cicciu, 2002).

However, it is now generally accepted that emotions as well as logic govern the way we act, learn and function throughout our lives. Emotions motivate us and affect the ways in which we make decisions and govern our actions. Goleman (1995) reminds us that we have two minds: a rational mind that thinks things through and an emotional one that feels; both these 'minds' store memories which will ultimately influence our responses within any given situation. In essence the effective leader should be aware of the preferred learning styles of their subordinates and be empathetic to these when directing them in their work, in order to get the best from the workers in reaching the overall goals of the organisation. This chapter will attempt to clarify the concept of EI, indicate how it 'fits' with current health care practice and how it can help to create an effective, efficient and successful team culture, thereby impacting on quality care delivery.

THE CONCEPT OF EMOTIONAL INTELLIGENCE

Gardner (1983) suggests that psychologists have identified a variety of intelligences over the years which can be grouped into three clusters: abstract, concrete and social. **Abstract Intelligence** is an ability to understand and manipulate verbal and mathematical symbols while **Concrete Intelligence** is deemed to be the ability to understand and manipulate objects. **Social Intelligence** is the ability to understand and relate to people; it is here that EI has its roots.

In 1986, Payne first referred to EI as 'the ability to express emotions' (Rankin 2013: 2719). This notion that EI is about free expression has however been debated by later authors. For instance, Salovey and Mayer (1990: 189) offered a definition of EI stating that it is 'a type of social intelligence, which involves the ability to monitor one's own and other emotions and to use this information to guide one's thinking and actions'. In essence they talk of EI having three elements:

- Appraisal and Expression of Emotion
- Regulation of Emotion
- Utilisation of Emotion.

Within each of these elements there are characteristics that include being aware of oneself and allowing oneself to respond more appropriately to a given situation. People in this 'category' tend to be talented in recognising others' emotional reactions and thus produce an empathetic response to them; they may appear warm and genuine, whereas those not possessing these skills may come over as being impolite or diffident. They claim that EI can be used effectively in problem solving because both positive moods and emotions enable a greater degree of flexibility in future planning, so making the most of future opportunities. In addition Salovey and Mayer claim that a good/positive mood is also very useful in creative thinking. Mayer et al. (2001: 234) identified EI as 'the ability to recognize the meaning and emotions and to use them as a basis for reasoning and problem solving'. Therefore, this has to support clinical judgements and thus effective patient care outcomes in health care. Shanta and Connolly (2013: 174) conclude that EI is a crucial component in the ability to provide holistic care in the wider context of patients, colleagues and themselves.

So EI is based on a long history of research into human behaviour and Social Psychology. Goleman's 'corporate' approach (1995) focuses on personality traits that imply such people are ambitious, enthusiastic and committed to achieving their goals, whereas Salovey and Mayer's 'academic' model (Figure 10.1) concentrates on the impact of emotions on actions, intelligence and the potential for learning, understanding, developing and growth (Hein, 2003).

Hein is quite sceptical about the value or use of EI; he offers the following definition: 'Emotional intelligence is the innate potential to feel, use, communicate, recognize, remember, learn from, manage and understand emotions.' He goes on to say that Goleman and others suggest that EI is the ability to feel good about doing whatever you are told, ordered, forced, convinced, or expected to do. It is the ability

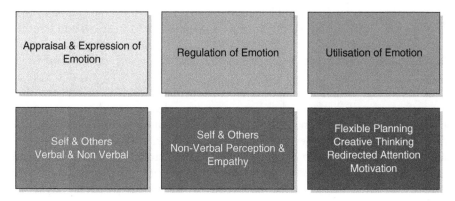

Figure 10.1 Elements of EI

Adapted from Salovey and Mayer, 1990

to keep doing it regardless of the level of stress or pressure you are put under. It is the ability to find ways to cope with your stress and thus keep doing it, regardless of your actual true desire to do it. In other words, EI is the ability to keep doing it despite all your negative feelings – even feelings which may be coming from your conscience. It is, therefore, the ability to go against your feelings and to not feel your emotional pain or discomfort. It is the ability not to listen to your conscience or your own inner voice, but to listen instead to external voices which tell you to study, achieve, perform, run, jump, buy, sell, shoot, kill. An emotionally intelligent leader, then, is one who can persuade others to do the same thing and to make them feel good about it, and want to wake up in the morning and keep doing it.

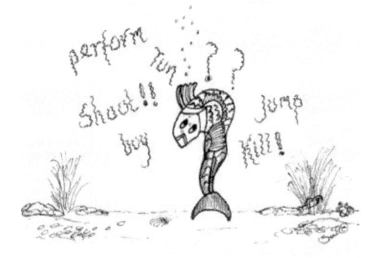

Boylan and Loughrey (2007) suggest that during the training of students time should be given to developing skills in emotional intelligence through experiential workshops. It has been proposed by Pau and Croucher (2003), in their research among dental undergraduates, that stress is related to the level of emotional intelligence; health care leaders would therefore benefit from skill development in this area. Littlejohn (2012) highlights the emotional scarring from stress and conflict in the workplace, particularly in the acute sector, where patient turnover is constant with now more highly dependent patients. She advocates for more training in emotional intelligence in order to reduce workplace stress but also to prevent more risks to patients and provide better quality care. McMullen (2003) also suggests that in order to foster a self-directed adult learning culture, leaders need to be emotionally intelligent themselves and encourage an atmosphere of respect and honesty. In line with this Akerjordet and Severinsson (2010) explored the state of science of EI related to nursing leadership and concluded that, despite controversy, nurse leaders need to have an in-depth knowledge of EI as it could contribute to improved professional identity and evidence-based nursing; these findings may then be extrapolated to include other health care professions.

> ◆ **Activity**
>
> Think of a situation where there were difficulties in interacting with a patient.
> Now imagine you are that patient in the middle of this situation.
>
> - What difficulties could you have with the interaction with the professional?
> - What feelings do you have concerning this interaction?
> - How would you like this difficult situation to be resolved?
> - How well do you think the health professional has dealt with your feelings?

Often when we interact with a patient who appears difficult it is because of a previous poor experience or they may be just plain frightened by the whole illness scenario. Many times we take on board the feelings and findings of others when we are going to care for the patient who appears difficult. It is, of course, much better to formulate your own opinion when you meet with the patient. I can remember many occasions where I was in this situation. Having talked to both colleagues and the patient, it was quite clear that for some reason my colleagues and the patient had not 'hit it off'. I found the patient was fearful of their proposed surgery and needed reassurance – we got on perfectly well.

In the context of the six Cs and the need for value-based practice and compassionate care for patients, Rankin (2013) undertook a longitudinal quantitative study with 307 student nurse applicants and found that there was a positive relationship between EI and practice performance, academic performance and retention. Although the study only went so far, further research was recommended to further the notion of a more positive link between EI and compassionate care. EI not only applies to patient relationships but can also apply to student experience in their placement areas; I am sure you will have been told that Sister so-and-so is an absolute tyrant but then found her to be a pussycat – I did often. We have to accept that we cannot always 'get on' with everyone but if we adapt our approaches we should be able to get the best out of people most of the time. I would like to think my approach – of putting myself in the other person's shoes – appears to work.

As a leader it is desirable that you are aware of the emotions of others and reflect on this in the context of how people perceive they can learn from the situation facing them. As a health care professional, understanding the differing preferred learning styles of individual patients, their relatives and members of the multidisciplinary team is essential.

PREFERRED LEARNING STYLES

Although we all learn constantly, we have a preferred way of learning. This is a 'learning style' and it is useful to understand your own preferred style and that of others in order to be effective in the team. According to Honey and Mumford (1982) there are four main learning styles (Activist; Reflector; Theorist; Pragmatist), each of which exhibits its own features. An examination of these styles reveals a range of characteristics attaching to each:

- Activists:

  o Are 'hands-on' learners
  o Get fully involved in new experiences
  o Are open minded and enthusiastic
  o Will 'try anything once'
  o Revel in crisis management, 'fire fighting'
  o Get bored by detail
  o Act first and consider the implications later.

- Reflectors:

  o Are 'tell me' learners
  o Prefer to stand back and observe
  o Look at all angles and implications
  o 'Chew it over' before reaching conclusions
  o Take a back seat in meetings and discussions
  o View the situation from different angles
  o Enjoy watching others and will listen to their views before offering their own.

- Theorists:

  o Are 'convince me' learners
  o Like to think problems through logically, step by step
  o Assimilate disparate facts into complex and logically sound theories
  o Rigorously question assumptions and conclusions
  o Don't allow their feelings to influence decisions
  o Are uncomfortable with subjectivity, creative thinking.

- Pragmatists:

  o Are 'show me' learners
  o Are keen to try out new ideas to see if they work
  o Like concepts that can be applied to their job
  o Tend to be impatient with lengthy discussions and are practical and down to earth
  o Emphasise expediency – 'the end justifies the means'. (Adapted from Mumford, 1997)

Based on these preferences, different activities are therefore likely to produce different responses and have implications not only for team management but also for therapeutic patient care.

You can take a test to see what kind of preferred learning style you have by completing any of the questionnaires available online and comparing your results with the

Table 10.1 Learning styles

Learning Style of Team Member	Example of Preferred Activity
Activist	May like the responsibility of leading a project relating to production of a clinical guideline
Reflector	May not contribute well in 'task and finish' scenarios but proposes innovative notions after the deadline and offers valuable insight into the evaluation activity
Theorist	May like to undertake a literature review related to a proposed innovation in clinical practice
Pragmatist	May have seen a new way of practice elsewhere and then want to change practice locally. Works without too much attention to detail or thinking the consequences of their actions through.

descriptors; www.educationplanner.org/students/self-assessments/learning-styles-quiz. shtml (accessed 15 May 2015) is one you could try. I tend to be multi-modal as, depending on the situation, I am able to adapt; however, my most preferred learning style is activist/pragmatist. My colleague on the other hand leans towards the theorist/reflector style so we complement each other well when working together. There are many other theories that can be taken into account, for example, VARK (Visual, Auditory, Reading, Kinaesthetic) highlighted by Fleming (2010) showing elements which reflect the Honey and Mumford ideology is just one of many. You may find you fit into a number of categories, as we do, or that you have a dominant style with far less use of the others; what is important is that you recognise that there is no 'right' mix and that your preferred styles are not fixed. You can develop ability in less dominant styles as well as further developing styles you already use. All these styles come back to the fact that we need to recognise different approaches both in ourselves and others.

◆ Activity

How do you remember a telephone number?

Try saying it aloud as though you are giving it to another person. Some of you will remember it in groups of three numbers (123 456 789) while others will remember it in groups of two numbers (12 34 56 78 9). Interestingly, I remember my house phone number in groups of two but my mobile in groups of three; I am not sure how to explain this but it does demonstrate that we think differently depending on the situation.

Using multiple learning styles and 'multiple intelligences' for learning is a relatively new approach; it is an approach that educators have only recently started to recognise.

Traditional schooling used (and continues to use) mainly linguistic and logical teaching methods and a limited range of learning and teaching techniques. Many schools still rely on classroom and book-based teaching, much repetition, and pressured exams for reinforcement and review, that is, theorist, reflector styles. A result is that we often label those who use these learning styles and techniques as 'bright'. Those who use less favoured learning styles (activist and pragmatist) often find themselves in lower streamed classes, with various not-so-complimentary labels and sometimes lower-quality teaching. This can create both positive and negative spirals that reinforce the belief that one is 'smart' or 'dumb'. By recognising and understanding your own learning styles, you can use techniques better suited to you which, in turn, will improve the speed and quality of your learning; it will also make learning in the workplace more meaningful. So in much the same way as teachers can use their knowledge of preferred learning styles in the classroom, to enhance the student learning experience by presenting information to the learner in different ways, so the effective leader can use these skills in the workplace in order to achieve the desired outcomes.

Your preferred learning style(s) have more influence than you may realise. Your preferred style guides the way you learn; it also changes the way you internally represent experiences, the way you recall information, and even the words you choose. Research shows us that each learning style uses different parts of the brain. By involving more of the brain during learning, we remember more of what we learn. Researchers using brain-imaging technologies have been able to find out the key areas of the brain responsible for each learning style. For example the styles described by Fleming (2010) may also be called:

- **Visual** The occipital lobes at the back of the brain manage the visual sense. Both the occipital and parietal lobes manage spatial orientation.
- **Aural** The temporal lobes handle aural content. The right temporal lobe is especially important for music.
- **Verbal** The temporal and frontal lobes, especially two specialised areas called Broca's and Wernicke's areas (in the left hemisphere of these two lobes).
- **Physical** The cerebellum and the motor cortex (at the back of the frontal lobe) handle much of our physical movement.

In some literature you will also see the following styles referred to:

- **Logical** The parietal lobes, especially the left side, drive our logical thinking.
- **Social** The frontal and temporal lobes handle much of our social activities. The limbic system also influences both the social and solitary styles. The limbic system has a lot to do with emotions, moods and aggression.
- **Solitary** The frontal and parietal lobes, and the limbic system, are also active with this style.

Being aware of these factors will mean that the effective leader will be able to get the most out of their workforce.

In this way clinical effective leaders would attend first to the social conditions that foster good team working by ensuring there is a stable, cohesive team; they can then logically provide the team with a clear direction for improving patient care through confident self-directed practice by individual members of the team. They also need to ensure that work practices empower the team rather than impede the work. Where necessary they will tweak the organisational structures and systems so that the support and necessary resources are available to complete the task. They arrange for (or provide themselves) expert coaching to help their team take full advantage of the situation. The leader will do all these things in their own way by using their own behavioural/learning style and strategies they have found have worked best in the past. The one thing that makes them stand out from the 'not so effective' leader is that they can adapt their style as they recognise the need to from the reaction of others.

THE VALUE OF EMOTIONAL INTELLIGENCE IN COMPLEX TEAM WORKING

Within teams there are individuals who work and think in different ways, each benefiting the overall progress of project work. Belbin (2000) talks of differing roles taken on within the team structure and how each of these roles enhances or detracts from the effectiveness of the team. Similarly, it can be argued that if the leader of a team knows about the best ways people work or take instruction, they can ensure that the team is effective in the way it works.

Shanta and Connolly (2013) linked emotional intelligence in nursing practice to King's *Interacting System Theory* (Figure 10.2) which has a focus on the dynamic interactions of humans through three interacting systems: personal, interpersonal and social realms.

Knowing how people work and think can serve to get the best out of them. One manager I have worked with asked a member of staff to sort out an issue. This member of staff reacts like a chicken whenever she is asked to do anything; you can

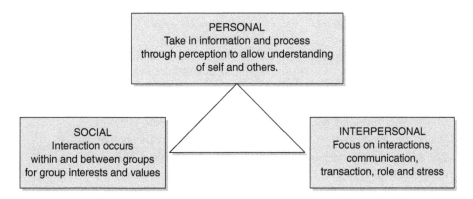

Figure 10.2   Representation of King's Theory of Interacting Systems (1981)

watch her ruffling up her feathers as she thinks through what might be required and what she feels she will not be able to achieve. A few well-chosen words to 'smooth' her feathers and she happily goes off to complete the task. Another member of staff was approached with the same issue by the manager who only had to say: 'I have had this idea ...'. The staff member said 'OK' and the next time the manager saw her the idea had been taken up and successfully planned out. For yet another member of staff who was passed the idea from the manager, the response would be: 'Oh that's *interesting*' but nothing further would be done. This member of staff requires a direct list of actions: first, do this; second, do that; third, do the other, and so on in order to attempt to complete the task.

Of course, as effective leaders we need to be flexible. One manager I knew preferred the direct, ordered chain of acts approach that worked for her; she assumed that it would work for everyone and consistently used that approach. Doing this she occasionally alienated new employees as they did not feel valued and this transactional approach allowed no recognition of the skills and experience they had which would allow them to deal with the issue in their own way. Part of my role was to let the new staff member know that it was just the manager's way and not directed at them personally.

Kite and Kay (2012) highlight that emotional intelligence is linked to better situational outcomes by linking intellect and emotional awareness to manage ourselves and our relationships better. They note ten characteristics of emotionally intelligent people and less emotionally intelligent people (Table 10.2).

Table 10.2   Characteristics of EI people and less EI people.

EI people	Less EI people
1 Continually striving for personal development	Assuming that something good will turn up
2 Unrelenting commitment to support others' interests	See things with their own eyes
3 Clarity of intentions	Are imprecise about their goals
4 Sustaining positive values	Follow the crowd before they follow their conscience
5 Listening and observation	Reject the opinion of those they perceive to lack authority
6 Objectivity	Don't want to believe they can change themselves or others
7 Challenging the status quo	Put status before authority
8 Taking the longer view	React on impulse not thought
9 Converting negative inclinations into positive thought	Are pessimistic in the face of change
10 Nurturing the team	Communicate what they think people want to hear

> ◆ **Activity**
>
> The debate of whether there are two types of people can be too simplistic and maybe the issue of context is more important.
>
> Can you suggest two recent situations when you have behaved in a 'less EI' mode and another occasion when your behaviour was more EI mature?

Maybe the notion of a polarised status of people is far from the truth; you may find that when reflecting on your own styles as in a force-field analysis you exhibit elements of both behaviours but a dominance towards one side or the other, which may change as you develop professionally. The idea that individuals can behave differently in specific situations is also more likely.

Considering styles of leadership alongside EI we can see that Transactional Leaders tend to be serious, value one-way communication, use emotional management and often delay gratification. Transformational Leaders value empathy and two-way communication; they tend to be friendly and use empathy to motivate staff. Both of these approaches are built on the Trait, Situational and Contingency models. So taking these different approaches into account will lead to effective team working. Clearly there is still a place for the more traditional leadership approaches in patient care, particularly within emergency care when the end goal is one of patient safety. The engaged leader with emotional competence should be able to use his or her knowledge to help members of their team to identify and reach their personal destiny; this type of leadership plays on the cognitive and behavioural knowledge and skills linked to the notion of neuropsychology.

POSITIVE PSYCHOLOGY

Positive psychology (PP) was a term summarised as the study of positive emotion, positive character, and positive institutions (Seligman and Csikszentmihalyi, 2000). This emerging science is based on the premise that we are capable of happiness, life satisfaction, and optimal performance by devoting our efforts to cultivating our strengths. Two main concepts are identified:

- Expressing gratitude: this has surprisingly wide ranging benefits to both the recipient and the person conveying appreciation, and
- Identifying and augmenting your signature strengths; this is a far more effective strategy to accomplish life satisfaction (authentic happiness) than exploring and trying to improve your weaknesses.

Considering these two elements it is clear that the successful leader will use praise and then thank the workforce when a task has been completed effectively. An overzealous commendation may appear false but demonstrating 'thanks for a job well done' will enhance the way the team works together and give the team members a sense of pride. By using its unique individual strengths, the team is also more likely to achieve positive and timely outcomes. There are said to be four corners of PP which uses a similar framework to the four elements of a SWOT analysis, as shown in Figure 10.3.

The science of optimal human functioning	Redresses imbalance and undue negative focus
Emphasises the study of what works	Learns from successes rather than studying failures.

Figure 10.3   The implications of neuroscience on leadership

By being aware of these 'corners' the effective leader can utilise the strengths of each member of the team in order to achieve the goals of the organisation. This adds to the value of good leadership. In terms of clinical health care professional leaders, this means moving from a *blame culture* to a *lessons learned* climate.

Activity

How would you assess the culture of your team, for instance with respect to:

- Near misses
- Medication errors
- Poor compliance to manual handling procedures.

There is a 'lessons learnt' climate (circle appropriately):

Strongly Agree   Agree   Neutral   Disagree   Strongly Disagree

---

NEURO-LEADERSHIP

Linked to PP is the notion of neuro-leadership which refers to the application of findings from neuroscience to the field of leadership. It is an emerging field of study focused on bringing neuro-scientific knowledge into the areas of leadership development; management training; change management; education; consulting; and coaching. It provides a new scientific framework for understanding and therefore enhancing the practice of leading others. An enhanced understanding of how the brain works has been able to shed light on ways those leaders can:

- Enhance their thinking
- Strengthen their ability to influence others *and*
- Help staff successfully work through change.

Rock et al. (2009: 1) highlight the notion of the neuroscience of engagement where they state that:

> understanding the neuroscience of engagement is more than just an interesting discussion; rather, it will open up insights for leaders to more accurately and effectively predict, measure and improve employee engagement across all types of organizations.

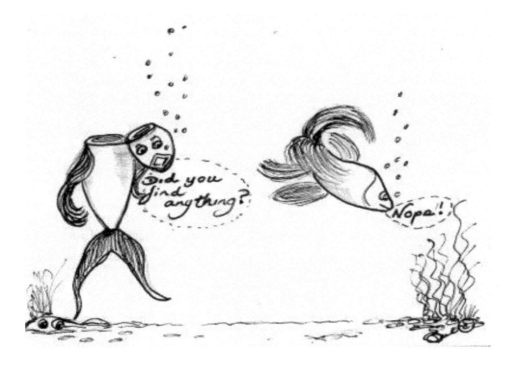

All health care professionals would require a high level of neural engagement which would refer to experiencing high levels of activation of their reward and self- regulation circuitry when at work and they would have high levels of dopamine in their system. These levels may be reduced through lack of sleep, boredom or job dissatisfaction. The idea of the threat and reward system links in to the social-cognitive and affective neuroscience literature. Rock (2008) identifies five SCARF domains (Status, Certainty, Autonomy, Relationships and Fairness):

- individual's self-perceived importance in relation to others (status)
- ability to predict the future (certainty)
- individual's perception regarding their sense of control over events (autonomy)
- safety with others, of being associated with an in-group (relatedness)
- the perception of fairness in the way people are treated (fairness).

This model could help health care professional leaders to positively influence the clinical or team environment and drive the workforce forward in a constructive manner. You may want to assess these issues in light of the strengths and weaknesses of people in your team.

Overall it can be seen from the literature that EI has almost as many followers as it has critics. Neuro-leadership is also not without its critics; it has been questioned whether having scientific brain data to back up what is commonly believed adds any value. Yet advocates suggest that neuro-leadership provides a scientific basis and language to management studies that managers and leaders can relate to. Further, it is believed that the relatively young field of neuro-leadership will continue to reveal new insights into how to lead effectively. It could be concluded that awareness of EI and PP can be of great use if working in the health care arena where to be 'tuned in' to patients' and clients' feelings may well enhance treatment. Similarly the notion of neuro-leadership will complement EI by supporting meaningful team leadership.

Summary of Key Points

This chapter has briefly looked at various aspects of emotional intelligence in order to meet the identified learning outcomes. These were:

- **Discuss the notion of emotional intelligence** While EI is not a new phenomenon, it can clearly be seen to be of benefit within the overall management of effective team working.
- **List a variety of preferred learning styles** Here we examined the notion of a variety of learning styles that can be recognised and used by the effective leader.
- **Identify your preferred learning style** Through examining our own preferred learning style we can appreciate how different people may react in given situations and how these learning styles may benefit patient/client care.
- **Critique the value of emotional intelligence in complex team working situations** EI can be used to provide a good stable base for the team to work from. It is also strongly linked to compassionate care.
- **Define the emergence and value of positive psychology in leadership** Positive psychology in leadership is said to aid the organisation in becoming a positive place to work so leading to a happier and more cohesive workforce.
- **Discuss the notion of neuro-leadership in the workplace** Valuing the workforce and developing a method by which all leadership strands are brought together is vital in the role of the effective leader.

FURTHER READING

Akerjordet, K. and Severinsson, E. (2008) 'Emotionally intelligent nurse leadership: a literature review study', *Journal of Nursing Management*, 16 (5): 565–77.
Bellack, J.P. (1999) 'Emotional intelligence: a missing ingredient?', *Journal of Nurse Education*, 38 (1): 3–4.

Chapman, M. (2005) 'The positive psychology of emotional intelligence and coaching', *Competency and Emotional Intelligence*, Winter 2005/06, 13 (2).

de Mio, R.R. (2002) 'On defining virtual emotional intelligence', *ECIS 2002*, June, Gdansk, Poland.

Freshwater, D. and Stickley, T.J. (2004) 'The heart of the art: emotional intelligence in nurse education', *Nursing Inquiry*, 11 (2): 91–8.

Harmes, P.D. and Credé, M. (2010) 'Emotional intelligence and transformational and transactional leadership: a meta-analysis', *Journal of Leadership & Organizational Studies*, 17: 5.

Skinner, C. and Spurgeon, P. (2005) 'Valuing empathy and emotional intelligence in health leadership: a study of empathy, leadership behaviour and outcome effectiveness', *Health Services Management Research*, 18: 1–12.

Visit the companion website at https://study.sagepub.com/barr3e for more resources.

PART 3

THE ORGANISATION

11 THEORY OF ORGANISATIONAL LIFE

> ## Learning Outcomes
>
> By the end of this chapter you will have had the opportunity to:
>
> - Understand the importance of the overall organisation
> - Discuss the importance of strategy, structures and systems within the organisation
> - Critically explore the notion of organisational culture
> - Reflect on the nature of organisational roles
> - Critically examine professional responsibility and accountability as well as the notions of authority and delegation
> - Develop an overview of Human Resource processes in organisations.

INTRODUCTION

Over the last few chapters, you have been encouraged to examine the individual as a leader and within the dynamics of the team. It is now useful to scrutinise the management of an organisation and its top leadership. The health industry has many different types of organisations: some lie within the 'not for profit' public sector, some organisations are run 'for profit' and some organisations are a combination of both of these models, such as General Practice. Other organisations are run through charity finance and the public purse, for example hospices or establishments for serious long-term conditions. This chapter will unravel the theoretical aspects of organisational life in order for you to learn more about the context in which health care delivery operates.

WHAT IS THE PURPOSE OF AN ORGANISATION?

Organisations can be a simple, collective group of people such as in a small General Practice or they can be more complex, reflected as enterprising entities like the National Health Service. Organisations are integral to our social, cultural, political, economic, technological and physical environment. Smith (1995: 11) defines an organisation as a 'group of people who invest something … in the expectation of getting something out'. An organisation can more precisely be defined as: 'A social unit of people, systematically structured and managed to meet a need or to pursue collective goals' (www.businessdictionary.com/definition/organization.html accessed 5 August 2014).

It is suggested that the purpose of an organisation is to:

- Help to achieve organisational goals
- Ensure the optimum use of resources
- Help perform managerial functions
- Facilitate growth and diversification *and*
- Ensure humane treatment of employees. (en.m.wikipedia.org accessed 8 August 2014)

> ◆ Activity
>
> Do you feel these ideas reflect the health organisation in which you work?
>
> How do they apply for;
>
> - the NHS
> - private hospitals
> - residential care homes
> - General Practice
> - St John's Ambulance/Red Cross?

You might have thought that the purposes listed above relate well to the current NHS even as it faces its biggest challenges since its inception in 1948. This may also hold true for the other health care organisations listed but smaller businesses are more focused in their goals and it may be argued are better able to care for their staff. However, it could also be argued that the ability to ensure humane treatment of NHS employees as a whole is compromised due to the pressures of throughput and dependency. It may vary according to which area you are currently working in and the philosophy of the employer, but discussions emanating from the North Staffs debacle (Francis, 2013) indicate that consideration of employees came low on the hierarchy of business needs.

The NHS is a statutory organisation that is governed by statute in the UK and steered under the direction of the government party that is in power. Over the last 40 years or so, the NHS has been driven by the following policy issues:

- The introduction of market-based mechanisms to allocate and distribute its finite resources to meet ever-growing health needs and demands
- 'Contracting out' of some of the peripheral services to the private sector
- Notions of private initiatives to support the fixed budget of the NHS.

This is not so very different for any other international health care organisation across the developed market economy; therefore these have been seen as a way of dealing with the complexity and increased demands placed on health care provision today. The study of organisational life is a specific discipline that is pertinent for leadership and requires knowledge from the social sciences, psychology, economics and possibly political science. Leaders need to have an awareness of how their own organisation works and the extent of its effectiveness and success. Leaders also need to be able to steer the organisation towards this, on a continuous basis, whether that organisation is a small team, a clinical ward, a directorate, an NHS Trust or even the whole NHS. The 2015 General Election has seen the Conservatives get back into power and lose their coalition basis. It may be assumed that continuity of government policy will continue to consolidate the past health reforms.

STRATEGY, STRUCTURE AND SYSTEMS

For an organisation to be regarded as effective and efficient, many elements have to be coordinated and managed, which means that leadership is vital. The McKinsey 7 'S' model (Peters and Waterman, 2004: 9) suggests the elements required are:

- Strategy
- Structure
- Systems
- Skills
- Shared Values
- Style
- Staff.

Leavitt's (1965, 1978) simple model helps leaders to reflect upon the interdependency of organisational elements. These interdependent elements are crucial and a good leader should be able to recognise the importance of all of them, especially when it is thought that the organisation is becoming less effective and efficient.

The Weisbord (1976) Six Organisational Model (Figure 11.1) offers another perspective but highlights the central importance of leadership.

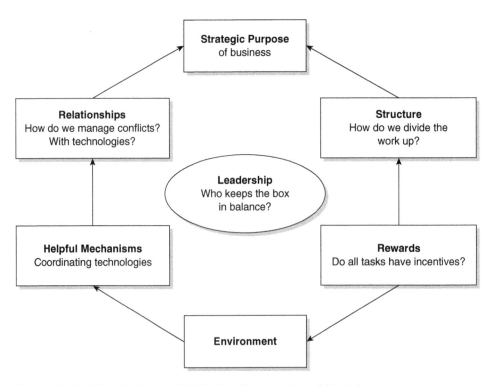

Figure 11.1   The Weisbord (1976) Six Organisational Model

Activity

Write down what you think about the strengths of these three models.

It is useful here to note the importance of strategy, structures and systems in all three models. Although other elements are relevant they have been covered elsewhere in this book.

STRATEGY

The concept of strategy is complex because it has various meanings. It could be seen as 'a course of action to achieve specific objectives' (CIMA, 1998). Mintzberg et al. (2003) noted it could also be used to mean:

- A plan
- A position
- A pattern of behaviour
- A perspective.

These ideas illustrate that a strategy is not always considered as rationally and proactively planned. Leadership requires strategic thinking; what does this mean for clinical leadership? Strategic decisions are seen to be based on the values, beliefs and expectations of those in power in an organisation. Clinical leaders need to be aware of their own power base but also that there is no single way of thinking strategically.

RATIONAL STRATEGY

Rational strategic decisions should relate to:

- The scope of the organisation's activity
- The long-term direction of the organisation
- The organisation's environment
- The available resources and resource allocation
- Present climate of change.

The rational approach involves strategic analysis, strategic choice and implementation. The basis of strategic analysis should come from a review of the organisational mission and goals followed by internal and external analysis. Iles and Sutherland (2001) point to a number of external and internal analysis tools that can be used in health care, particularly when planning new developments and as a form of project management for clinical change:

- **PEST** (Political, Environmental, Sociological, Technological factors)
- **PESTELI** (including features above but also Ecological, Legislative and Industry factors)
- **SWOT** (Strengths, Weaknesses, Opportunities and Threats)
- **PROCESS MODELLING** (for example a 'patient journey').

Iles and Sutherland not only looked at rational strategic tools but also highlighted a number of creative analysis tools. The rational approach to strategy formation has been criticised because of the need for futuristic forecasting, planning being separated from the operational side of the organisation and the formalisation of the activity. Health policy could be seen as a rational form of strategy. Simon (1960) felt that the best strategic decisions were not always made (optimisation). Strategic decisions were more likely to be based on least effort (satisficing – a decision making strategy that entails searching through the available alternatives until an acceptability threshold is met). This was seen as 'muddling through'. In terms of change, small-scale adjustments are the usual strategic focus in order to avoid major errors (Lindblom, 1959).

EMERGENT STRATEGIES

Emergent strategies arise from patterns of behaviour, which are exhibited, and strategically significant operational episodes. For instance, there may have been no conscious overall plan to utilise European hospitals for surgical care but, through the marketing of their services, it was felt by some British health care managers that this may have been a useful solution to reducing waiting lists. The 'logical incrementalism' strategy is seen as a compromise between the rational approach, 'muddling through' and emergent strategy. Strategy is seen as a process of learning within an overall organisational direction and small-scale ideas are seen as experiments or projects within a learning culture (CIMA, 1998).

VISION, MISSION AND GOALS

Organisational top leaders need to identify what is their future vision, what is their mission statement and what are the goals and objectives, in order to drive their people through to the same outcome to meet demand. Health care organisations now need to set annual goals and objectives that can be regularly measured or evaluated. In the past it was usual to set five–ten-year aims and goals in the NHS; now, however, it appears that the political and external pressure for change is too dynamic. The difficulty of communicating and driving through annual organisational goals for change is one for debate. In terms of the variety of goals there are probably four basic models (Table 11.1).

Table 11.1   Four models of organisational effectiveness (CIMA, 1998)

	Human Relations Model	**Open Systems Model**
Flexible Structure	*Goals:* People orientated skills	*Goals:* Growth focus, good environment relationship
	Internal Process Model	**Rational Goal Model**
Stable Structure	*Goals:* Stability, efficient communication, change avoidance	*Goals:* Productivity, efficiency

According to Mintzberg (1998) there are seven types of forces that drive the vision, mission, goals and objectives of an organisation:

- Direction
- Efficiency
- Proficiency
- Competition
- Concentration
- Learning
- Cooperation.

Mission statements are formal statements that communicate the vision of the organisation. They are usually brief and cover the following areas:

- The purpose of the organisation
- The strategic intent
- Policies and standards
- Organisational values.

> ### ▶ Activity
>
> Has your Health Trust communicated their mission to you? Try to find out where this is and check whether you feel it represents what is happening in your health industry. What about your own clinical area – do you have an identified mission statement? Does it need revising? Do your team members know about it?

Often the mission statement is now found on an organisation's web page. The goals, objectives and future plans are there for public scrutiny. Policies, procedures and guidance can be found on the organisational intranet. These should be accessed as it includes information pertinent to the smooth running of the organisation, and is used as a benchmark by which to assess quality of delivery when the organisation is being inspected.

LEADERSHIP AND HEALTH POLICY

Health policy can be seen as a rational strategic plan to distribute scarce resources. There are two main economic issues concerning the health service industry in all countries:

- Rising expectations and demands for health care – infinite demand
- Finite resources to deal with these needs, demands and wants.

Health policy reflects how political leaders shape the distribution of these finite health funds and resources to deal with the presenting infinite health service demands. Policy also denotes the strength of belongingness within a society to achieve solutions and a commitment to trying new ways of coping with the underlying issues.

Palfrey (2000) suggests health policy is therefore about:

- A desire to improve people's quality of life
- An attempt to improve a nation
- A perceived need to reduce costs/save money
- A perceived need to stabilise expenditure but improve the standard of services
- A practical concern to retain power/authority.

Not all countries' governments have the same commitment to health care as each other and the amount of money put into a system varies widely across the world. However, a higher percentage of funding to a health system does not necessarily equate to healthier populations. New health policy focuses on changing and challenging the status quo. This can relate to the following:

- Changes to the perception of health needs
- Changes to health care structures and systems
- Changes to health care processes
- Changes to roles and responsibilities
- Changes to power bases.

GLOBAL LEADERSHIP

It could be said that the World Health Organization (WHO) leads out on health issue policy. The WHO (2014) defined health policy thus:

Health policy refers to decisions, plans, and actions that are undertaken to achieve specific health care goals within a society. An explicit health policy can achieve several things: it defines a vision for the future which in turn helps to establish targets and points of reference for the short and medium term. It outlines priorities and the expected roles of different groups; and it builds consensus and informs people. (www.who.int/topics/health_policy/en/ accessed 14 November 2014)

Griffiths (2014: 163) identifies that due to world ageing populations, lifestyle-related disease and environmental issues, public health concerns are increasing on a global basis. Health leaderships across the world are thus facing a huge challenge to put policy into practice particularly in the areas of obesity, smoking and reducing alcohol consumption.

NATIONAL HEALTH LEADERSHIP

Besides the Department of Health's role in national leadership there are also the main professional statutory regulatory bodies. These are the General Medical Council (GMC), The Nursing and Midwifery Council (NMC) and the Health and Care Professions Council (HCPC) and they have a public protection role through their standards and practice codes for their members involved in care. A recent 2014 review of these professional regulators indicated that their role in public protection could well be improved and proposed 125 recommendations for change. A response to this report from the government has yet to be produced but you might want to check out the review at http://lawcommission.justice.gov.uk/areas/ Healthcare_professions.htm_accessed 15 November 2014.

The Health and Care Professions Council (HCPC) stated that 'holders of public office should promote and support ... principles by leadership and example'. This Council state:

We are a regulator, and we were set up to protect the public. To do this, we keep a Register of health and care professionals who meet our standards for their training, professional skills, behaviour and health. (www.hcpc-uk.org, accessed 11 August 2014).

All health professionals are thus presently governed by their standards of proficiencies or competences and their codes of practice. Pre-registration standards of proficiency highlight the importance of care delivery, management and leadership. The Department of Health's publications *Modernising Nursing Careers* (DH, 2006c) and *Modernising Medical Careers* (DH, 2004b, 2008c) also highlighted the importance of the role of health professionals in improving the nation's health in the context of modern society. Scott (2014: 3) also has noted a proposed new NMC code of professional conduct in response to the concerns raised by the Francis

Report (2013) and the need for responsibility at all levels for escalating concerns 'promptly and appropriately' will be embedded into the Code.

CHANGING GOVERNMENT STRATEGY

The NHS Plan (DH, 2000a) and *A First Class Service* (DH, 1998) were strategies about improving the quality of the health service and target setting was high on the last government's agenda. The role of the National Institute of Clinical Excellence (NICE) and the National Service Frameworks for quality (NSFs) became established under these policies. The Darzi reforms (DH, 2008a) in 'High quality care for all' laid out further demands for health care improvements.

The coalition government's *Equity and Excellence: Liberating the NHS* (DH, 2010a) built on the past modernising policy but with an added focus on:

- Patient and public involvement
- Improving health care outcomes
- The empowerment of accountable professionals
- Improving efficiency by cutting bureaucracy.

The 2012 Health and Social Care Act has since further developed health legislation and came into effect in 2013. Strategic Health Authorities and Primary Care Trusts were disbanded while NHS England, Clinical Commissioning Groups (CCGs) and Public Health England were established. *Understanding the New NHS* (DH 2014) provides an excellent overview of the new structures and roles, as well as strategic leadership and quality issues from a policy perspective.

Activity

Review the document *Understanding the New NHS* from the DH website on the companion website. What are your first thoughts?

I think this document illustrates how complicated the NHS really is. For those who are new to the NHS, it can appear irrelevant and 'stuffy'. I have many of my own student notes that were taken over the years relating to 'The structure of the NHS' which at the time seemed miles away from our worlds. However as you progress in your health career, the knowledge of these NHS structures and functions becomes more relevant to you and helps you to attune your leadership perspectives. So be patient!

Commissioning in the NHS

An important aspect of the NHS is that since the 1990 reforms, a market driven NHS has become the dominant model. Different organisations are seen as service providers and other organisations in the NHS are purchasers of those services. This model has been felt to have improved the quality of the services and to have set health care priorities for local communities. It is the CCGs that are now the organisations who identify the services that are needed and they commission and monitor these services.

The process of commissioning involves:

- Profiling the needs of the local community: use of demographical and epidemiological evidence
- Identifying the health care priorities and outcomes
- Commissioning and developing services
- Monitoring, reviewing and evaluating.

There is still controversy regarding some of the Darzi reforms (DH, 2008a) and whether some initiatives have not really proved worthwhile such as CQUIN (Mays, 2013). The loss of PCTs and SHAs and the introduction of the CCGs are still under debate. Some feel there is a slide towards privatisation of the NHS and it may take some time to bed down a clear NHS structure and strategy for the future.

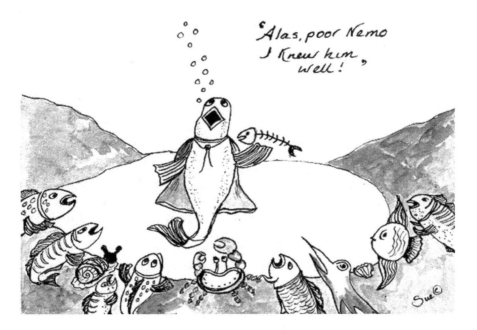

A decade ago, Wanless (2002, 2004) highlighted the important role of technology in the NHS. He noted that the following needed to be considered:

- The initial replacement cost, with running costs, of technology such as scanners, over time
- The pace of technology in the UK (in comparison to other countries)

- That new technology may tend to result in an increase in activity and widening population access
- The importance of the role of NICE to review the impact of technology on patient outcomes
- The possibility of seeing some key diseases (such as cancer) being managed as chronic diseases
- Use of genetics and stem cell technology.

The development of an assessment process for health service evaluation of technologies is also an important feature of the effectiveness and efficiency of NHS treatments and it is recommended that you access the companion website to see the work of the National Institute for Health Research and (www.hta.ac.uk accessed 14 November 2014).

PUBLIC HEALTH, HEALTH PROMOTION AND POLICY

Public health as an aspect of overall health policy has been an important feature of the health service in Britain in recent years. This is deemed as the 'new' public health as opposed to traditional public health which was more focused on eradicating infectious diseases and social welfare. The World Health Organization set out the 1977 *Health for All* strategy and went on to draw up the Ottawa Charter in 1986, which has set the scene for the new public health ideology.

UK public health policy in the shape of *Our Health, Our Care, Our Say* (DH, 2006a) identified the importance of people getting access to good health care, particularly those who are considered as socially marginalised, that is, those in prison, poverty, or who are disabled or housebound. This policy reflected the importance of patient power, and participative and inclusive health care as well as the need to address the inequalities of health as illustrated in the Acheson Report (1998). *Healthy Lives, Healthy People: Our Strategy for Public Health* (DH, 2010c) gave a new direction and new service proposal for 'joined up' services across local authorities and the NHS. More recently Public Health England (PHE) and the relevant Health and Wellbeing Boards have been established to attempt to join up services between health and local authorities where the determinants of health, such as housing, education and social services, can provide a more cohesive, joined-up approach to address the health and social inequalities of the nation. Whether these public health developments will be recognised as 'joined up' is still being debated. The health of people in Ireland, Scotland and Wales is maybe felt as marginalised. More concerning is the impact of the recent economic downturn and the need to cut public services – particularly in local authorities.

It appears that as one health strategy is brought into focus, there is a tendency for other policies to be marginalised. For instance, a focus on people who are more likely to get heart disease or cancer may take precedence over those who have learning disabilities or those susceptible to childhood accidents. It is debated whether health policy is seen as a planned strategic activity or whether it is a result of lobbying from various sections in society, where whichever lobby 'shouts' the loudest gets the most attention. The products of raised consciousness and community action are often seen as the essential building blocks to force the legislators and regulators to act.

▶ Activity

- What would you consider as the most important elements of public health policy?
- Suggest ways your own team could influence public health policy.

The team might want to get together with others to campaign for their own protected meal breaks; maybe encourage the setting up of a food bank to help less fortunate people in their area. Protests at a Birmingham supermarket, by parents and health professionals, led to a change in the policy of having sweets and crisps stacked at supermarket checkouts.

It has been suggested that health care professionals are generally good at health education with patients but rarely are able to make their voice heard in policy-making related to health promotion (Whitehead, 2006). As a leader, it is important to try to help your team understand that other groups (for example, the homeless, the unemployed, those in prisons, people with mental health problems) in society also find it difficult to influence policy-making themselves. Making them aware of the valuable ways in which they could influence health and health services on a broader basis can be very powerful in bringing a team together, whatever clinical area they work in.

Policies are formulated at various levels and it should not be assumed that influencing overall health policy at government level is what is always expected. Policy at ward, clinical or Trust level is also important for leaders to support and encourage staff to get involved with their own local policy-making clinical groups.

INVOLVEMENT IN THE POLICY-MAKING PROCESS

There are four main stages that staff teams can get involved in. Leaders could make their teams aware of these areas and the need for utilising evidence or research-based information.

- Agenda setting: problem identification and recognition of issues for policy
- Communicating the development of health care options by appraisal: setting of alternatives, forecasting, cost–benefit analysis
- Helping in choosing policy and its implementation
- Evaluation and review of policy.

Policy is often concerned with getting the right messages over and setting up the right structures for implementation. It is now useful to look at the issue of structures within an organisation.

STRUCTURE

The way an organisation structures its people or functions is important in order to understand how the communication flows from one organisational area to another. Another perspective concerning structures may be that the way an organisation plans its structure relates to the way it plans to *constrain* and *control* its people. Generally, a hierarchical organisational structure is seen within the health service. Task allocation, supervision and coordination generally are undertaken through the organisational structure.

 Activity

Can you briefly draw your own immediate structure within your organisation?

Drucker (1989) suggests that organisational structure should satisfy the following tests:

- The structure should be geared for future performance, not on a historical basis
- The structure should have the minimum number of management levels
- The structure should reflect *upward training and development* towards the top of the organisation.

TYPES OF STRUCTURES

The most usual structure that is represented is the hierarchical vertical structure (Figure 11.2). This hierarchy can be quite 'flat' but it can also contain many more levels – a 'tall' hierarchy. This is true within the NHS. Another structural form may be seen as a cross-functional team under several project managers (Figure 11.3). This is usually seen as a complex matrix form of structure. Smaller matrix forms of project teams may be less hierarchical, such as those community teams who work together depending on the needs of specific patient groups. Generally, however, within the health service most professionals have a hierarchical structure of accountability as well.

   There are many other shapes and forms of structures influenced by international and historical factors. The European Community as an organisation is a highly

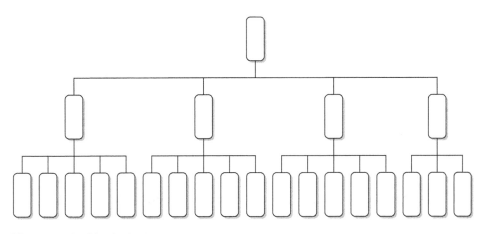

Figure 11.2   Vertical structure

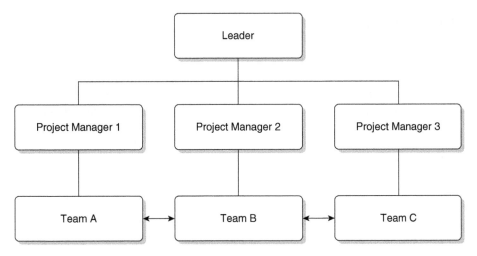

Figure 11.3   Complex matrix structure

complex structural entity that bears no resemblance to a hierarchy. However, Leavitt (2005: 2) argues that hierarchies pervade all life, 'in democracies, theocracies, oligarchies, monarchies and autocracies'. He went on to note that there were even heavenly hierarchies. In rank order these are:

1. Seraphim
2. Cherubim
3. Dominations
4. Thrones
5. Principalities

6. Potentates
7. Virtues
8. Archangels
9. Just plain Angels.

Leavitt (2005) suggested that human hierarchies were far from being angelic and we do not always like what they do to people and productivity. He went on to argue that hierarchies are, however, inevitable. Within each level of the hierarchy, job and role descriptions and span of control are important elements of the organisational structure. Leaders need to recognise the boundaries of job descriptions and the ability of some people to expand these. For others there may be difficulty in fulfilling all the elements of their job description. The span of control reflects the number of subordinates who report to a single supervisor. The 'flat' hierarchy may mean that a supervisor may have a broad span of control whereas a 'tall' hierarchy may reflect a very narrow span of control.

ORGANISATIONAL ROLES

In order that an organisation may meet its goals, the work of individual people must be achieved by the variety of roles. A 'role' is regarded as an 'expected pattern of behaviour associated with members occupying a particular position within the structure of an organisation' (Mullins, 2005: 538). Role expectations change and develop from the time someone takes on a new role until they leave that role. Most *health care students* are allocated to clinical placements in order to learn their professional role during their training and it is here that they become socialised to their own sphere of work. Learning outcomes, aims and objectives, as laid down by the professional benchmarks, will drive this learning. The management of learning for their professional role is dependent on the learning environments – the place where learners interact with clients, patients and practitioners. Students will then qualify and take their turn in teaching, mentoring and assessing students.

Buckenham (1988) found that the perceptions of students changed during training, in that first-year students thought more about the actual delivery of health care while third-year students thought that the clinical aspects of the job were less important than the effective management aspects. Whatever course you undertake, it appears that many qualified practitioners still feel unprepared for the management aspect of the role. Back in 1974 Kramer called this feeling the 'reality shock'; the feeling of dread, terror and fear abound (Kramer, 1974). Schmalenburg and Kramer (1979) further identified four phases of role transition from student to practitioner:

• Honeymoon
• Shock
• Recovery
• Resolution.

It is important that leaders and experienced staff recognise the difficulties that face novice practitioners and help to set up formal and informal support mechanisms. The inclusion of a management and leadership module within pre-registration training gives the newly qualified practitioner an insight into expectations. It is through the exposure to leadership/management knowledge and supervised exposure to practice that new health care professionals can take on leadership roles more effectively. Butler and Hardin-Pierce (2005) note the importance of collaboration between educationalist and service leaders to influence the transition process positively. They recognise the challenges in health care today where there are staff shortages, increased patient acuity and early patient discharges in the acute sector.

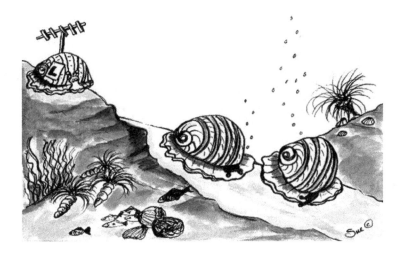

Whenever you take up a post as a new staff member in any of the health care professions, the expectations from your employer will relate to your ability to engage in and maintain high standards of health care. There will be an expectation to develop excellent communication skills, both verbal and written. In addition, you are expected to keep yourself up to date with your evidence-base elements of care delivery; however, self-confidence within these expectations may be low at times and it may be difficult for you to recognise the support needed. Feedback on your professional, managerial, educational and administrative skills will help to develop you through a preceptorship and appraisal system. Appraisals are often carried out yearly and a Personal Development Plan (PDP) is agreed between yourself and your supervisor.

Robinson and Griffiths (2009) in their Scoping Review for the King's Fund explored the impact, facilitation and constraints of preceptorship on clinical practice. Preceptorship now involves supervised practice for a fixed length of time (Gopee and Galloway, 2014: 250) dependent on the identified needs of the preceptee. The NMC (2006) have indicated that support and guidance from an experienced professional colleague is invaluable for newly qualified nurses, those returning to practice and for nurses from abroad entering into UK practice.

Preceptorship may be seen as a means of improving patient care through workforce retention and development of clinical skills, but more research is needed in these areas. The care delivery expectations of your role will be dependent on the philosophy and culture of the organisation and the particular type of health care activities that your course has prepared you for within that context. You will be expected to assess, plan, implement and evaluate care within the standards and philosophy of the organisation. Therefore, it will be important for you to be familiar with policies, procedures and systems that are operationalised in the workplace. There is an expectation that you will contribute to a high standard of care and develop effective relationships at all levels, including those with clients/patients and relatives.

In another part of your role you will be responsible for the care management of a group of patients or clients. However, there should be support from senior colleagues. In your role, your decision making and problem solving skills will be applied and tested. You will have to decide on priorities of care and on the use of resources within your control and disposal. The organisation and management of the care of a group of clients/patients is going to be your direct responsibility. In that pursuit you will be expected to cope with some aspects of change as well as being able to delegate, monitor and supervise junior staff who are working in your team. You may also be invited to participate in clinical audit and other activities, which involve collecting information and reviewing care.

There are some expectations that all employers have of their new recruits. Therefore, they have been categorised as general. These include the following behaviours: punctuality, reliability, responsibility, accountability and showing enthusiasm for the post. The importance of authority, accountability, responsibility and delegation is seen within the formal job or role description. This formal contract reflects the ability of the organisation to achieve its mission.

ACCOUNTABILITY, RESPONSIBILITY, AUTHORITY AND DELEGATION

It is useful at this point to distinguish between the terms 'accountability', 'responsibility', 'authority' and 'delegation' and what this means to you and your team.

> ### Activity
>
> See if you can define the following:
>
> - Accountability
> - Responsibility
> - Authority
> - Delegation.

It is important to recognise the various definitions of these concepts, which often get confused. Here are some suggested meanings:

- **Accountability** means being able to explain and justify actions or non-actions for a responsibility given to you. This is seen as an important part of a quality system.
- **Responsibility** involves an obligation to perform certain duties or make certain decisions and having to accept any reprimand from the manager for unsatisfactory performance.
- **Authority** is the right to take action or make decisions that legitimises the exercise of power within an organisation.
- **Delegation** means the conferring of a special authority from a higher authority. It involves a two-part responsibility. The one to whom authority is delegated becomes responsible to the superior for doing the job, but the superior remains responsible for getting the job done.

Marquis and Huston (2006: 689) give a broad moralistic view of the term when they define accountability as: 'Internalised responsibility whereby an individual agrees to be morally responsible for the consequences of his actions'. This definition implies a personal thought process, which is more than just an expectation of a job or a position. Martin (2001b) confirms that accountability and responsibility go together. In leading or managing team activities, you may be asked to account for the areas of work for which you are responsible. Accountability is thus more than responsibility. In being accountable, it is now assumed that evidence can be provided for the way the responsibility has been carried out. Accountability within the health service is influenced by professional regulation and civil, employment and criminal law (Table 11.2).

We have seen that, over the years, the public's expectations of their health service have been raised. Improved health technology, media coverage and the availability

Table 11.2 Features of responsibility, authority and accountability terms

Responsibility	Authority	Accountability
• Allocated and accepted • Implies ownership • Implies outcomes • At least a two-way process	• Right to act in areas of given and accepted responsibility • Levels of authority: 1 Gathers data/ information 2 Gathers data/ information and makes recommendations 3 Gathers data/ information, makes recommendations and initiates action 4 Informs others how to act/ delegates	• Ability to reflect and evaluate actions/ non-actions/ decisions • Aids learning for future events

of the Internet has meant that the public has had more information on medical and therapeutic advances. Accountability in a civil sense must be seen within this context. The health service is made up of many large organisations where there are numerous people who manage others. The chief executive of a large health Trust is seen to be *accountable* for the total performance and clinical governance of his/her organisation.

◆ Activity

Why do you think it is important to have a stringent level of accountability in health care?

Patients may not actually know whether they are receiving good or poor care, particularly when they are very ill or disabled. The public have become very aware that they have particular rights and expectations from their health service; they are now demanding more accountability for public health services especially in the light of Francis (2013) and other reviews. Health care professionals, in particular, work in a very privileged position of trust and need to respect confidences and privacy and use their integrity when managing the care of individuals. The public put a great deal of trust and value in health care personnel when they encounter them in the health service and are often vulnerable when they are in a highly dependent state.

DUTY OF CARE

The concept of 'duty of care' is also important. Cox (2010) in Scrivener et al. (2011) highlights that the law imposes a duty of care on practitioners in circumstances where it is 'reasonably foreseeable' that they may cause harm to patients through their actions or their failure to act. Scrivener et al. also equate the duty of care with responsibility, whatever the task.

Professional accountability on an individual level is laid down within the requirements of each health professional's regulating and registering body, such as the GMC, NMC and HCPC. The term 'professional' is used in this context to convey the notion that health care workers who have a specific qualification which includes registration with a statutory body are expected to display behaviours that are consistent with their specific code of conduct. In this sense, professional behaviour which would be expected of you will include being courteous, non-judgemental, respectful and objective with patients and relatives all the time. In addition to your behaviour, there is also an expectation that your knowledge base and practice will be supported by evidence derived from research and good practice.

> ### ◆ Activity
>
> Look at the following dilemma where professional accountability and responsibility feature.
>
> Mr P, a patient in a ward, is very anxious the evening before his operation. The doctor has prescribed Mr P's usual night sedation but unfortunately, there is no stock of this drug in the drug trolley for the 10 p.m. drug round.
>
> - What could be done?
> - What action should the nurse on duty take, remembering she is accountable for acts of commission and omission?

The nurse could take a reasonable period to try to locate the drug from another ward. If she has no staff to send to look for the drug, she could ask the nurse manager. If the drug was considered 'non-urgent' she may have to make a decision on whether the drug could be safely omitted and ordered the next morning or whether it was important enough to contact the House Officer. Can you think of some 'non-urgent' drugs? Some bowel preparations such as Lactulose may be considered to be non-urgent, however if it is part of the pre-operative preparation it may be considered as vital. However, as night sedation is important, the nurse should telephone the doctor if the drug cannot be found in the hospital, particularly as it is the night before the operation and it is best practice that the patient has a good night's sleep in preparation for the forthcoming event. The doctor may wish to prescribe something else to ease the patient's anxiety.

EMPLOYMENT ACCOUNTABILITY

Employment accountability is set out under a contract of employment, so all employees will be held accountable to their employing organisation. This is true even for the top person in an organisation, such as the Chief Executive. However, in order to be held accountable for managing large organisations it is necessary that the top people are effective, so effective delegation is necessary right down the hierarchical line. Registered practitioners are accountable to their line manager for their own actions and the actions of their subordinates in getting the 'job done to the expected standard'. Their subordinates, such as physician's associates or health care assistants, are responsible for doing the job required of them while on duty and will be contractually accountable to the registered practitioner. Students may also be held to account for their 'professional' behaviour to both a university and the NHS Trusts involved but, unless they have an employment contract, they will not have a specific line manager. Leaders need to be fully aware of the accountability, responsibility and authority issues that are interrelated with the teams of staff they work with.

ORGANISATIONAL CULTURE

The culture of an organisation has an important part to play in its success. It is a concept that is difficult to define: Handy (1985: 186) defined organisational culture as 'sets of values and beliefs – reflected in differing structures and systems'; while Mullins (2005: 891) defined an organisational culture as 'the collection of traditions, values, policies, beliefs and attitudes that constitute a pervasive context for everything we do and think in an organisation'.

Cultures are affected by:

- The past
- The climate of the present
- The involved technology
- The type of work
- The aims
- The kind of people who work there.

> ### ◆ Activity
>
> Can you make some notes about the culture in your own clinical area, paying attention to these aspects?

The hospice area I work in has a relatively short past; it has only been around for about 30 years, it is a well-respected and valued organisation in the community, and its foundations lie in the charity that started it and contributes to its maintenance today. The climate of today is one of expansion: day centre, hospice at home and new hospice provision in another city and town reflect a changing organisation. The technology involved is one of palliation, medication, doctoring, nursing and allied health care, inpatient technology of beds, mattresses and home comforts as well as therapeutic alternatives such as counselling, aromatherapy and reflexology. The type of work is generally of a slower pace than in an acute hospital. There is very little rushing around. Work centres on drug rounds, medical rounds, meals and choices that the patients make – be it activities such as bathing, talking with visitors or other patients and a range of activities in the day centre. The aim of the hospice is to provide palliative care for those who have a progressive deteriorating health condition. The kind of people who work there have to be particularly able to cope with the difficulties of bereavement but also be active in rehabilitation skills to empower patients to take as much control of their lives as possible. There is a kindness and caring personality of staff whom I have seen that is in-built and they demonstrate care throughout the whole organisation, be they doctors, nurses, catering staff or volunteers – almost as though they are all potential 'hospice customers'.

An organisation's culture is important in the way it influences the process of socialisation for team members and shapes organisational behaviour. French and Bell (1990: 19) have modelled organisational culture on the structure of an iceberg, where there are formal (above the sea) and informal (below the sea) aspects of the organisation (Figure 11.4).

	The formal (overt) aspects	The informal (covert) aspects
	• Stated goals • Technology • Structure • Policies and procedures • Products • Financial resources	• Beliefs and assumptions • Perceptions • Attitudes • Feelings • Values • Informal interactions • Group norms

Figure 11.4 Formal (above the sea) and informal (below the sea) aspects of an organisation

There are many models of types of organisational cultures. We will reflect on three models (Handy, 1985; Schein, 1985; Johnson and Scholes, 1989). Handy (1985) identified four types of organisational culture (see Figure 11.6).

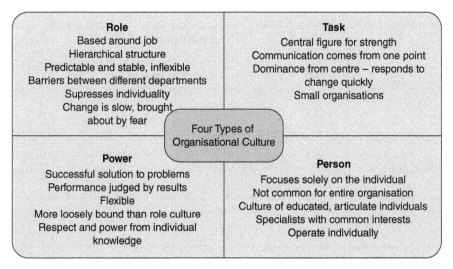

Role
Based around job
Hierarchical structure
Predictable and stable, inflexible
Barriers between different departments
Supresses individuality
Change is slow, brought about by fear

Task
Central figure for strength
Communication comes from one point
Dominance from centre – responds to change quickly
Small organisations

Four Types of Organisational Culture

Power
Successful solution to problems
Performance judged by results
Flexible
More loosely bound than role culture
Respect and power from individual knowledge

Person
Focuses solely on the individual
Not common for entire organisation
Culture of educated, articulate individuals
Specialists with common interests
Operate individually

Figure 11.5 Types of organisational culture. Adapted from Handy, C.B. (1993) *Understanding Organisations* (4th edn). Oxford: Oxford University Press

> ### ◆ Activity
>
> Can you give an example of each of these types that may be seen in health care?

The NHS as a whole may be seen as a role culture. Small project teams may be working in a task culture. Research teams, high dependency, theatres or educational units may be seen as having a power culture, and consultancy may be one of person culture.

Another model of culture types is from Schein (1985), who identified two continuums. One is not better than the other; they are simply different. Schein noted that leadership should be seen in context and in the culture of that context highlighting the relationship between leadership and culture formation (Table 11.3).

Table 11.3   Schein's (1985) relationship between leadership and culture formation

←————————————————————————————————→

Operate independently	Ideas valued from older, wiser and higher status individuals
Ideas valued from any individual	
People are responsible, motivated and capable of governing themselves	People are capable of loyalty and discipline in carrying out directions
Conflict is OK and can be sorted out through groups	Relationships are lineal and vertical
Group members will care for each other	Each individual has a place in the organisation
	The organisation is responsible for taking care of its members

The third model is that highlighted by Johnson and Scholes (1989) (Figure 11.6). It is one of an organisational cultural web, which portrays the complexity of organisation culture in reflecting how the different components all influence each other.

> ### ◆ Activity
>
> Can you write five words about each of the components seen in the web and your organisation?

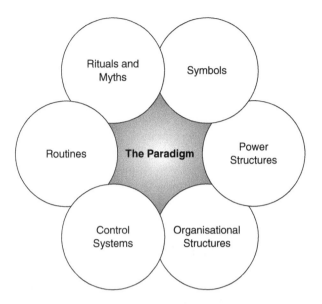

Figure 11.6 Johnson and Scholes' (1989) organisational cultural web

You may have thought about many elements within your practice area. Coming from a nursing background my thoughts are:

- **Rituals and myths:** community staff using newspaper as a barrier to infestation
- **Symbols:** wearing a uniform
- **Power structures:** visibility of Ward Sisters, Charge Nurses or Advanced Practitioners
- **Organisational structures:** salary bandings; Agenda for Change structures
- **Control Systems:** appraisals; Personal Development Reviews
- **Routines:** bathing and dressing everyone before 11 a.m.; Heath Visitors to leave the office and commence visiting homes starting late morning.

HEALTH SERVICE SYSTEMS

There are many systems within a health care organisation such as the NHS and a variety of ways of looking at the nature of different systems. An organisational system is said to be concerned with flows of processes through the organisational structure (Handy, 1985). The NHS systems could refer to a:

- Strategic controlling system
- Marketing system
- Financial system

- Information, research and technology system
- People management system
- Operational system.

All of these systems are interrelated and are as important as each other. Clinical leaders need to recognise these different valuable parts of the organisation and work at networking with different personnel within these systems so they can seek clarification and advice, as necessary, on a broader scale to help with their own decision making. The relevance of collaboration with the human resource management (HRM) system, however, cannot be overstated. If leaders are responsible for dealing with and influencing people, the skills of the HRM should offer the best support.

HUMAN RESOURCE MANAGEMENT (HRM)

Foot and Hook (1996: 4–5) identify the breadth and function of HRM through a space ship model proposed by the Employment and Occupational Standards Council (EOSC). They note that the way to enhance the performance of people in an organisation is through standards of employee relations, staff development, staff reward and employer relation (see Figure 11.7). Leaders need to be able to identify the importance of having the right staff to provide health care delivery and how they are formally managed within their employment contract. So the skills and knowledge are centred around:

- processes of workforce planning
- recruitment and selection
- induction, training and development
- performance management
- employer well-being and support
- outsourcing.

These are all seen within the context of legislation relating to health and safety, equal opportunities, discrimination and rights of the individual. From a leader's perspective, it may be important to end the focus of this chapter on the induction, training and development needs of their team members.

INDUCTION OF NEW STAFF

Induction is seen as an important process in helping new staff and students settle into the existing culture, such as a clinical environment, to help them to understand what is expected from them. It is the first part of a staff development process for new employees and may be closely followed by the period of preceptorship

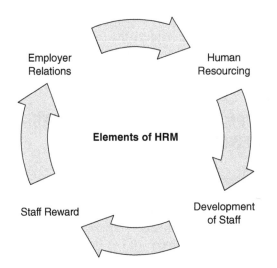

Figure 11.7   Elements of HRM based on Foot and Hook (1996)

identified earlier. In the health service, important health and safety information needs to be conveyed, such as where the fire alarms are, how the fire alarm system works, and emergency resuscitation and accident procedures. Induction, however, is more than just passing on procedural rules. It is seen as an important part of socialising people into an organisation. Marquis and Huston (2011) even suggest that induction is the first part of the *indoctrination* process and highlight the link with induction, retention and productivity.

> ▶ **Activity**
>
> Can you relate to the feelings you had as a newcomer to an established team?

It is difficult to try to 'fit' into an already socialised work team and the structure of that organisation. It is, therefore, important that new individuals get a sense of support and friendship when they first join a new team, as well as knowing how to deal with procedural emergencies. Cable and Parsons (2001) found that informal rather than formal types of socialisation had more effect on helping people settle into a new area. Culture is an important aspect in induction. Due to the difficulty of recruiting health care staff, solutions involving recruiting from abroad have meant there have been extra challenges for induction programmes as well. There have been discriminatory stories of the difficulties facing our international recruits who have come in to support our health service. The variations in practice abroad, the language and jargon differences as well as the non-verbal messages that relate to acceptance of staff

from abroad have been barriers to the integration of our internationally trained colleagues. Recently the government (DH 2014) have issued guidance related to the
level of spoken and written English together with the adaptation of practice to meet
UK standard expectations.

TRAINING, DEVELOPMENT AND THE NHS KNOWLEDGE AND SKILLS FRAMEWORK (KSFS)

Once staff have been recruited, it is important to value their contribution and motivate them towards achieving a sense of belonging and progression. The Department
of Health has produced a framework (DH, 2004a) to highlight the variety of levels
of skills and knowledge that health care staff reach within the hierarchy of the
organisation. It was a complex framework but has been much simplified and now
focuses on six dimensions:

- communication
- personal and people development
- health, safety and security
- service improvement
- quality
- equality and diversity. (www.nhsemployers.org/SimplifiedKSF accessed 14
  November 2014)

This is a useful framework which can help leaders work with their teams to develop
higher order skills and knowledge. The use of regular appraisal, yearly Development
and Performance Reviews (DPRs), and training and development plans are essential
in order to help staff to move 'upwards' in the organisation. This ultimately can only
enhance better patient care that will fit into the clinical governance perspective of
the organisation (Chapter 12).

Summary of Key Points

This chapter has briefly looked at various aspects of organisational life in order to meet
the identified learning outcomes. These were:

- **Understand the importance of the overall organisation** By understanding the
  organisation in terms of structures and processes you can more easily see an overall
  picture rather than just a small functioning part.
- **Discuss the importance of strategy, structures and systems within the organisation**
  From a broad NHS policy to a practice perspective we have seen how the health

service sets about achieving its goals. Strategies are vital in order to cope with the pressures of effective service provision. Varieties of strategies were highlighted in order to demonstrate organisational direction and its communication through mission statements and policy.

- **Critically explore the notion of organisational culture** This highlighted overt and covert aspects of any organisational climate, be it the NHS as a whole or a small team organisation.
- **Reflect on the nature of organisational roles** This involved examining the expectations of staff and students in a health care organisation and the importance of effective leadership in helping people attain their full potential.
- **Critically examine professional responsibility and accountability as well as the notions of authority and delegation** Effective leadership requires an understanding of these aspects in terms of supporting boundary management for team members.
- **Develop an overview of Human Resource processes in organisations** By examining the importance of human resources, leaders should be able to manage effective recruitment and retention strategies. This was looked at in the context of the NHS Knowledge and Skills Framework within the health service.

FURTHER READING

Department of Health (2005) *A Patient-Led NHS*. London: DH.

Easterby-Smith, M., Burgoyne, J. and Arunjo, L. (1999) *Organisational Learning and the Learning Organisation*. London: Sage.

Schein, E. (1997) *Empowerment, Coercive Persuasion and Organisational Learning: Do They Connect?* Henley on Thames: Henley Management College.

Senge, P.M. (2006) *The Fifth Discipline* (2nd edn). London: Random House Business.

Visit the companion website at https://study.sagepub.com/barr3e for more resources.

12 QUALITY

Learning Outcomes

By the end of this chapter you will have had the opportunity to:

- Identify the importance of quality in the health service for better patient outcomes
- Discuss the historical developments that led to the present quality agenda

- Critically explore the importance of patient safety in the context of quality health care
- Discuss the importance of clinical governance, audit, effectiveness and risk management
- Compare a variety of quality models to inform effective leadership for continuous improvement of health care delivery
- Relate the importance of leadership in clinical supervision as a method of developing professional learning.

INTRODUCTION

The White Paper *A First Class Service: Quality in the New NHS Health Services* (DH, 1998) demonstrated the commitment of past governments to providing quality health services and its features are still pertinent today, particularly the relevance of clinical governance and lifelong learning. We are concerned about quality in health care because it ultimately affects patients and staff. There is also an assumption that a quality health service will improve the health of the nation. This chapter will examine what is meant by the concept of quality and how it has developed over time. Models such as *The EFQM© Excellence Model* (European Foundation for Quality Management (EFQM), 2014), Total Quality Management (TQM) and clinical governance will be highlighted. There will also be a focus on patient safety in the light of the Francis Report (2013) which highlighted the NHS's neglect of patient safety and care. The impact of quality and the necessary human factors within the health service will also be examined in the context of how this enhances the overall quality of care delivery to patients/clients. There will be limited reference to the idea of cost effectiveness for leaders but it is seen as an important aspect in quality management.

HISTORICAL CONTEXT OF QUALITY MOVEMENT IN HEALTH CARE

In the 1970s and early 1980s, the concept of quality became more important in industry. Quality as a valued commodity began to be associated with manufacturing industry, where products were inspected for their worth. Dowding and Barr (2002) noted the development of quality from the 1960s until the beginning of the twenty-first century (see Table 12.1).

However, this emphasis on quality was rarely associated with the service industries and not particularly with health care. Health care was felt to be in business for the good of society, not profit, and thus closed to quality scrutiny. The British government launched the National Quality Campaign in 1984 for both private and public industries, with the NHS being strongly encouraged to put a quality control system in place. There was initial resistance and scepticism from professionals who

Table 12.1 Development of quality

	Traditional pre-1960	Technocratic 1960s and 1970s	TQM 1980s and 1990s
Definition	La crème de la crème	Fitness for use Meeting requirements	Satisfying and delighting the customer
Who defines quality?	Everybody knows what it is	Experts	Customers
Nature of quality	Attributes of product or service	Attributes of product or service	Process and outcomes
What produces good quality?	Good people and materials	Good people and materials	The right processes
Relationship to cost	Top quality is the most expensive	Quality can be found at all prices but improving quality implies raising costs	Quality is free

felt that they already gave a quality service. From these initial developments, the NHS worked through concepts such as quality assurance, then moved through to the Total Quality Management concept (which focuses on meeting and satisfying the needs of customers), towards the idea of continuous process improvement. The latter idea focuses on an active journey of not only meeting customer needs but on 'delighting the customer'. Whether this phrase can be seen as appropriate in health service delivery is debatable but at least it reflects that quality is not just about complacency and 'standing still'.

A *First Class Service* (DH, 1998) set out a statutory 'duty of quality' for all providers of NHS services. The statutes introduced the National Performance Framework, clinical governance and quality structures such as the National Institute for Clinical Excellence (NICE) and the Commission for Health Improvement (CHI). Specific plans were launched to improve the health service, especially in terms of effectiveness, efficiency and excellence, through Primary Care Trusts and technological communication networks. The drive for quality was seen through the indicators of partnership and performance. NICE, as the agency for establishing which overall treatments and interventions work best, has the remit of making sure clinicians know about them. CHI is responsible for monitoring clinical governance in the NHS and is able to investigate organisations that fall short of providing adequate care (Garbett, 1998).

Quality management has now been encompassed by the wider care sector and the Care Quality Commission (CQC) was set up in 2009 as a new health and social care regulator for England. Their aim is to ensure better joined up care provision for everyone in hospital, in a care home and at home. They assess and inspect health and social care and work to improve health and social care services with specific work around people affected under the Mental Health Act.

Leadership and innovation is seen as an important feature of modernising the health service in order to bring in a better service delivery that is more responsive to the needs of the public. A quite funny but informative cartoon (An Alternative Guide to the NHS) can be found on the companion website.

TOTAL QUALITY MANAGEMENT (TQM)

Total Quality Management is a business philosophy based on customer satisfaction and the notion of continuous improvement. TQM is a strategy aimed at the whole organisation in order that resources are better managed; people cooperate so that the organisation is more flexible and responsive to what are seen as internal and external customers. It was Deming who first introduced this quality model very successfully to manufacturing in Japan in the 1950s (Deming, 1986). One feature concerning the importance of 'customer focus' meant that organisations started to think very differently about their products and how they met with buyers' expectations. The notion of 'customers' as a feature within the health industry creates a difficulty. In business, customer growth is seen as an ideal and healthy. If patients are seen as customers in the NHS, their growth would infer greater cost to an already stretched service. However, this aside, the use of 'customer' within the concept of quality has got a wider interpretation. Mosadeghrad (2014) sees that TQM is not without its difficulties. His literature review research points to the following barriers: insufficient education and training, lack of employees' involvement, lack of top management support, inadequate resources, deficient leadership, lack of a quality-oriented culture, poor communication, lack of a plan for change and employee resistance to the change programme. Mosadeghrad (2014) concludes that organisations need to better understand these quality barriers issues in their quality management focus.

Customers are seen as individuals or groups of people who need a product or a service. The breadth of this definition means that customers can be our patients and clients, or *external customers*, as they are outside the organisation. In broader terms, it could also relate to any external agency that purchases a service from any health provider such as a NHS Trust or a Strategic Health Authority. There are also internal customers within an organisation, reflecting the interdependent relationships between organisational departments. All internal departments are affected by the quality of each other and no department/ discipline works in isolation. If the X-Ray department did not come up with their services on time, then this would affect surgical and medical decisions. Similarly, if there was a poor catering service, medical and therapy staff may feel more disgruntled and this may influence the quality of interpersonal communications with patients.

QUALITY OF DEVELOPMENT IN HEALTH CARE

Quality is a relative concept and although we all have some idea what is good and what is bad, identifying what is acceptable is not so straightforward. Quality could be seen as being effective and efficient. Drucker (1967) defined efficiency simply as 'doing things right' and effectiveness as 'doing the right things right'. The questions to ask though are 'what is right?' and 'how do we know we are doing the right things right?' It may be very difficult to know what is right in emotional support, for example, so we can only 'best guess' initially and then later reflect on the outcomes in order to see how well the patient reacts. In other cases, we know that using an ABC approach to first aid is the right approach to use, based on evidence and research. So, effectiveness and efficiency may not tell the full story of quality within health care. Health care quality could be seen in terms of meeting the health needs and expectations of the population at the lowest cost (Øvretveit, 1992). The question of defining quality is difficult and it is probably more important to focus on the elements of quality.

The World Health Organization (1983) identified the four main principles of quality assurance in health care as:

- Professional performance (technical quality)
- Resource use (efficiency)
- Risk management
- Patient satisfaction with the service provided.

Goetch and Davis (2014: 3) give the analogy of the three legged stool relating to

- **People:** empowered staff, quality is expected not inspected
- **Processes:** cultural improvement; good enough is never good enough
- **Measures:** benchmarking, quality tools and target setting
- **The 'seat'** is then the customer focus.

They explore the continued importance of 'Total Quality' and internal and external customer focus for survival. Moullin (2002: 13) examined health and social care quality in terms of 'meeting customer requirements and expectations at an acceptable price'. This was set against three other notions of quality:

- Fitness for purpose
- Conformance to specifications
- Conformance to requirements.

Fitness for purpose originated from the work of the quality guru Juran (1986), in asking whether a treatment or intervention is appropriate. For example, some new technologies may give very accurate health data but if the technology is difficult for patient attachment, causes them discomfort, or is difficult for health professionals to read and interpret then it is not fit for purpose. **Conformance to specification** originates from the work of another quality guru, Levitt (1972), where customers set the specifications of the health service they require and how well it is addressed and measured. However, it is unusual for patients to get involved in this activity. It is more likely to be PCTs (now in the process of merging into NHS Trusts) or GPs who do this and, although it is hoped that they try to reflect the ideas of patients, it is not necessarily easy to represent all patient views. **Conformance to requirements** arises from the work of Crosby (1984) and involves looking at meeting needs, demands or requirements of the customers. However, this does not address the infinite patient needs and the costs of meeting these health needs. Moullin's (2002) idea of quality in 'meeting customer requirements and expectations at an acceptable price' addresses the relationship between requirements of customers and costs. There is still some question that our customers in health provision do not always bear the full cost of their care as patients. Therefore patients do not always have the leverage to drive up quality.

PATIENT SAFETY AND HUMAN FACTORS

The Health and Social Care Act 2012 set up the Care Quality Commission (CQC) in order to act as a regulator for health and social care in England. Their remit is to ensure safe and high quality services are provided to patients. Glasper (2014: 110) highlights that the inspection system previously used by the CQC is set to be replaced by a more focused inquiry into hospitals, care homes and other health and social care institutions. The focus will be in five areas:

• Is it safe?
• Is it effective?
• Is it caring?
• Is it responsive to people's needs?
• Is it well-led?

This approach hopefully will prevent the poor state of care like that delivered at Mid Staffordshire NHS Foundation Trust. This new approach does however demonstrate the link between good care, safety and good leadership. McCaughan and Kaufman (2013) in their comprehensive review of patient safety knowledge note the different 'patient safety' terminology:

• Harm – where health care negatively affects a patient/client's health or quality of life. This may be due to errors or to those known possibilities such as surgical complications, adverse drug reactions or hospital acquired infections
• Errors or mistakes – due to faulty judgements, decisions or problem solving

- Slips and lapses – errors caused by lack of attention or distraction
- Adverse events – unintended harm by medical management
- Patient safety incidents – i.e. unintended or unexpected incidents
- Near misses – i.e. potentially harmful but prevented
- 'Never' events – e.g. wrong limb amputation.

Adverse events can be related to primary, acute or tertiary care. Common adverse events may often be preventable. Some common examples may be:

- Development of pressure ulcers
- Chest infections
- Poor catheter care
- Medication errors
- 'Failure to rescue': unrecognised patient deterioration maybe resulting in cardiac arrest, suicide.

Mollon (2014) analysed the concept of 'feeling safe during hospitalization' using Walker and Avant's attributes, antecedents and consequences model. From the qualitative literature the analysis can be seen in Table 12.2. The conclusion was that more patient-centred care models and the creation of more positive environments were needed for patients to feel safe.

Table 12.2   Concept analysis of 'feeling safe' (Mollon 2014)

Attributes	Antecedents	Consequences
• Trust	• Relationship	• Control
• Cared for	• Environment	• Hope
• Presence	• Suffering	• Relaxed/calm
• Knowledge		

Power et al. (2012) identify the contribution of the Commissioning for Quality and Innovation (CQUIN) framework in raising the standards of health care based on a target system for providers where inductive financial payments are seen as rewards. The nature of these incentive schemes can be seen as either helpful or unnecessary, unwarranted bureaucracy-building in a culture competitive with the NHS. The NHS Safety Thermometer was one of the CQUIN schemes launched in 2012 to take a snapshot measure of four common 'harms' in the NHS. These are:

- Pressure ulcers
- Falls
- Urinary infection (catheterised patients)
- Venous thromboembolism.

The *prevalence* data is gathered by frontline staff on one day per month from clinical records, patient examination and patient or carer interview. Buckley et al. (2014) explored their Trust's implementation plan to use the Safety Thermometer. They used the opportunity of gathering data from 160 student nurses who were 'harm free care' trained for the process and raising their awareness of patient safety and in 2012, the DH recognised this initiative of one of three 'best practice' examples.

The context of health care delivery and patient safety has over the years been challenged by the reduction of senior and more experienced staff available at weekends, evenings and nights in order to contain the staffing costs in unsocial hour payments. Moore (2014) notes the new strategy to transform hospital care for a more consistent care 24 hours, seven days a week. She notes the national research showing patients admitted during the weekend have a significantly higher risk of dying within 30 days than those admitted on a Wednesday. This new approach means the 'manic Mondays' of ward rounds, discharges and requests for new diagnostics will be evened out over the week. This may also mean more extended and expanded practice with more experienced nurses taking the place of junior doctors in training during the unsocial periods. This will also influence the need to increase community health services to a 24/7 provision, for instance in district nursing service, nursing and care homes. The difficulties with this are whether funding can be found for more health care practitioners.

Patient safety and medication prescription/administration are also significant. Around 1,800 patient prescriptions in three general practices across three primary

Table 12.3 Models of patient safety (after McCaughan and Kaufman, 2013)

Person Model (Person and Behaviour Characteristics)	System Model (Organisational Focus)	Human Factors (Combination of Person and System Models)
• Individual characteristics: knowledge, skill and competence	• Financial and environmental resources: staffing levels, administrative and managerial support and available equipment	• The individual
• Task complexity for individuals	• Management priorities	• The job
• Team factors: leadership communication and supervision	• Policies and standards	• The organisation
	• Culture of support or blame	• Ergonometric and environmental technology to enhance better health care judgements

care Trusts were examined in a retrospective case-note review and Avery et al. (2012) noted that around one in 20 prescriptions contained a mild to moderate error and that one in 550 were seen to be serious. These were seen to be missing information on dose or essential monitoring. Many factors were associated and more research is needed.

McCaughan and Kaufman (2013: 51) identified three relevant models for health professionals assessing patient safety.

HUMAN FACTORS

The case of 37-year-old Elaine Bromiley, who died during a fairly minor surgical treatment in 2005, was investigated and it was found that she was being treated by two experienced anaesthetists, two operating department practitioners, an ENT surgeon and two recovery nurses in an emergency situation. Emergency equipment was all at hand including the tracheostomy kit that could have saved her life (Reid and Bromiley, 2012). The Harmer (2005) inquiry found that the surgical team were not neglectful but that there was a lack of discussion between the team about the best course of action and there was confusion about the use of different pieces of equipment. It appears there was a lack of appreciation of human behaviour under the stressful situation and everyone lost sight of the escalating deterioration and the leadership and contribution of all in the team was poor. The husband of Elaine, a pilot, has campaigned to understand the human factors and the absence of these non-technical skills that affected the emergency care needed for his wife. The similarities between the surgical context and aviation industry highlighted the need for more simulation training in the health industry. The UK Clinical Human Factors Group (CHFG) was set up. It is a broad coalition of health care professionals, managers and service users who have partnered with experts in human factors from health-care and other high-risk industries to campaign for change in the NHS.

The CHFG (2014) note that 'Human factors encompass all those factors that can influence people and their behaviour in a work context, human factors are the environmental, organisational and job factors, and individual characteristics which influence behaviour at work.'

They also note Catchpole's (2011) relevance of clinical human factors for

Enhancing clinical performance through an understanding of the effects of teamwork, tasks, equipment, workspace, culture, organisation on human behaviour and abilities, and application of that knowledge in clinical settings.

The role of human factors in medical care linked to patient safety is therefore seen as being different from the neglectfulness and incompetence of certain health care practitioners, which is often the worldview and subject of media attention when things go wrong in clinical care. The latter brings about a blame culture which can be unhelpful in moving the organisation to learn from past mistakes. Flin and Maran (2004) and White (2012) identified that in health care, cognitive, interpersonal and social non-technical skills are as important as technical skills.

Cognitive skills include:

- Situation awareness
- Decision making
- Task management.

Interpersonal and social skills include:

- Leadership
- Followship
- Effective communication.

It is these non-technical skills that may affect health outcomes for patients when teams are under stress and do not perform at their most effective. This is also true where there is an authority or hierarchical difference in the multiprofessional teams as well as between regulated and unregulated members of staff.

Accountability and having the confidence to speak up are essential at all levels of care-giving. Health care professionals need to engage all those in the team, at whatever level, to have a voice for the safety of patients. In 2004 the National Patient Safety Agency (NPSA) produced the 'Seven steps to patient safety' model (Table 12.4). Specific publications for mental health, primary care and general practice teams have also been produced. These are invaluable leadership issues for developing any team culture.

Table 12.4 Seven steps to patient safety for health care teams (NPSA, 2004)

Step 1: building a safety culture	Create a culture that is open and fair
Step 2: leading and supporting the practice team	Establishing a clear and strong focus on patient safety throughout your organisation
Step 3: integrating risk management activity	Developing systems and processes to manage your risks and identify and assess things that could go wrong
Step 4: promoting reporting	Ensuring staff can easily report incidents locally and nationally
Step 5: involving and communicating with patients and the public	Developing ways to communicate openly with and to listen to patients
Step 6: learning and sharing safety lessons	Encouraging staff to use root cause analysis to learn how and why incidents happen
Step 7: implementing solutions to prevent harm	Embed lessons through changes to practice, processes or systems

The role of patients and the public in monitoring the quality of their health services is not new but there is an agenda to increase their voice being heard. Coulter (2011: 185) has suggested that patients and citizens are an untapped resource and have an important contribution in eight policy areas:

1. Improving care processes
2. Building health literacy
3. Selecting treatments
4. Strengthening self-care
5. Ensuring safer care
6. Participating in research
7. Training professionals
8. Shaping services.

Shapiro et al. (2013), for instance, highlight the role of patients in the USA in being more in control of checking on the quality of their surgical procedures. However the public are often not well equipped to know how to determine what it is they should be checking when they are obviously concerned about their own health and pending treatment. Research has shown that coronary care nurses are more likely than any other health care professional to recognise, intercept and correct errors that are life threatening (Rothschild et al. 2006). Mansour (2014) notes that nursing education therefore has to address how to prepare students with knowledge and skills related to patient safety from early on in their courses. His quantitative research into student perceptions of patient safety is a useful start in raising awareness to influence practice and he notes the value of the WHO (2011) Patient Safety Curriculum which is globally recommended for embedding into all nurse education.

Moller (2013: 506) notes the importance of accountability and transparency in medical error reporting. Health service cultures must change from a blame culture where staff are reluctant to admit near misses or mistakes to a culture of fairness and understanding of the connection between human factors and system failures. She highlights a quote from a 2009 safety report:

'To err is human

– To delay is deadly'

Effective leadership, accountability and the quality of the organisational culture are therefore vital to maintain patient safety (McCaughan and Kaufman, 2013; Moller, 2013).

MODELS OF QUALITY IN THE HEALTH SERVICE

There are numerous and possibly contentious ways of identifying what overall quality means in the health service. In reality, we probably see health care quality models merging into an eclectic model communicated by government policy today but, depending on the audience, one may enjoy more emphasis than the others.

Table 12.5 Quality models characteristics

Model	Characteristics
Biomedical	Addressing biological dysfunction
	Appropriate relief of symptoms and ability to cure diseases
Teleological	From the perspective of patient's holism. Offering dignity, privacy, empathy, confidentiality and information to help them understand their needs and health choices
Preventative	Offering services which prevent ill health
Business	Offering a growth in services in primary care with more convenience, acceptable waiting times and clinical environments

The EFQM Excellence Model (European Foundation for Quality Management Model of Excellence (EFQM®), 2014) has been helpful in offering a 'whole system' overview (Figure 12.1) of the health service and is valuable because it recognises that people and leadership are so much a part of success and getting good results.

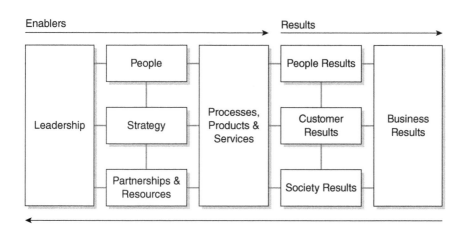

Figure 12.1 EFQM Excellence Model © EFQM, 2014

Ringrose (2013) conducted research which reviewed a variety of global quality models, then engaged a number of management consultants through the research and finally developed the 'Organisational Excellent Framework'. This can be seen in Figure 12.2.

You may want to check out the website for more details on this research-based model and see if it helps you understand the dimensions of patient health care quality (http://organizationalexcellencespecialists.ca/products-and-services/). Other

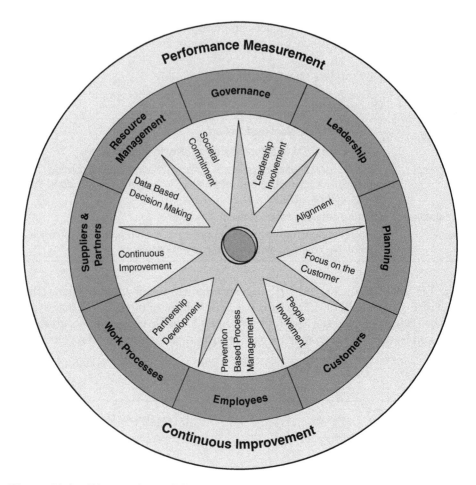

Figure 12.2 Ringrose's model

research has involved exploration of what quality dimensions would be important to the health service. Interestingly Greaves et al. (2012) recently explored the 'cloud experience' of patients to unconventionally unearth how blogs and social media sites such as Twitter can be used to detect poor healthcare experiences in patients' own narrative. This development appears to be gaining momentum in recognizing how important the internet and social media has changed the lives of the population and thus giving them a more public voice. The early research work of Berry et al. (1988), who used in-depth interviews with a number of 'customer' groups, concluded that the groups highlighted several dimensions of quality (Table 12.5).

Table 12.6 Dimensions of quality

Quality Dimension	Best Practice	Poor Practice
Reliability	Good IT health information	Failure to contact service user if that was agreed
Responsiveness	Staff who are able to address issues that arise unexpectedly	Long waits without direct action/ no explanations from issues that arise unexpectedly
Competence	Skilled staff	Staff inadequately trained for tasks required
Access	Ease of access to facilities or staff. Good signposting and attention to those with disabilities	Poor signposting/ limited parking
Courtesy	Polite and helpful staff	Patronising and unhelpful staff
Communication	Staff who explain a diagnosis and alternative treatments/ interventions without jargon	Lack of information about what is happening or what could happen
Credibility	Staff you can trust and depend on	Staff who don't appear to have the full information about individuals
Security	A feeling of safeness/ confidentiality	Unlit access to facilities
Understanding	Staff who make an effort to understand them as individuals	Staff who don't recognise a regular service user
Tangibles	Pleasing physical appearance of facilities	Poor/ out of date equipment/ accommodation

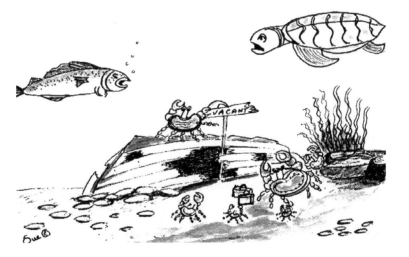

You may feel that these are very important dimensions to all of us as patients. In a way, they point to the expected standards of a good service delivery whether we are looking at buying a second-hand car, a home or a piece of jewellery. In terms of the NHS, there can be difficulties in always reaching the standard required by patients, a professional body or by health service managers; it is important to identify how well a service measures up to each of their standards. So what are standards? What do they mean for health practitioners? The setting of local standards of all kinds of professional care is seen as vital to assuring quality. The Royal College of Nursing use a definition of a 'standard' as:

> a level of quality against which performance can be measured. It can be described as 'essential' – the absolute minimum to ensure safe and effective practice, or 'developmental' – designed to encourage and support a move to better practice. (DHSSPS, 2006)

Barr and Dowding (2012: 228) offer the following notions that standards:

- describe the desired quality of performance
- have been agreed
- be clearly written
- contain one major thought
- be measurable
- be concise
- be specific
- be achievable
- be clinically sound.

There are eight prerequisites for a successful standard:

- A philosophy
- The relevant skills and knowledge
- The authority to act
- Accountability
- The control of resources
- Organisational structure and management style
- The professional relationships
- The management of change.

Standard statements should be related, descriptive, free from bias, suitable for quantification, valid and reliable so that they are unambiguous. There have been several Quality Assurance models for standard setting proposed. Donebedian's (1966) approach to quality evaluation has been regularly used within the NHS and serves as a reminder of the different domains that affect health care (see Table 12.7).

Table 12.7 Donebedian's approach to quality evaluation

STRUCTURE

The factors within the organisation that enable work to be carried out. These may be environmental facilities, equipment, staffing, educational facilities and management factors.

PROCESS

The performance or activity required to achieve the outcome, i.e., the care given to an individual, group or community.

OUTCOME

The result of care and performance or the effect of care on an individual, group or community.

However, Keighley (1989) argued against the Donebedian approach and identified two elements of a quality standard: the technical performance and the expressive performance. Technical performance is something that the customer expects the NHS to deliver consistently. Good technical performance is achieved through knowledge that is required in training, in the use of supplies, the use of facilities and, most of all, is dependent on the number of staff available to deliver the service. In contrast, expressive performance is concerned with attitudes of staff – in their relationships and interactions with customers, with each other – and the manner in which the staff deliver the service. This 'fits' well with the notion of 'non-technical skills' mentioned earlier and the findings proposed by Berry et al. (1988) but it is also true to say that it is more difficult to say what constitutes 'good expressive performance', as this can be quite subjective to the individual giving or receiving it. In terms of measuring quality in the NHS as a whole, Maxwell (1984) first introduced a framework of the dimensions of quality in health care:

- **Acceptability:** Services are provided such as to satisfy the reasonable expectations of patients, purchasers, providers and the community.
- **Equity:** A fair share for all the population. The service or procedure is what the individual or population actually needs.
- **Efficiency:** Resources are not wasted on one service or patient to the detriment of another.
- **Effectiveness:** Achieving the intended benefit for the individual and the population.
- **Accessibility:** Services are not compromised by undue limits of time or distance.

> ◗ **Activity**
>
> Think about your own clinical care delivery. Jot down how each of these aspects can be applied to your service.

Maxwell's model, although useful as a checklist, has largely been encompassed into the modern NHS quality initiatives through the NHS performance framework. However, in 2008 the World Health Organization (2008a: 48) reaffirmed the basic concepts of quality in European Health Care as being:

- **Effectiveness:** delivering health care that adheres to an evidence base and results in improved health outcomes for individuals and communities, based on need
- **Efficiency:** delivering health care in a manner which maximises resource use and avoids waste
- **Accessibility:** delivering health care that is timely, geographically reasonable, and provided in a setting where skills and resources are appropriate to medical need
- **Acceptable/patient-centred:** delivering health care which takes into account the preferences and aspirations of individual service users and the cultures of their communities
- **Equitable:** delivering health care which does not vary in quality because of personal characteristics such as gender, race, ethnicity, geographical location, or socioeconomic status
- **Safety:** delivering health care which minimises risks and harm to service users.

It appears then that there is general consensus on what health care quality means and how it can be measured.

CLINICAL GOVERNANCE

The notion that public services had a responsibility for monitoring and improving their provision, in the context of health care, was coined clinical governance. Scally and Donaldson (1998) and McSherry and Pearce (2011) noted that clinical governance is to be the main method of improving the quality of patient care in the NHS.

Clinical governance needs organisation-wide transformation, clinical leadership and positive organisational cultures. There is a need for learning from past failures such as variations in standards of care, particularly with respect to breast and cervical screening programmes. Poor quality is often detected through complaints, audit, untoward incidents or routine surveillance. Scally and Donaldson (1998) proposed the key to success being a more open, participative and shared culture, with good leadership, team training and working, as well as evidence for good practice.

The government defined clinical governance (DH, 1998) as:

A framework through which NHS organisations are accountable for continuously improving the quality of their services and safeguarding high standards of care by creating an environment in which excellence in clinical care can flourish.

Bassett (1999: 5) suggests clinical governance can be best summarised as:

A protective mechanism (umbrella) for both the public and healthcare professionals, ensuring that their hospitals and community trusts are actively developing structures to improve the quality of care in the hope of preventing any recurrence of the Bristol Case 1998.

Lilley (1999), as the Director of the Clinical Governance Research and Development Unit at the University of Leicester, concurred that clinical governance:

- Is everyone's business
- Involves patients and service users
- Ignores departmental and service boundaries and works across them
- Involves everyone in developing their professional capabilities
- Is continuous and evolving in its quest for improvement
- Is about finding out what works best and doing it every time
- Is based on evidence
- Is transparent and open.

He highlighted that the responsibilities of NHS Trusts were to:

- Establish leadership, accountability and working arrangements
- Carry out quality assessments
- Formulate action plans
- Clarify reporting arrangements.

Health practitioners have to accept responsibility for developing and maintaining standards of care within their local service. Ultimately, health care needs to be evidence-based, and professionals need to identify the rationale for treatment and care being effective as well as efficient.

In terms of clinical practice, Crinson (1999) noted five key components for a system of clinical governance:

- Clinical audit
- Clinical effectiveness
- Clinical risk management
- Quality assurance
- Staff development.

More specifically the National Audit Office (NAO) (2007), in reviewing clinical governance progress in primary care, noted the components of clinical governance in improving quality and safety as relying on:

- Improving services based on lessons from patient safety incidents/near misses
- Improving services based on lessons from complaints
- Ensuring the quality of patient experiences
- Involving patients and the public in the design and delivery of health services
- Involving professional groups in multi-professional audit
- Collecting 'intelligent' information on clinical care
- Proactively identifying clinical risks to patients/staff
- Measuring the capacity and capability to deliver services
- Ensuring effective clinical leadership.

The NAO made future recommendations to strengthen clinical governance for the Department of Health, Strategic Health Authorities and PCTs with respect to guidance, monitoring, better systems of accountability and development of staff for evidence-based care, audit and service involvement. McSherry and Pearce (2011) have proposed a future evolution of clinical governance towards what the Department of Health (2006b) term 'integrated governance' which is:

> systems, processes, and behaviours by which Trusts lead, direct and control their functions in order to achieve organisational objectives, safety and quality of service and in which they relate to patients, carers, the wider community and organisations.

Despite a decade of rhetoric regarding quality patient care, governance and costly policy publications, the media continue to inform the public of poor standards of care and patient outcomes.

CLINICAL AUDIT

Dunitz (1995) identifies audit as a measuring, evaluation or study process which should improve the medical care a patient should receive. There have been many attempts to do more than set standards. The idea of measuring quality implies that there will be some benchmark of quality acceptability. The definition of a benchmark is 'a standard of best practice and care by which current practice and care are measured'. Benchmarking is defined as a systematic process in which current practice and care are compared to, and amended to attain, best practice and care (DH, 2010d). BS5750 or the ISO9000 were examples of awards (or reaching a certain quality benchmark in organisations, but they are often seen as quite administratively mechanistic). However, all health practitioners have a responsibility to make sure audit of key benchmarking policy is on their agenda. *Essence of Care* (DH, 2001b) set out standards for the quality of fundamental or essential aspects of care.

> ### ◆ Activity
>
> What do you know about the benchmarks set out in *Essence of Care*?

Essence of Care (DH, 2001b) set out eight benchmarks for patient care:

1. Continence and bladder and bowel care
2. Personal and oral hygiene
3. Food and nutrition
4. Pressure ulcers
5. Privacy and dignity
6. Record keeping
7. Safety of clients with mental health needs in acute mental health and general hospital settings
8. Principles of self care.

More recently, in 2010, the document *How to Use the Essence of Care* revisited the benchmarks for best practice in care (DH, 2010d) (see Table 12.8).

Table 12.8 Essence of Care

1 Bladder, bowel and continence care
2 Care environment
3 Communication
4 Food and drink
5 Prevention and management of pain
6 Personal hygiene
7 Prevention and management of pressure ulcers
8 Promoting health and well-being
9 Record keeping
10 Respect and dignity
11 Safety
12 Self care

> **◆ Activity**
>
> Go to the Department of Health website (www.gov.uk/government/publications/
> essence-of-care-2010) and review the impact this document has on your own clinical
> care. Identify how leadership is dealing with the monitoring and audit that is suggested.

Monitoring quality is often confused with the terms 'audit' or 'evaluation'. The following definitions may help differentiate the terms:

- **Monitoring:** The continuous or regularly repeated observations or measurements of important parts of the service related to structure process output or outcome.
- **Audit:** A discrete activity composing of a detailed periodic review of part or whole of a service or a procedure. In audit, there is an explicit search for improvement. This means that the importance of an audit extends beyond monitoring into developing the service.
- **Evaluation:** Refers to the judgements concerning information arising from a monitoring system.

On the clinical side, there has been a move towards multidisciplinary team audits (clinical audit). These audits focus more on the patient experiences or 'journey' rather than on the various individual services provided.

CLINICAL EFFECTIVENESS

This is about whether patient outcomes are achieved by the right health care interventions. Research is needed to identify what the relationship between outcomes and interventions may be. However, some health care professionals do not always see themselves as scientists or researchers but as 'action orientated doers' (Parkin and Bullock, 2005). Those who use the health service are looking to see the effectiveness of health care, more so than ever, and so research is important. Hunt (2001) notes that the main key advances in the last century have depended on professionals working with the public to advance practice through research. Nurse/midwifery consultancy is seen as a key driver for some professional research-mindedness in nursing and midwifery.

There are many questions about certain health care interventions where even the research is ambiguous. However, Muir Gray (1997) points to key questions about the use of research as evidence for health care. These are related to the relevance of the research, the range of outcomes and effects, generalisability, and whether any intervention does more harm than good. This must be taken in the context of a traditional science background, and generalisability may not always fit with the nature of qualitative research. Effective therapeutic care on an individual basis is often difficult to measure. This, therefore, has to be balanced against the context of the centralising management of the health service. Hamer and Collinson (2005: 92) highlight the present-day sophistication in quality management with the developing NHS Performance Management Framework, 'Star Rating', and embedded clinical effectiveness in every field of practice.

THE NHS OUTCOMES FRAMEWORK

The Department of Health through its Executive proposed the NHS Performance Assessment Framework in 1999, which provided a range of performance measures for the benefit of all health service stakeholders. Performance Indicators (PIs) in the Health Service have been valued for the following reasons:

- To ensure that NHS goals are achieved
- To be accountable to a growing range of stakeholders
- To survive through competition.

More recently the Department of Health has developed the NHS Outcomes Framework which focussed on improving health and reducing health inequalities through five domains

- Preventing people from dying prematurely
- Enhancing quality of life for people with long term conditions
- Helping people to recover from episodes of ill health or following injury
- Ensuring that people have a positive experience of care
- Treating and caring for people in a safe environment; and protecting them from avoidable harm.

The NHS Outcomes Framework (2013/14) defined that high quality care comprised of effectiveness, patient experience and safety; this is enshrined into the Health and Social Care Act (2012).

HEALTH EQUITY AND HEALTH EQUALITY

Equity concerns fairness, impartiality and treating like cases alike. It could be seen as a separate entity or as a sub-criterion of effectiveness. It is concerned with treating patients and clients equally when they are in similar situations. Health equality is seen as the condition of being equal and concerns the removal of disadvantage.

Health inequality relates to differences in health experience and outcomes between different population groups; health inequity relates to differences in opportunities for different population groups, which result in unequal:

- life chances
- access to health services
- nutritious food
- adequate housing, etc.

The policies *Equity and Excellence* (DH, 2010a, 2010b) join up the ideas of quality and equity by cutting bureaucracy and improving efficiency. Buck and Jabbal (2014), through The King's Fund and the Joseph Rowntree Foundation, proposed a 'poverty focused' NHS through a public health, system leadership and culture approach; for example deprived children and young people in Derbyshire were targeted through the development of care being offered nearer to home or school increasing access mainly through Health Visitors and School Nurses.

CLINICAL RISK MANAGEMENT

In order to minimise errors and complaints in the health service, risk management is a very important aspect of the drive to prevent litigation. Lugon and Secker-Walker (2006: 102) note the seven pillars of establishing clear and effective patient and professional partnerships as:

- clinical effectiveness
- risk management effectiveness
- patient experience
- communication effectiveness
- resource effectiveness
- strategic effectiveness
- learning effectiveness.

The foundations of these pillars include systems awareness; communication; ownership and leadership. Lilley and Lambden (1999) identify three aims to risk management that can broadly be seen as:

- Reducing or eliminating the harm to the patient
- Dealing with the affected patient and supporting clinical staff
- Safeguarding the organisational assets.

In terms of a risk assessment for moving and handling, you will see the importance of these aims for patients who are not able to move themselves easily. If every bed in hospital had a slip sheet, maybe more nurses would use them and avoid discomfort/injury to the patient and risk of back injury to themselves, and reduce high absenteeism and even litigation for the Trusts.

Lilley and Lambden (1999) also identified the four principles of risk management:

- Risk identification
- Risk analysis
- Risk control
- Risk cost.

Risk management does involve the ability of all staff to report adverse problems and events without fear of being made a personal scapegoat. This will require courage and more positive support for 'whistle-blowing', which is not always easy for new staff who may not understand the organisational culture and the impact of them acknowledging any problems.

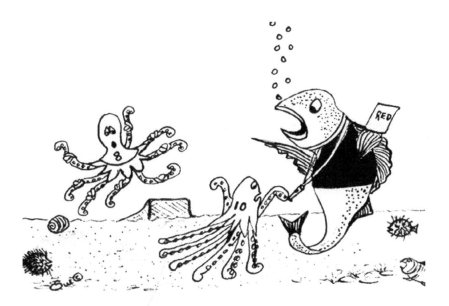

QUALITY ASSURANCE

The ability of the health service to assure quality is an important means of building public confidence but must be taken in the light of what staff feel are important standards. The use of care pathways is one example of what patients/clients will expect and what commissioners will expect to build into their contracts. While this is only an example of how quality might be assured it is also a method of establishing an evaluative process, which is what quality assurance, clinical audit and clinical governance is really all about.

STAFF DEVELOPMENT

Ultimately, quality relies on well-trained and critical practitioners who are well motivated and enthusiastic about improving care continuously. Clinical governance,
therefore, relies on professional regulation and lifelong learning. The importance of
staff development is clear but it does depend on health organisations having the
finances to deal with this. In NHS Trusts with high financial deficits, training budgets
are the first to go. Therefore, the question of who funds staff development is an
important issue as, ultimately, this aspect of quality underpins the health service
clinical governance theme.

PROFESSIONAL DEVELOPMENT AND CLINICAL SUPERVISION

Health care professionals are expected to engage in professional development
activities within their sphere of work. Leadership is key to this engagement in learning; through encouragement and direction staff can be motivated to recognise and
utilise alternative learning activities in order to keep up to date and fulfil professional body requirements. Learning can cover a spectrum of activities which relate
to direct involvement with clients/patients, relatives as well as colleagues and other
members of their health care team.

     Clinical supervision as an aspect of quality, which allows professional and team
growth, is generally influenced by two main issues:

- The nature and scope of the post and the intrinsic demands for giving information and helping others to understand, apply and use information
- Supporting and facilitating the learning and development of junior colleagues
and students.

There are many definitions of clinical supervision; one such definition, given by
Cassedy (2010: 5), is:

> A regular and formal agreement to engage in a professional working relation-
> ship, facilitated by the supervisor to support the supervisee to reflect on practice,
> with the aim of developing quality care, accountability, personal competence and
> learning.

Hawkins and Shohet (2012: 5) however go further to explore the wider aspect of
the notion of clinical supervision between the practitioner and client relationship
development, the quality of work and enhancement of self, practice and profession.

     The NMC (2008) noted that clinical supervision enabled registrant nurses to:

- Identify solutions to problems
- Increase understanding of professional issues
- Improve standards of patient care
- Further develop their skills and knowledge *and*
- Enhance their understanding of their own practice.

However, some professions allied to medicine see clinical supervision in a different light: a method of monitoring performance on an individual or team basis in order to establish that response times are being achieved in the case of paramedics, or that all vulnerable children are seen appropriately by social workers, and midwives have a system of statutory supervision through their Midwives Rules and Standards (NMC, 2010).

The clinical supervisor has an important role in helping the clinical supervisee achieve developmental growth through:

- Creating a context of curiosity for the supervisee
- Generating multiple perspectives on a situation
- Inviting supervisees to arrive at their own solutions
- Giving positive feedback
- Confirming a supervised person's ability
- Creating new perspectives on professional–patient relationships.

A contract for clinical supervision can clarify the expectations of this activity for both parties.

ACCOUNTABILITY AND QUALITY

Accountability for practice involves 'moving with the times' and not just relying on what was taught during initial training. Knowledge and skills from the past will not be adequate to meet the demands of today and the future. Therefore, professional responsibility involves being accountable for updating these areas and being research minded. The various professional bodies expect everyone to maintain a portfolio of evidence in order to demonstrate exactly this. Professional leaders should be able to assess whether individuals in the team are keeping up to date with current developments in order to maintain credibility and accountability. Accountability is about a personal and team philosophy of continuous improvement in order to improve patient care so that patient-centredness is embedded in professional day-to-day work. Martin (2001a, 2001b) identifies that quality care standards are linked with top decision making and highlights the role of health and social service bodies, which are accountable for strategically shaping the quality of our services for patients at present.

CONCLUSION

The main emphasis of this chapter has been to examine the concepts of quality and attempt to relate them to professional practice. An overview of quality in health care has been offered, and some of the historical developments and policy in quality have been highlighted – and then taken into the context of the contemporary health service, towards the concepts of patient safety, clinical governance, clinical audit, clinical effectiveness and clinical risk management. A number of quality models have been briefly explored. Finally, the importance of staff development and clinical supervision has been examined to reflect the relevance for leaders of developing and motivating their teams towards self-mastery – for the benefit of patients/clients and improvements in care.

Summary of Key Points

This chapter has identified the importance of leadership and quality in the health service in order to meet the identified learning outcomes:

- **Identify the importance of quality in the health service for better patient outcomes** This was discussed in the context of present quality agendas through a variety of policy drivers.
- **Critically explore the importance of patient safety and the aspect of human factors associated with safe care.** This was discussed in the context of the Care Quality Commission remit.
- **Discuss the historical developments that led to the present quality agenda** The historical developments towards the present quality NHS agenda related to a number of quality gurus and their influence on the health service and health care delivery.
- **Discuss the importance of clinical governance, audit, effectiveness and risk management** These aspects of contemporary policy were explored and debated within the finite resources of health services.
- **Compare a variety of quality models to inform effective leadership for continuous improvement of health care delivery** A number of models of quality including TQM, EFQM and the NHS Outcomes Framework were examined within the context of current patient care delivery.
- **Relate the importance of leadership in clinical supervision as a method of developing professional learning** The notion of leadership and clinical supervision, as elements of clinical governance, highlighted the requirement for identifying learning needs and planning for professional development.

FURTHER READING

Parsley, K. and Corrigan, P. (1999) *Quality Improvement in Healthcare: Putting Evidence into Practice* (2nd edn). Gloucester: Stanley Thornes (Publishers) Ltd.

Peters, T. and Waterman, R. (1988) *In Search of Excellence*. London: Harper Collins.

Stephens, L. (2010) 'Improving the service: working together to promote normal birth', *British Journal of Midwifery*, 18 (6): 348.

Williamson, G., Jenkinson, T. and Proctor-Childs, T. (2008) *Contexts of Contemporary Nursing* (2nd edn). Exeter: Learning Matters. Chapter 9.

Visit the companion website at https://study.sagepub.com/barr3e for more resources.

13 LEADERSHIP FOR CHANGE

INTRODUCTION

This chapter attempts to draw together the various notions of leadership and examine their effects on leading for change. Leadership during periods of change can be extremely difficult so it is important to know just how the information in the preceding chapters and the theories of effective change management can be used together in order to work in an effective and harmonious environment. Well-handled change is seen to be for the benefit of all rather than something that is imposed upon the workforce. Organisational change is also a complex and well-researched area. This chapter will explain the process of change management and discuss the behaviours that might be seen in the organisation during change. Experience dictates that in many situations the process of change is not given enough attention to ensure that it is as successful and painless as possible. It may seem difficult, at times of change, to think about the future – particularly when there appears to be government legislation-induced change after change. Few periods of history can be thought of as transforming but currently we appear to be living through one of those periods, particularly in health care. We are facing two major conflicting challenges: control of health care costs *and* the provision of quality care to all patients and clients.

These two factors are fundamentally altering the health care delivery system and so impact on the ability to lead effectively during change.

DEFINING CHANGE

Although change appears constant and indeed a frequent event in health and health care, it is not always clear what it means. There are a number of definitions of change. The BNET Business dictionary states that change is 'the coordination of a structured period transition from situation A to situation B in order to achieve lasting change within an organization' (www.change-management-coach.com accessed 11 November 2014). However Clarke and Copcutt (1997: 2) noted more complexity to the concept:

Change is not a single process or group of processes: It ... does not exist at all. It is an ideal, a story made by everyone who is experiencing discontinuity. Viewed as a cause of events, by others as a consequence, it can be the disease, diagnosis and the cure.

> ### ▶ Activity
>
> What do the above definitions mean to you?
>
> How could they relate to a recent personal change you have encountered?

The first could infer that change is about *moving* – like a house or a job move from one place to another. Or it could be more complex and depend on how you perceive it. A recent personal change involved the installation/movement of a new printer in my office. By the second definition, it involved buying a new printer with difficulty finding the ink cartridges (cause of events) and new printer cartridges being easily available and a scanning function as an added extra (consequence). There was a concern and indeed stress about learning how to use the printer and its connection to the Internet (disease). The benefit of taking time to read the manual and trying out various options means that there is an improved printing function but scanning and faxing is now possible – success (cure). From simple to complex definitions it appears that there will be some form of movement along a continuum which could be either linear (Figure 13.1) or cyclical (Figure 13.2).

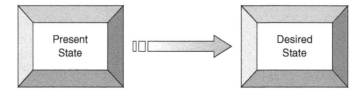

Figure 13.1   Linear continuum

However Freshwater (2014: 97) noted that 'change is not only inevitable and is also a fundamental aspect of being human'. She also alludes to the fact that change does not always equate to improvement and that the evidence and research for best practice for managing change appears to miss the *context* of how leaders facilitate a successful change and focus instead on the *process* of managing change.

LEADING CHANGE

There may be many examples of change in health care (see Table 13.1). Some involve very large projects such as changing NHS Trust structures and thus cultures

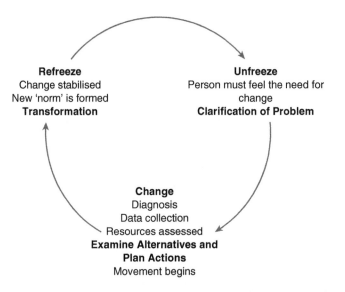

Figure 13.2 Cyclical process model. A combination of Lewin (1951) and Lippet et al. (1958)

Table 13.1 Some examples of changes in health care

- Advanced surgical, anaesthetic and medical treatments
- Cardio-pulmonary resuscitation techniques
- Rapid response treatment for patients with suspected stroke along with early discharge rehabilitation services
- Introduction of nursing led units in hospitals
- Innovation of wireless point of care systems. Clinical information systems are individualized in the electronic patient record (EPR) and the longitudinal electronic health record (EHR). The use of personal digital assistants (PDAs) and voice-over Internet protocol (VoIP) is developing.
- Diabetic, respiratory and cardiac care management by practice nurses
- Development of walk-in centres in the community
- SMS/ texting/ social media services to reduce rates of defaulted appointments or enhance health education
- How2trak software to improve wound care outcomes
- Online booking for better general practice access
- Development of skills such as Cognitive Behaviour Therapy (CBT), solution focused, promotional and motivational guidance therapies to enhance mental health of wellbeing in adults and children
- Setting up new local services to improve breast feeding rates, reduce post natal depression and address poverty and child protection issues through access to professional/ peer support.

and on the other side, others are quite small but all may have resonance with the health benefits for patients, clients and families. Ultimately these changes are about addressing *need* especially in an era of 'information revolution' and aligned health technology.

This array of examples are just a few in the changing world of health care innovations. If you get the opportunity to attend a professional conference, there are often a range of new ideas, research, health industry products and services that have been recently developed that you may want to consider in your own field of practice. As we develop professionally we are charged with the notion of improving care through innovation. MacPheem and Suryaprakash (2012) through project analysis research of 133 nurse leaders' year-long projects concluded that first-line nurse leaders were well able to successfully manage projects beyond their traditional scope of responsibilities. This highlights the nature of developing autonomy and responsibility in professional care.

From the plethora of published material on issues of change management, many models might seem relevant in the area of health and social care.

Ackerman (1997) identified three types of change:

- **Developmental change:** Planned or emergent incremental change focusing on the improvement of skills and processes
- **Transitional change:** Planned and more radical organisational change (based on the work of Lewin, 1951; Kanter, 1983)
- **Transformational change:** Radical organisational changes of structure, processes, culture and strategy based on learning and adaptation.

One widely recognised model of change, which is perhaps simplistic but well understood as in our first definition, is described by Lewin (1951), who suggests that there are three key stages to any change. These changes are:

1. **Unfreeze** or unlock from the existing level of behaviour
2. **Change** the behaviour or move to a new level
3. **Refreeze** the behaviour at the new level.

Lewin's three-stage model can be applied to almost all change situations in order to analyse the success and failure of the whole process. In 1958, Lippet et al. suggested a three-phase model to enhance Lewin's model:

- The **clarification** or diagnosis of the problem
- The **examination** of alternatives and establishing a plan of action for the change
- The **transformation** of intentions into actions to bring about change.

These two models jointly (Figure 13.2) create a useful cyclical process model that is applicable to the situation undergoing or requiring change. However, it should be noted that change in any health service is not always seen as being this simple.

Swansburg and Swansburg (1998) note other theorists, such as Havelock (1973) and Rogers (1983), who suggest more comprehensive staged models for change and innovation (Table 13.2).

Table 13.2 Rogers' (1983) vs Havelock's (1973) models of change

Rogers' (1983) Five Stage Diffusion of Innovation Model	Havelock's (1973) Six Stage Model
1 Awareness	1 Build Relationship
2 Interest	2 Diagnose Problem
3 Evaluation	3 Acquire Resources
4 Trial	4 Choose Solution
5 Adoption	5 Gain Acceptance
	6 Stabilisation and Self Renewal

Activity

Do you have any preference for Rogers' or Havelock's models?

It appears that Havelock, despite being an earlier model, has integrated the importance of relationships and people into the model. This reflects a focus on whether people in the team will actually identify with a need for change, which reinforces the importance of the leader in a changing situation.

Global leadership for developing multinational industries involves great change. Global managers, for example in banking, pharmaceutical, retail or car industries, face the arduous task of catalysing and steering change efforts and aligning extremely large and far-flung multinational corporations and certainly do this amidst ethical concerns. Change interventions that work in one country do not always work in another so health leaders must be aware of cultural beliefs, values and expectations when suggesting changes in their own organisation.

However it must be said that global and even national research and development in health care delivery is important and may trigger innovative ideas for developing, rather than directly importing, in a different context.

Activity

Have you read any recent clinical literature concerning your own specialism from abroad such as Europe, the USA, Australia or Asia?

You may have dismissed it as it was 'irrelevant or foreign'. Reflect on the relevant assumptions you held.

Time is always a problem for busy health care professionals working in practice and keeping up to date with literature and evidence. Bullen et al. (2014) note the challenge of conducting and integrating research into clinical practice and the difficulty of time constraints for practitioners engaging in research.

Having attended a few global and national conferences as well as procuring an RN licence abroad, the bigger picture is really helpful and I now appreciate there is much to learn from a broader global perspective. Health-related experience abroad helps us with the 'helicopter view of our own practice' and can proceed to plan for innovative changes. I remember being surprised with seeing whiteboards over patients' beds in the USA where nurses wrote and agreed the 'simple daily collaborative care plans/ goals' (this would follow a daily nursing health assessment). This felt 'patient agreed and centred' but was challenging for me against the backdrop of a reserved British and NHS culture. However I thought the alternative might be that UK patients/ families are often unaware of any informal/ formal daily assessment and plans for the day/ weeks. So now I question the notion of how we really involve patient and public communication in all health contexts. In retrospect, the USA and UK health cultures are so very different but I now believe a more open and transparent care partnership really is the way forward and opening myself to global evidence-based health care can advance medical and care innovation and change.

THE LEADER AS AN INSTRUMENT OF CHANGE

In previous chapters, we discussed the benefits of knowing about your leadership/ followership style (Chapter 1) and also your problem solving style (Chapter 2). Now we can take the perspective of the leader being an instrument of change. You, as a change leader, at any level, need to play to your strengths rather than your weaknesses/blind spots and use a reflective approach within your team when driving through change. It is important to remember that you will be seen as a role model and others will look to you for direction, motivation and commitment. The way you handle the process of change, the stress involved and the way you interact with others will determine the success or failure of the change project.

In order to ensure a successful change, then, the present situation must be considered and information gathered in order to set the direction for improvement. Galbraith's *star* model (2001) highlights the complexity of change within organisations, how change should 'fit' within a number of elements in the organisation and the interaction between all elements (see Jay Galbraith's article and model on his web page www.jaygalbraith.com/images/pdfs/StarModel.pdf). For example, changing the way tasks are carried out has implications for the organisational objectives, people, information, structures and rewards. Denison's (2009) model is maybe more advanced/ comprehensive, acknowledging the importance of culture and stability as well as the internal and external influences in complex change environments. Its elements of an internal and external focus as well as the features of:

- strategic mission/goals
- adaptability
- consistency and
- team involvement

are worthy of exploring to understand the relevance in your own analysis of any improvement, change or innovation you wish to consider.

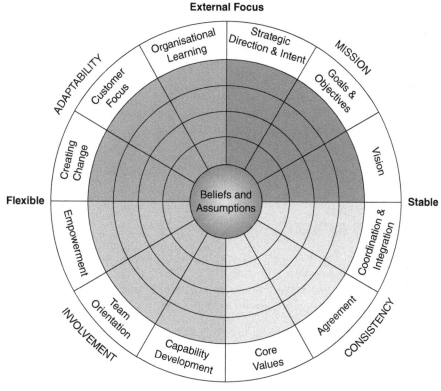

Figure 13.3   Denison's model of cultural change (2009)

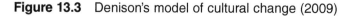

🔺 **Activity**

These models can be seen as very complex.

If you are new to your health care profession, do you agree?

(Continued)

(Continued)

What do you make of these for your own new leadership role?

If you have experience as a health care professional, what do you make of these for your own leadership role?

What action can you take to ensure you are considered a change leader?

It is useful to think of any new change in your clinical area and make notes about the wider aspects of change identified in these models; it may be that you would have liked more involvement or more development opportunities than have recently been promoted.

The NHS Institute for Innovation and Improvement (2009b) document relating to change in the health service noted five key areas for consideration for leaders when taking a team on an organisational or cultural change:

- Organisational Performance and Health
- The Discovery Process
- The Influence Model
- Change Architecture
- The Benefits Hierarchy.

This is really useful for the larger changes in health and is worth considering for smaller projects of innovation and change too. However the models above appear to have a top-down perspective. The 7-step RAPSIES model of change (Gopee and Galloway, 2009) may be a really useful 'step' framework for managing any change effectively.

The RAPSIES model focuses on the following steps:

- Recognising the need for an improvement in practice
- Analysing options for change-setting, identifying people involved
- Preparing for change – identifying change agent, the intended outcomes and education required
- Strategies for change process
- Implementing the change: piloting and timing
- Evaluation against intended outcomes
- Sustaining the change.

This change model gives more detail than Lewin's staged model and can be seen as a more democratic approach to change with a wide interpretation of where in the health industry this process may originate. So for instance a hospital porter who thinks there are too many patients waiting for hours on trolleys can provide a catalyst for change, as can a newly qualified health visitor who sees that there are conflicting health education messages for a 'back to sleep' policy from a paediatric orthopaedic department, or a health care assistant who is concerned that the speedy breakfast trolley routines in her ward do not allow enough time for more vulnerable older patients to be supported in helping them enjoy and eat their food.

RESPONSE TO CHANGE

Kramer (1974) identified a phenomenon described as the 'Reality Shock' that was seen to occur when a student nurse becomes a registered nurse. A conflict between the student nurse's expectations of the role and its reality in the work setting emerged. The four phases of role transition from student to professional identified in Chapter 11 are:

1. Honeymoon phase
2. Shock phase
3. Recovery phase
4. Resolution phase.

While Kramer's work related to a nursing scenario, these findings are well-known stages expected of any project change. It is natural that when a change is proposed there will be some reaction to the event. The point where the need for change becomes a desire to change is accepted as being pivotal and, therefore, the start of the movement process. If we take as an example the changes to moving and handling procedures, it was during the 1990s that the great risks of poor moving and handling practices in clinical care were identified. The RCN initiated change for professional groups amid little or no debate with external organisations. Due to the lack of involvement of care organisations, acceptance of change was not easy; there was no clear starting point and it is difficult to identify when the 'need for change' became a 'desire for change'.

Reactions to change are often surprising to change leaders because of the wide spectrum of emotions involved. Kubler-Ross (1970) identified ten potential reactions to bereavement. While her work examined the reactions to death and dying, the emotional features can be applied to all change – as those who experience the change are being drawn away from their comfort zone into an unknown area. The ten phases are highlighted in the resource on the companion website.

There are many reasons why resistance to change occurs, and leaders need to try and anticipate these and understand them as natural phenomena. Kotter and Schlesinger (1979) identified four key reasons:

- **Self interest:** People resist change if they perceive that they may lose out in some way. This could be as simple as loss of power or input in decision making. There are many individuals who simply resent being told what to do. Similarly, staff tend to think that their own approach is the best with sayings such as 'this is how it has always been done so why change' and 'if it ain't broke, don't fix it'.

- **Misunderstanding and lack of trust:** Strangely, efforts to create safer working systems can be negatively received and not trusted. It is vital that the leader engenders enthusiasm for the proposed change, letting all the team know what is happening at each stage in order to combat this element and take on board their individual issues into the change plan.
- **Low tolerance to change:** Some people are concerned with stability and security and find change daunting.
- **Different assessments or expectations:** There are often different perceptions of the change process held by the people involved and the costs of that change will be higher or lower for different groups. Indeed, the cost of the proposed change must be considered in influencing the outcome. The force-field analysis plays a large part in determining where change is needed and the cost of that change will lead to success. Conflict is seen when the benefits of a proposed change are biased towards one group's needs at the expense of another group. So if the change is seen to benefit only the organisational management structure but add further work for the workforce there is likely to be little cooperation with the process.

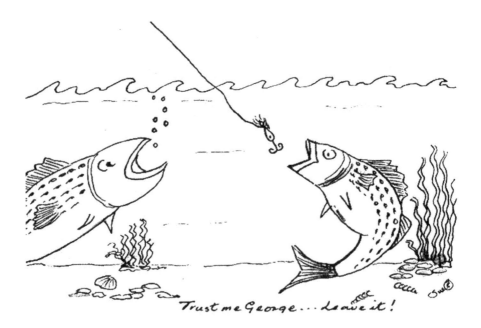

Trust me George... Leave it!

LEADING THE TEAM THROUGH CHANGE

Leaders need to assess the willingness of each individual to take on board change. There will be some people in the team who, inherently, do not like any sort of change and will demonstrate a low tolerance to any new initiatives. Within some areas of the health service there has been constant change over recent years and team members may exhibit signs of change fatigue in these rapidly developing areas due to constant patterns of change. However, there may be many levels of change makers and change resisters; within any team, there will be individuals who react to change in many different ways (Table 13.3).

This might seem quite a simplistic view and tends to categorise individual team members in relation to how they may react to change at one point in time rather than seeing individuals as changing as the process progresses.

◢ Activity

Think back to Chapter 2 (Leadership/Followership and MBTI® exercises) to see if you can spot any trends. Then ask yourself the following questions:

- Which behavioural pattern (below) do you most often adopt in response to change?
- Does your behaviour always fit this pattern or does it change depending on the situation or your maturity?

Table 13.3   Types of individuals (adapted from Rogers and Shoemaker, 1971)

Change (Progressivism) Innovator (Change Maker)	Proactive during the process of change, e.g. implements new policy or procedure
Early Adopter	Readily accepts the change, e.g. another professional adapts to the change
Early Majority	First group to follow early adopter, e.g. local team becomes involved in the change
Later Majority	Other groups follow suit, e.g. other teams introduce the policy
Laggards	A reticent group who tend to remain sceptical, although not openly hostile to change, e.g. colleagues who compare but do not take part
Rejecters (Change Resister) Status Quo (Traditionalism)	Openly oppose change, e.g. individuals resist becoming involved in the implementation of the policy

You will not be surprised to know that your attitude towards change depends on a number of factors; the situation you find yourself in has a great part to play together with whether you see the change as having a positive influence on your employment position. You might think of other factors that have influenced you in the past and made you behave like a laggard rather than an early adopter. It is now prudent to explore the effects of successful and unsuccessful change and the ways in which a leader can affect outcomes.

SUCCESSFUL vs UNSUCCESSFUL CHANGE

In health care provision, the need for change has never been greater, both in practice and management systems. The effective leader will recognise that change brings with it a number of feelings, including a sense of achievement, loss, pride and stress. As a leader, it is important that you understand the change development because leaders must be able to give a rationale for it and communicate an understandable plan to those who must manage the change and incorporate it into their lives (Malloch and Porter-O'Grady, 2005). Effective leaders will embrace change and lead health-care delivery forward; they will exhibit exceptional planning skills and be flexible in adapting to the change they have directly initiated.

As previously discussed, the feelings generated when change is imminent are similar to those experienced during bereavement or loss (Table 13.2). Unplanned change may be accidental or change by drift (Marquis and Huston, 2006: 171) – this is particularly noticeable when the *change is imposed* and a selection of obstructive behaviours may be seen. By contrast, during a change that is expected, rehearsed and informed, the behaviours exhibited are more complementary and positive in their manner. Planned change occurs because of an intended effort by the change agent. As a leader, you will need to be that change agent and make efforts in planning change carefully.

It is clear that initiating and coordinating change requires well-developed leadership and management skills. Dye (2000) goes as far as to say that one of the most fundamental values that differentiates effective leaders from average ones is the desire to 'make a difference'.

UNPLANNED CHANGE

> ### ◆ Activity
>
> Try to remember a time in your life that involved unnecessary or unplanned change.
>
> Why did you think it was unnecessary?
>
> Did it follow Lewin's or Lippet et al.'s model?
>
> What could have been done to make the change more acceptable?

A colleague told me about her shift patterns at work, in a local GP practice, being changed overnight and without any consultation. When she spoke to her manager, she was told that her contract allowed this to happen and that there was no need for consultation. My colleague was not happy and felt that she had to find new employment as there was no way the employers were going to change their minds.

Following her resignation, channels of negotiation were opened and an agreement was reached. Clearly when this situation is related to Lewin's model one can see that there was no opportunity for 'unfreezing', whereby the situation is recognised as requiring change, but the managers went straight to the 'change' element with very little success. Had the situation been handled differently, with discussion and information being offered throughout, there may not have been as much resistance to the change, thereby leading to greater success.

All too often leaders of change have a plan but do not share it or encourage input from others. They might not see the importance of effective communication. For example, if the plan/change is seen as short term, the leader can become short-sighted; if it is someone else's idea and is not 'owned' by the leader, communication can be weak. Whatever the situation we must all recognise that change occurs and so we must be able to plan in order to manage that change. One example of this could be government deliberations related to the recent amalgamation of the small regional ambulance services into larger organisations in order to deliver better care to the patient (DH, 2005a). The thinking supporting this change was of increasing efficiency and cutting costs, due to fewer people being paid at the higher end of the salary scale. The White Paper noted the opportunity to build on the significant improvements of the previous few years and a statement was made to improve radically the services provided. It set out how ambulance services can be transformed from a service focusing primarily on resuscitation, trauma and acute care towards becoming a mobile health resource for the whole NHS. The object was to improve leadership – both clinical and managerial – so that the organisational structure, culture and style matched new models of care. Unfortunately, in terms of communication to the people involved 'at the rock face', it was not sufficiently detailed. Ambulance personnel perceived the real change issue as being the effect on job security during and after the change. As such, the change took place in an atmosphere of distrust and uncertainty, which lasted for many months. Figure 13.4 depicts the effects on people when change is not handled well and very few people know what is happening, why it is happening, or how long the change will take.

All change cannot be contained, directed or managed. Unplanned change will continue to happen in a haphazard way but planned change will be targeted and purposeful. When managers make decisions that appear to be unrelated to current work practices it can be unsettling for the workforce. The uncertainty of the whole process means that decisions may be based on unspoken, sometimes unconscious assumptions about the organisation, its environment and future (Mintzberg, 1989), so resistance may be high. The common mistakes made when change is difficult or unsuccessful are:

- Inappropriate time scales
- Unclear aims
- Inadequate resources
- Ignoring knock-on effects
- Contamination in trying to change too many things at once

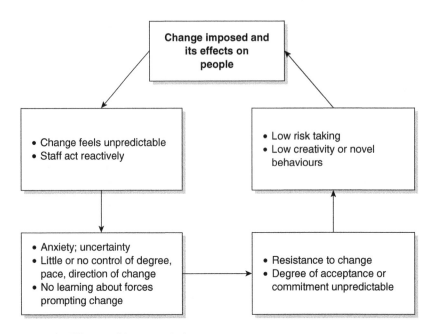

Figure 13.4 Effects of imposed change

- Hijacking – where someone who may wish to settle an old score tries to sabotage the new project
- Incorrect diagnosis – limited force-field analysis or knee-jerk reaction to solving the problem
- Lack of ownership.

PLANNED CHANGE

Planned change is well thought out, timely and necessary. The rhetoric of planned change features all the positive aspects of informing the workforce of what is happening and why. It is a reasoned and well-thought-out activity which will have a positive benefit for care delivery. In reality, the change might be thought to be well planned but there may be pockets of the workforce who have a less rosy view of it. Figure 13.5 depicts the effects on people when the change is handled well and everyone knows what is happening, why it is happening and how long the change will take.

Kotter and Schlesinger (1979) described a broader range of strategies a leader of change might consider in order to facilitate a more successful process. They are:

- Education and persuasion
- Participation and involvement
- Facilitation and support

- Negotiation and agreement
- Manipulation and co-option
- Implicit or explicit coercion
- Review and monitoring.

> ### ▶ Activity
>
> Can you think of a well-planned change in your practice area? Jot down which elements within Figure 13.5 were successful.

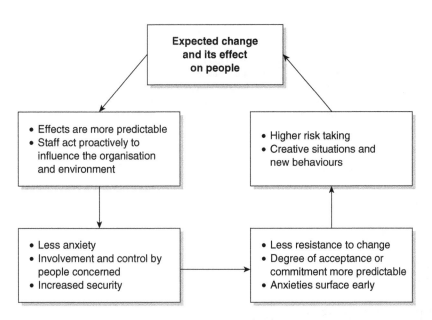

Figure 13.5   Effects of planned change

You might have thought of many instances where change was discussed and started well but hit difficulties, and the whole process became confused due to slippage or various interpretations of people's expectations. In hindsight you may have thought that those leading the change could have managed the change approach better. Bennis et al. (1985) identified three simple strategies to promote organisational or group change (see the resource on the companion website).

The diagram in Figure 13.6 depicts the notion that integrating all elements of change strategies is useful for successful change and no one strategy would achieve effective change alone.

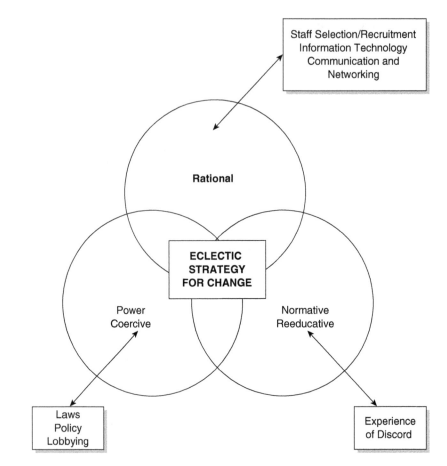

Figure 13.6　Strategies for change

EDUCATION AND PERSUASION

One of the most frequently used ways of minimising resistance to change is through educating people about the need for change. Education is vital during the 'unfreezing' stage of the change process. However, persuasion is required within the approach. There are a variety of approaches to education and persuasion that might be of help:

- The legal argument
- The ethical argument
- The financial argument
- The evidence argument
- Meeting professional standards.

PARTICIPATION AND INVOLVEMENT

It is important that staff, carers and those receiving care are involved in the decision-making process.

Facilitation and support

If negative feelings towards the change are exhibited then it is important to consider the empathetic and sympathetic approaches of facilitation. Training is usually seen as a good start to the support process, moving on to co-working and effective supervision during the change. Skilled facilitators should spend time preparing as well as understanding the factual content of the change.

Negotiation and agreement

As part of acceptance of the new methods and behaviours there may be issues for group agreement. In order to reach a consensus and agreement, it may be necessary to negotiate the way forward in small steps to allow the 'later majority, laggards and rejecters' to reach an acceptable outcome. However you reach the desired outcome you – as leader – must ensure that undue pressure is not placed on any single individual.

MANIPULATION AND CO-OPTION

If the change process is not working, it may be necessary to resort to a more subversive method in order to manipulate people to agree. Co-opting a hesitant member of staff to assist in the process may give them ownership and can be very effective in getting them 'on side'. Once this has been achieved they may bring others with them, so assisting in the smooth running of the process. Should you have a group member who is strongly opposed to the change, they may try to hijack the outcome and affect the dynamics of the group; the infiltration of a key supportive individual might assist in changing the views of that person.

IMPLICIT OR EXPLICIT COERCION

When all else fails, creating a power base where the change leader could offer some sort of reward for adhering to the change or punishment for resisting it can be resorted to. Some care organisations resort to considering disciplinary actions if the change is not implemented. This can only be considered as a last resort. It must be remembered that if punishment is the driving force behind the change then there is a very real possibility that, once these threats are removed, the resisting group will go back to their old ways.

REVIEW AND MONITORING

As with all changes there must be an evaluative period to conclude. The change should be measured and related to how well it has been accepted and adopted. The review needs to be ongoing in order to ensure that the old practices are not reverted to.

> ### ➤ Activity
>
> Have you been involved in a change situation where there was resistance to a particular change?
>
> Consider the way this resistance was overcome and make notes on the effect the change had on the group.

I can remember a time where we wanted to introduce 'pre-operative visiting' for all our patients so that they would know what to expect in the anaesthetic room. We did not want to tell the patients about the details of surgery in case of raising anxieties. At the time, it was felt that all patients would want to know what was going to happen to them in the anaesthetic; they were shown photographs of the anaesthetic environment, briefly told about the monitoring equipment to be used and any questions they wanted to ask were answered. Clearly, for one anxious patient this was too much information and he declined the operation. Following this episode the surgeon forbade the anaesthetic nursing staff from going near his patients. We had to write a script so that the surgeon could see what his patients were being told, but for a while we only went to see the patients if requested. The change had been implemented without full communication with all involved but, fortunately, a compromise was reached which served the needs of all concerned.

PROJECT MANAGEMENT

The activity of planning a project for change is a vital skill for experienced healthcare professional leaders. Project management can be defined as the discipline of planning, organising, securing and managing resources to bring about the achievement of objectives within a project. There are various models for project management, depending on the industry involved. Within health care the use of models ranging from the very simple (such as Assess, Plan, Implement and Evaluate) to quite complex ones (such as Prince2) is prevalent. In Prince2 there are clear procedures for roles and tight management of resources. The overall corporate management oversees the starting up, initiation, controlling of stages, managing boundaries, and project closure as separate entities.

In the early stages of your career, once qualified, you may be asked to lead out on a practice innovation or service improvement. You may well then link this request with change management and initially consider a simple approach to a project management activity. Buttrick (2005) noted the stages of project management are seen as:

- Initiating
- Planning
- Executing
- Monitoring
- Closing.

It is important, in all these stages, to communicate with a wide group of stakeholders in order for success to occur and become more externally as well as internally focused. Initially you will need to liaise and network with patients, colleagues and interested parties – in both an informal and a formal manner prior to perhaps writing a report proposing your ideas for the project to gain support from senior colleagues. These activities require a number of management tools, some of which may be new and some quite challenging. Iles and Sutherland (2001) provided a wide range of useful suggestions in supporting change in the NHS. One of the first useful activities is to examine the project issue using PEST (Political, Economic, Social and Technological) and SWOT (Strengths, Weaknesses, Opportunities and Threats) analyses with various stakeholders.

PEST ANALYSIS

Upton and Brooks (1995) note various perspectives related to change management which help in trying to see the need for change. These perspectives can be viewed as:

1. Very broad trends at a national and international level
2. Regional and localised changes that affect patterns of service delivery
3. The leader as an instrument of change.

The first two perspectives are very important in understanding why change may be necessary, but the third is vital if you are to lead change effectively. Without this understanding it would be very difficult for you as a leader or manager to ensure that what you are doing fits with prevailing trends in society and healthcare delivery.

POLITICAL CONTEXT

Recent policy changes concerning NHS Trusts and community-led services in a market health economy continue to focus on quality, performance standards and patient power. Public accountability, while still allowing for local decision making, is still on the agenda but a reduction in the bureaucracy of health service management is planned. All these changes are purported to squeeze more out of the NHS while devolving accountability and responsibility away from central government to a level closer to the patient.

ECONOMIC CONTEXT

Most of the developed world's governments are looking at ways in which they can contain health care expenditure by rationalising or prioritising treatments, setting ceilings on procedure costs and achieving cost improvements. There are attempts to integrate cost, quality and outcome in order to aid decision making by policymakers and planners.

SOCIAL CONTEXT

As the population lives longer, the cost of care is increasing for the vulnerable and chronically ill. This, alongside global mobility from countries with poorer health-care provision, is out of line with other demographic factors. There are also higher consumer expectations about the breadth and quality of services that are received. In addition, there is greater public sophistication in terms of understanding and choosing what is needed or wanted. All of these factors add to the overall cost of health and social care.

TECHNOLOGICAL CONTEXT

Discoveries in the fields of health care interventions, medicine and total health systems continue to reshape the NHS and look likely to accelerate. Of course, this aspect is harder to predict but potentially may have the greatest impact on health-care delivery. Overall, it requires a high degree of flexibility and ability to respond quickly and effectively to change within the service.

SWOT ANALYSIS

This tool was discussed in Chapter 2 for personal development. It was documented by Ansoff in the 1970s and 1980s; although the originator is uncertain, it is useful in all project management in its assistance in reviewing the internal environment of the local organisation.

Activity

Considering your own clinical team, populate the SWOT grid below.

Strengths	Weaknesses
Opportunities	Threats

You might have considered as strengths your team's commitment to high quality patient care and that you have a full complement of staff; under weaknesses you may identify occasional team conflict around duty rostering. Opportunity for clinical updates for both students and staff may be recorded and threats may come from the amalgamation of services across acute and primary care.

PLANNING FOR CHANGE

Once the broad view of the internal and external environments has been explored, the impact of the project needs to be seen in the context of the strength of the drivers for change. Lewin's (1951) force-field analysis is another useful tool to review the sustainability of any change envisaged.

Using a force-field analysis that includes both hard (quantitative) and soft (qualitative) factors, it is possible to depict how important the proposed change might be and to predict its success. An example of a part analysis might be seen when a new 12-hour working shift pattern is suggested (Figure 13.7).

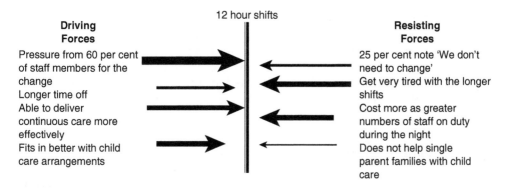

Figure 13.7 Force-field analysis for change related to implementing a 12-hour shift pattern

You can see from the strength of the arrows that some of the forces are much stronger than others, so that the overall need for change appears to be the stronger argument and it would, therefore, be useful to continue to plan for change. This change must be planned effectively and initially should be considered as a pilot project – with an evaluation date to see whether the change should continue.

> ◆ **Activity**
>
> Think of a situation, within your clinical area, where a change may be necessary and draw up a force-field analysis of the need for that change.

You might have found this relatively easy. Did it give the results you expected? Did it highlight the need for the proposed change? Often the results of such an exercise demonstrate that the proposed change is not quite as strongly required as first thought. It also helps to identify the restraining factors, so that appropriate strategies might be considered, but it is important to gather together a project team if you can so that you get a good picture of the current situation. This will help the team develop a sense of ownership of the proposed change. You could ask some of the following questions to indicate how ready for change the workplace team is:

1. How ingrained are the various forces?
2. Which ones are the most open to reduction?
3. What influence can we use to help overcome difficulties or constraints?
4. Are there things we need to find out in order to get a clearer picture of the local influences?

It is therefore prudent to consider the following when driving through a change in the workplace: direction, timescales, communication, resources, making change real, and job security (Table 13.4).

The GANTT chart was developed by Henry Laurence Gantt in the 1910s and is used to illustrate a schedule of activity, usually against a timeline. We probably do not realise that we use them in everyday life, for example when planning for a holiday or shopping for Christmas. There are many examples of GANTT charts on the Internet; Google the term and surf around the wide variation offered – most work on an Excel application principle which may be the easiest method for starting.

ACTION LEARNING SETS

More and more, action learning sets are utilised to facilitate change in the health service, although they can be seen as taking valuable resources in a time-strapped health service environment (Malloch and Porter-O'Grady, 2005: 153). Action learning sets help individuals see the need for change and bring their own personal

Table 13.4 Considerations for driving through change

Direction	Everyone clearly understands what is happening. There is a sense of purpose.
Timescales	Clear and relevant – may be achieved by using a GANTT chart.
Communication	If ineffectual then there are clear grounds for rumour, innuendo and gossip. Gets rid of hidden agendas.
Consultation	Staff need to be informed and involved at every stage of the change.
Resources	Time, money, people, materials – where will they come from and how will they be paid for? Increasingly, employers rely on goodwill that may lead to employee resentment.
Making change real	Involve yourself and behave in ways consistent with the change you are trying to bring about.
Job security	During organisational mergers and reconfigurations, people need to know their place in the new structure. They will not commit to change if their personal place is not secured.

relationship into the change process. Action learning is seen in the context of learning and reflection, supported by colleagues, with the purpose of change. It is based on the following principles of team working:

- Meeting regularly
- Consistent membership
- Addressing members' problem tasks
- Sharing, support, questioning
- Group success
- Review
- Facilitation.

In order for action learning to succeed, there is a need to agree the following ground rules:

- Confidentiality
- Commitment and continuity of attendance
- Clarity of objectives
- Constructive challenge
- Work as a group of peers
- Recognise individual strengths/limitations
- The role of the facilitator is clearly defined.

Scenarios for change are set up and the facilitator assumes a questioning stance. The whole group engages with helping individuals face their particular change difficulty. The elements in Figure 13.8 could be potential frameworks in order to ensure all involved recognise the change issues and have ownership of that process.

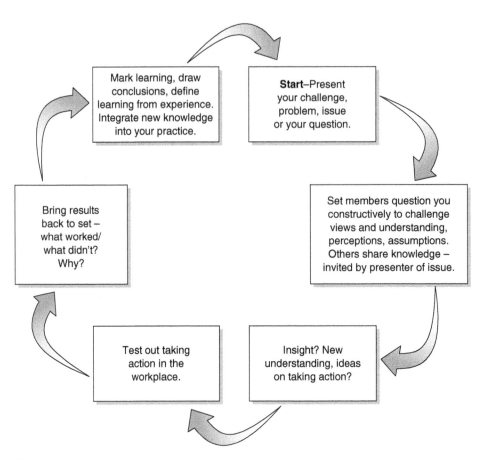

Figure 13.8 Action learning model

(*Source*: Revens, 2011)

Rayner et al. (2002) identify that action learning offers a unique opportunity to develop leadership skills in a safe, non-threatening situation. The ability of leaders or facilitators to analyse problems, gain personal confidence and identify solutions for change for the benefit of clinical effectiveness is paramount. Douglas and Machin (2004) emphasised the value of action learning sets for interdisciplinary collaboration in their grounded theory research in mental health.

The skills, knowledge and experience of the individuals whose responsibility it is to bring about change are varied and complex. It is vital that they consider the intricacies of people's response to change and how that might make the path to change difficult, full of barriers and pitfalls. Good preparation and planning of the process and involvement of interested parties at all stages helps to ensure appropriate support, encouragement and action, thus increasing the potential for successful change.

Summary of Key Points

This chapter has explored a variety of strategies that can lead to successful change. These are:

- **Explore change theory** A number of definitions, theories, models and perspectives have been utilised to reflect a breadth of theory underpinning the concept of change.
- **Discuss the need for effective leadership throughout the change process** The importance of leadership to shape change and lead people through the process of change was explored and there were a number of strategies proposed for effective leadership in this area.
- **Recognise effective change environments** Planned and unplanned change outcomes were discussed and the implications for success and difficulties were explored.
- **Debate the effects of change on individuals, groups and organisations** The varieties of effects of change on health care teams and individuals were debated and the impact on improving and changing care for patients and clients was highlighted.
- **Explore the value of Action Learning Sets in supporting change** This model of change was linked to the notion of team learning, problem solving and reflection using a facilitative approach.

FURTHER READING

Baulcomb, J.S. (2003) 'Management of change through force-field analysis', *Journal of Nursing Management*, 11: 275–80.

Butler, L. and Leach, N. (2011) *Action Learning for Change: A Practical Guide for Managers.* Cirencester: Management Books 2000 Ltd.

Davies, C., Finlay, L. and Bullman, A. (2000) *Changing Practice in Health and Social Care.* London: Sage/The Open University.

Gerrish, K. (2000) 'Still fumbling along? A comparative study of newly qualified nurses' perception of the transition from student to qualified nurse', *Journal of Advanced Nursing*, 32 (2): 473–80.

Gough, P. (2001) 'Changing culture and deprofessionalisation', *Nursing Management*, 7 (9): 8–9.

Paton, R. and McCalman, J. (2000) *Change Management: A Guide to Effective Implementation* (2nd edn). London: Sage.

Visit the companion website at https://study.sagepub.com/barr3e for more resources.

14 CONCLUDING THOUGHTS

INTRODUCTION

Malloch and Porter-O'Grady (2005: 180) state:

> Like any other pursuit, leadership is a journey. The only difference with regard to leadership is that leadership is a journey with no permanent destination.

This book has demonstrated how we might embark on that journey, support actions with theory, and successfully arrive at our individual and collective destinations. The leadership role reflects the journey of life and as such is not only confined to our professional role but also to how we conduct ourselves in the community as a whole. This chapter, therefore, attempts to highlight the discussions from all chapters and draw together elements of the leadership process through a variety of activities. By doing this you will be able to practise an integrative approach to leadership for yourself and perhaps change the behaviour of others around you.

Leadership is often seen as a cure for all difficulties in any organisation experiencing challenges and the health care industry is no different. Antrobus and Edmonds (1997) tell us that when change is imposed on the health service it reacts. Some health care professions have been seen traditionally to lack leaders. *The Future of Nursing* report from American research highlights the need for determined, visionary and skilled leadership from nurses able to access and influence at the highest level (Jasper, 2011: 419). The four key messages developed in the report are:

- Nurses should practise to the full extent of their education and training
- Nurses should achieve higher levels of education and training
- Nurses should be full partners with physicians and other health care professions in redesigning health care
- Effective workforce planning and policy-making require better data collection and information infrastructure.

Clearly while this focuses on the role of nursing in the USA there are important messages for all professions globally. It is, therefore, prudent to consider ways in which each of us can develop as potential leaders in the world of today and for tomorrow. Changes are occurring on a scale as important as those of the Industrial Revolution, and the health service needs to anticipate and respond to these changes. Education and training are vital to the plethora of changes (Health Education England (Lord Wills), 2015).

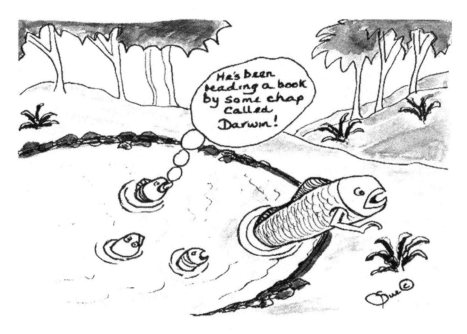

LEADING HEALTH CARE IN THE FUTURE

The speed of economic, political, social and technological change in today's world has implications for changing health services that are 'fit for purpose'. It is easy to look back to some glorious era, say, when the NHS was 'born' and believe that with a few adjustments we can go back to this health service where people were only too glad to be able to get their glasses provided by the NHS. The health services of the future will need to be very different and this requires leaders to push these developments through. Leaders need to have an 'eye' for the future and some literature evidence has tried to capture the notion of 'future building' exercises. This is seen as more than just crystal ball gazing, now being a management discipline in its own right. Rogers (1997: 1) signals that 'the future is a part of the consciousness of every human being', but highlights the assumption that 'Futures' studies are not predictable and it is not an exact science. Warner et al. (1998: 8) identify a number of reasons why it is important to look to the future. These are to:

- predict developments in the future
- provide early warning of potential opportunities as well as threatening developments
- stimulate a learning environment for creative ideas
- enable people to determine their own preferred future
- explore options
- support policy formation.

It is also important to note some of the following global trends:

- Information industry replacing manufacturing
- Increasing urbanisation
- More migration of peoples
- More fragmented family lives
- Persistence of economic inequalities
- Increasing elderly and also carer populations
- Declining birth rate and deferred child rearing
- A growing interest in environmental issues
- Increasing expectations – gerontocracy (power of older people) and better informed people requiring more health choices
- Various forms of health care privatisation
- Changing health care professional structures – more flexibility and more team working towards a generic workforce, providing better transparent accountability.

A new 2020 vision of health care environments explores the changing face of health care and the need to recognise the variety of possible environments where health care can be delivered, which moves away from a traditional and expensive model of care provision (Building Futures, 2001). A still relevant PSI Report, using multiple methodology research for forecasting, found that important medical developments from biotechnology were expected that would affect the food we eat, the ability for genetic profiling (Northcott, 1991: 217) and expected environmental issues in Britain. The PSI Report also highlighted the specific information technology revolution that would influence health services, through:

- Storage of patient records
- Diagnostic aids including kits for self diagnosis, based on computed tomography (CT scanning) and monoclonal antibodies and biosensors
- Epidemiological analysis
- Drug monitoring
- Surgical and medical interventions – use of fibre optics, lasers and lithotripters
- Aids for handicapping conditions
- Health care education, especially in distance learning applications.

However, it was noted that these developments would be constrained by budgets, information technology security, technical skills of staff and the culture in health and social care. Warner et al. (1998) also forecast that the following health challenges will present themselves:

- Increasing non-communicable diseases, for example, circulatory, cancer, gastrointestinal and metabolic disorders
- Increasing communicable diseases
- Nutritional issues
- Increase in mental ill health
- Increase in reproductive technologies.

The PSI report (Northcott, 1991: 303) also noted that accidents and violence were now seen as the main causes of morbidity in the under-30 age group. From these trends it is clear that there are going to be tensions in how health care services will cope with the demands on it. Will there be greater emphasis on primary care or acute care? Will cure and palliation override preventative services? How will those with a quiet voice get their health care services when those with a louder voice shout for their demands? What will be the impact of caring on families, especially as family life is more diverse and fragmented? How will the health care professional roles evolve?

Future scenarios for health care provision will be influenced by the wider global economy and also the national policies of the time. The increasing technological advancement noted by Wanless (2004) and Darzi (DH, 2008a) reports key health care drivers and now the delivery of the promised human genome may become more of a reality. Leaders need to consider these drivers for change and monitor the directions of the health service they provide.

Activity

- A leader has a role in ensuring the success of any change in the workplace by supporting participants of that change and challenging them to extend their practice.
- Consider how you would support your colleagues while developing your leadership role.
- List the attributes you feel are necessary to ensure you complete this role effectively.
- Consider which attributes you feel are strong in your leadership style.
- List and suggest how you can address the weaknesses you identified.

You may have considered a number of requisites highlighted when you completed the leadership/followership styles questionnaire (Chapter 2). Essentially you need to demonstrate awareness with regard to enhancing and developing leadership roles within your team, and develop the professional respect of colleagues together with the necessary expertise and experience to carry out the role. There are many other examples you might have identified. It is important to remember that when leading, effective goal setting must be applied and communicated so that everyone involved knows what is expected of them and can fulfil their potential. You may think of your role in terms of a flow chart like the one depicted in Figure 14.1, either cyclical or linear, so ensuring that all participants are 'kept in the loop'.

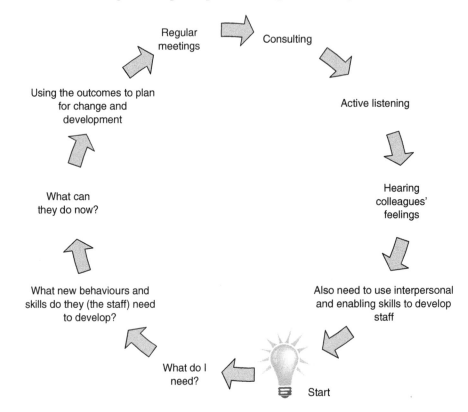

Figure 14.1   Forward planning and developing a leadership role

> ▶ **Activity**
>
> Drawing on all the concepts discussed within this book we can attempt to look to the future. Consider the changing role of the health care leader.
>
> - How would you design the basic competencies of the leader to reflect the needs of the twenty-first century in a technology healing context?
> - What knowledge would be essential for the processes of rework?
> - What protective skills would be necessary for the leader?
> - What would you leave behind that would not compromise the future value of health care provision?

Letting go of the past is a difficult exercise and requires careful analysis of what should be retained and what might be given up. If we consider the basic competencies of the health care leader we recognise that there is a need for better communication skills, so that everyone in the organisation knows what is happening and why. Similarly, there may be a case for changing work priorities; in the past, evidence suggested that 'holism' was the way forward rather than task orientation. It would be interesting to debate whether the constant demands put on health care services means this notion of holistic care is something of a luxury.

Ask the following questions in order to evaluate how you perform as a leader personally and as a leader within your clinical environment:

For me:

- How well am I doing?
- How do I compare with highly effective leaders – how should I be doing?
- What more should I aim to achieve to make it happen next year?
- What must I do to make it happen?
- What is my timetable for action and how shall I monitor progress?

For my clinical area:

- How well are we doing?
- How do we compare with similar clinical areas – how well should we be doing?
- What more should the clinical area do to make it happen?
- What must the clinical area do to make it happen?
- What should the clinical area's timetable for action be and how should progress be monitored?

The models of excellence enable you to set the results of your own diagnostic data against the evidence from highly effective leaders in other clinical areas. By asking these questions and then answering them, you should see more clearly the links between personal and clinical target setting and achieve a more coherent approach to your role in clinical improvement and leadership.

It is vital that effective health care leaders in the future take cognisance of the theories related to leadership. This book has attempted to demonstrate how this can be done in a variety of situations; it offers some solutions and ways in which you can apply theory to practice in a variety of health care settings. In the words of Nelson Mandela:

It is better to lead from behind and to put others in front, especially when you celebrate victory when nice things occur. You take the front line when there is danger. Then people will appreciate your leadership.

(Cited at: www.nelsonmandelas.com/mandela-quotes.php
accessed 21 November 2014)

REFERENCES

Acheson, D. (1998) *The Independent Inquiry into Inequalities in Health*. London: HMSO.

Ackerman, L. (1997) 'Change in development, transition or transformation: the question of change in organisations', in D. Van Eynde, J. Hoy and D. Van Eynde (eds) (2004) *Organisation Development Classics*. San Francisco, CA: Jossey-Bass.

Ackoff, R.L. (1981) 'The art and science of mess management', in C. Maby and B. Mayonwhite (eds) (1993) *Managing Change* (2nd edn). London: Paul Chapman, Open University, pp. 47–54.

Ackoff, R.L. and Greenburg, D. (2008) *Turning Learning Right Side Up*. Mahwah, NJ: Pearson Prentice Hall.

Adair, J. (1997) *Decision Making and Problem Solving*. London: Institute of Personnel and Development.

Adair, J. (2003) *The Inspirational Leader. How to Motivate, Encourage and Achieve Success*. London: Kogan Page.

Adair, J. (2006) *How to Grow Leaders*. London: Kogan Page.

Adair, J. (2010) *Develop your Leadership Skills*. London: Kogan Page.

Agor, W.H. (1986) 'Intuition: the new management tool', *Nursing Success Today*, 1: 23–4.

Akerjordet, K. and Severinsson, E. (2010) 'The state of the science of emotional intelligence related to nursing leadership: an integrative review', *Nursing Management*, 18 (4): 363–82.

Almost, J. (2006) 'Conflict within nursing work environments: concept analysis', *Journal of Advanced Nursing*, 53 (4): 444–53.

Almost, J., Doran, D., McGillis Hall, L. and Spence Laschinger, H.K. (2010) 'Antecedents and consequences of intra-group conflict amongst nurses', *Journal of Nursing Management*, 18 (8): 981–92.

Alvesson, M. and Spicer, A. (eds) (2010) *Metaphors We Lead By: Understanding Leadership in the Real World*. Abingdon: Routledge.

Anonson, J., Walker, M.E., Arries, E., Maposa, S., Telford, P. and Berry, L. (2014) 'Qualities of exemplary nurse leaders perspectives of frontline nurses', *Journal of Nursing Management*, 22: 127–36.

Ansoff, H.I. (1987) *Corporate Strategy* (revised edn). London: Penguin Books.

Antrobus, S. and Edmonds, J. (1997) *Nursing Leadership: Study Guide*. MSc Nursing Module NUM63U. London: RCN Institute.

Apekay, T.A., McSorley, G., Tilling, M. and Siriwardena, A.N. (2011) 'Room for improvement? Leadership, innovation culture and uptake of quality improvement methods in general practice', *Journal of Evaluation in Clinical Practice*, 17 (2): 311–18.

Armstrong, M. (1990) *How to be a Better Manager* (3rd edn). London: Kogan Page.

Askey, D. (2011) 'Best practice in audit', *Nursing Standard*, 25 (19): 51.

Avery, A.J., Barber, N., Ghaleb, M., Franklin, B.D., Armstrong, S., Crowe, S., Dhillon, S., Freyer, H., Howad, R., Pezzolesi, C., Serumaga, B., Swanwick, G. and Talabi, O. (2012) *Investigating the Prevalence and Causes of Prescribing Errors in General Practice*. Available at: www.gmc-uk.org/Investigating_the_prevalence_and_causes_of_prescribing_errors_in_general_practice___The_PRACtICe_study_Reoprt_May_2012_48605085.pdf (accessed 9 November 2014).

Bach, S. and Ellis, P. (2011) *Leadership, Management and Team Working in Nursing*. Exeter: Learning Matters.

Baker, S. (2007) 'Followship: the theoretical foundation of a contemporary construct', *Journal of Leadership and Organizational Studies*, 18 (1): 50–60.

Bales, R.F. and Strodtbeck, F.L. (1951) 'Phases in group problem solving', *Journal of Abnormal and Social Psychology*, 46: 485–95.

Bandler, R. and Grindler, J. (1990) *Frogs into Princes: Introduction to Neurolinguistic Programming*. London: Eden Grove Editions.

Barge, J.K. (1996) 'Leadership skills and dialectics of leadership in group decision making', cited in P.G. Northouse (2001) *Leadership: Theory and Practice* (2nd edn). London: Sage.

Barr, H. (2002) *Interprofessional Education Today, Yesterday and Tomorrow: A Review*. London: LTSN HS&P.

Barr, J. and Dowding, L. (2008) *Leadership in Health Care*. London: Sage.

Barr, J. and Dowding, L. (2012) *Leadership in Health Care* (2nd edn). London: Sage.

Barzey, S. (2005) 'Dealing with difficult people and situations', *Nursing Times*, 101 (16): 62–3.

Bass, B. (1985) *Leadership and Performance Beyond Expectations*. New York: Free Press.

Bass, B. and Avolio, B.J. (1990) 'Developing transformational leadership: 1992 and beyond', *Journal of European Industrial Training*, 14: 21–7.

Bassett, C. (ed.) (1999) *Clinical Supervision – A Guide for Implementation*. London: Nursing Time Books.

BBC (2012) 'Which is the world's biggest employer?' Available at: www.bbc.co.uk/news/magazine-17429786 (accessed 20 January 2015).

Beauchamp, T.L. and Childress, J.F. (2001) *Principles of Biomedical Ethics* (5th edn). New York: Oxford University Press.

Belbin, R.M. (2000) *Beyond the Team*. London: Routledge.

Bender, M., Connelly, C. and Brown, C. (2013) 'Interdisciplinary collaboration: the role of the clinical leader', *Journal of Nursing Management*, 21: 165–74.

Benner, P. (1984) *From Novice to Expert – Excellence and Power in Clinical Nursing Practice*. Reading, MA: Addison Wesley.

Benner, P. and Tanner, C. (1987) 'Clinical decision making: how expert nurses use intuition', *American Journal of Nursing*, 87 (1): 23–31.

Bennett, M. (1986) 'A development approach to training for intercultural sensitivity', *International Journal of Relations*, 10: 179–96.

Bennis, W.G. (1999) 'The leadership advantage', *Leader to Leader*, 12: Spring.

Bennis, W.G. and Nanus, B. (1985) *Leadership Leaders: Strategies for Taking Charge*. New York: Harper & Row.

Bennis, W.G. and Nanus, B. (2004) *Leaders: Strategies for Taking Charge* (2nd edn). New York: Harper Collins.

Bennis, W.G. and Shepherd, H.A. (1956) 'A theory of group development', *Human Relations*, 9: 415–37, in P. Hartley (1997) *Group Communication*. London: Routledge.

Bennis, W.G., Benne, K. and Chin, R. (eds) (1985) *The Planning of Change* (4th edn). New York: Holt, Reinhart, Winston.

Bennis, W.G., Parikh, J. and Leesom, R. (1994) *Beyond Leadership: Balancing Economics, Ethics and Ecology*. London: Blackwell.

Bergman, E. (2014) 'Managing conflict in clinical health care with diminished reliance on third party intervention forging an ethical and legal mandate for effective physician–patient communication', *Cardozo Journal of Conflict Resolution*, 15, 473–9.

Bernhard, L.A. and Walsh, M. (1995) *Leadership: Key to Professionalization of Nursing* (3rd edn). St Louis, MO: Mosby.

Berry, L., Zeithaml, V. and Parasuraman, A. (1988) 'The service quality puzzle', *Business Horizon*, Sept.–Oct.: 35–43, in M. Moullin (2002) *Delivering Excellence in Health and Social Care*. Buckingham: Open University Press.

Berwick, D. (2013) *A Promise to Learn – A Commitment to Act: Improving the Safety of Patients in England*. London: Department of Health.

Bishop, V. (2009) *Leadership for Nursing and Allied Health Care Professionals*. Milton Keynes: Open University Press.

Blake, R.R. and McCanse, A.A. (1991) *Leadership Dilemmas – Grid Solutions*. Houston, TX: Gulf.

Blake, R.R. and Mouton, J.S. (1985) *The Managerial Grid 111*. Houston, TX: Gulf.

Bloom, B. (1956) *Taxonomy of Educational Objectives, Handbook I: The Cognitive Domain*. New York: McKay Company.

Bolam v Friern Hospital Management Committee [1957] 2 All ER 118 [1957] 1.

Borton, T. (1970) *Reach Touch and Teach*. London: Hutchinson.

Borrill, C., West, M., Shapiro, D. and Rees, A. (2000) 'Team-working and effectiveness in the NHS', *British Journal of Health Care Management*, 6: 364–71.

Boylan, O. and Loughrey, C. (2007) 'Developing emotional intelligence in GP trainers and registrars', *Education for Primary Care*, 18 (6): 745–8.

Bradbury-Jones, C., Sambrook, S. and Irvine, F. (2007) 'Power and empowerment in nursing: a fourth theoretical approach', *Journal of Advanced Nursing*, 62 (2): 258–66.

Brake, T. (1997) *The Global Leader: Critical Factor for Creating the World Class Organisation*. Chicago, IL: Irwin Professional Publishing.

Buchanan, D. and Badham, R. (2008) *Power, Politics and Organizational Change: Winning the Turf Game*. London: Sage.

Buchanan, D. and Huczynski, A. (2004) *Organizational Behaviour* (5th edn). London: Prentice Hall.

Buchanan, D. and Huczynski, A. (2010) *Organizational Behaviour* (8th edn). London: Prentice Hall/Financial Times Management.

Buckenham, M.A. (1988) 'Student nurse perception of the staff nurse role', *Journal of Advanced Nursing*, 13: 662–70.

Buckingham, C. and Adams, A. (2000) 'Clarifying clinical decision making: interpreting nursing intuition, heurists and medical diagnosis', *Journal of Advanced Nursing*, 32 (4): 990–8.

Buckley, C., Cooney, K., Sills, E. and Sullivan, E. (2014) 'Implementing the safety thermometer tool in one NHS Trust', *British Journal of Nursing*, 23 (5): 268–72.

Bucknall, T. (2000) 'Critical care nurses' decision-making activities in the natural setting', *Journal of Clinical Nursing*, 9 (1): 25–36.

Building Futures (2001) *Building a 2020 Vision: Future Health Care Environments*. Available at: www.building futures.org.uk/assets/downloads/pdffile_1.pdf (accessed 31 May 2011).

Bullen, T., Maher, K., Rosenberg, J.P. and Smith, B. (2014) 'Establishing research in a palliative care clinical setting: perceived barriers and implemented strategies', *Applied Nursing Research*, 27 (2014): 78–83.

Burns, J.M. (1978) *Leadership*. New York: Harper and Row.

Butler, K.M. and Hardin-Pierce, M. (2005) 'Leadership strategies to enhance the transition from nursing student role to professional nurse', *Nurse Leadership Forum* 2005, Spring, 9 (3): 110–17.

Buttrick, R. (2005) *Project Workout* (3rd edn). Harlow: Pearson Education.

Cable, D.M. and Parsons, C.K. (2001) 'Socialisation tactics and person–organisation fit', *Personnel Psychology*, 54 (1): 1–24.

Cardwell, M., Clark, L. and Meldrum, C. (1996) *Psychology for A-Level*. London: Collins Educational.

Carlyle, T. (1841) *On Heroes and Hero Worship and Heroic in History*. Boston, MA: Adams.

Carnes, K., Cottrell, D. and Layton, M.C. (2004) *Management Insights: Discovering the Truths to Management Success*. Dallas, TX: Cornerstone Leadership Institute.

Cassedy, P. (2010) *First Steps in Clinical Supervision*. Maidenhead: Open University Press/McGraw-Hill Education.

Castledine, G. (1998) *Writing, Documentation and Communication Skills for Nurses*. London: Quay Books.

Catchpole, K. (2011) *Towards a Working Definition of Human Factors in Healthcare*. Available at: http://chfg.org/definition/towards-a-working-definition-of-human-factors-in-healthcare/ (accessed 18 September 2014).

Centre for the Advancement of Interprofessional Education (CAIPE) (1997) 'Interprofessional Education: A Definition.' CAIPE Bulletin 13.

Cemi,T., Curtis, G.J. and Colmar, S.H. (2012) 'Cognitive-experiential self theory and conflict-handling styles', *International Journal of Conflict Management*, 23 (4): 362–81.

Chan, J.C.Y., Sit, E.N.M. and Lau, W.M. (2014) 'Conflict management styles, emotional intelligence and implicit theories of personality of nursing students: a cross sectional study', *Nurse Education Today*, 34: 934–9.

Chartered Institute of Management Accountants (CIMA) (1998) *Organisational Management and Development* (3rd edn). London: BPP.

Clarke, J.E. and Copcutt, L. (1997) *Management for Nurses and Healthcare Professionals*. London: Churchill Livingstone.

Clawson, J. (2009) *Level Three Leadership: Getting Below the Surface* (5th edn). Upper Saddle River, NJ: Prentice Hall.

Clinical Human Factors Group (CHFG) (2014) *What is Human Factors?* Available at: http://chfg.org/what-is-human-factors (accessed 18 September 2014).

Collins, J. (2001) 'Level 5 leadership: the triumph of humility and fierce resolve', *Harvard Business Review*, January: 67–76.

Commissioning for Quality and Innovation (CQUIN) (2013): *2013/14 Guidance*. London: NHS Institute.

Cooke, H. (2006) 'Scapegoating and the unpopular nurse', *Nurse Education Today*, 27: 177–84.

Cooper, S., Kinsman, L., Buykx, P., McConnell-Henry, T., Endacott, R. and Scholes, J. (2010) 'Managing the deteriorating patient in a simulated environment: nursing students' knowledge, skill and situation awareness', *Journal of Clinical Nursing*, 19 (15–16): 2309–18.

Cortis, J. (2003) 'Managing society's differences and diversity', *Nursing Standard*, 18 (14, 15, 16): 33–9.

Coulter, A. (2011) *Engaging Patients in Healthcare*. Maidenhead: Open University Press/McGraw Hill.

Council of Europe/European Court of Human Rights (2010) *European Convention of Human Rights*. Strasburg: European Court of Human Rights and Council of Europe.

Covey, S. (2004) *The Seven Habits of Highly Effective People: Powerful Lessons in Personal Change* (15th anniversary edn). London: Simon and Schuster.

Cox, C. (2010) 'Legal responsibility and accountability', *Nursing Management*, 17 (3): 18–20.

Crainer, S. (1996) *Key Management Ideas*. London: Pitman.

Crinson, I. (1999) 'Clinical governance: the new NHS, new responsibilities', *British Journal of Nursing*, 8 (7): 449–53.

Crosby, P.B. (1984) *Quality Without Tears*. New York: McGraw-Hill.

Cunningham, I. (1986) 'Leadership development – mapping the field' (unpublished paper). Ashbridge Management College, Berkhamstead.

Cyert, R.M. and March, J.G. (1963) *A Behavioural Theory of the Firm*. London: Prentice Hall.

Dackert, I. (2010) 'The impact of team climate for innovation on wellbeing and stress in elderly care', *Journal of Nursing Management*, 18: 302–10.

Daft, R., Kendrick, M. and Vershina, N. (2008) *Management*. Hampshire, UK: South-Western Cengage Learning.

Daft, R.L. (2005) *The Leadership Experience* (3rd edn). Canada: Thomson South-Western.

Daft, R.L. (2006) *The New Era of Management* (international edn). Canada: Thomson South-Western.

Daft, R.L. (2008) *The Leadership Experience* (4th edn). Canada: Thomson South-Western.

Daft, R.L. (2010) *The Executive and the Elephant*. San Francisco, CA: John Wiley and Son.

de Bono, E. (1990) *Lateral Thinking: Creativity Step By Step*. New York: HarperCollins.

Deming, W.E. (1986) *Out of the Crisis*. Cambridge: Cambridge University Press.

Denison, D.R. (2009) *Denison Model*. Available at: www. denisonconsulting.com/knowledge-center/model (accessed 11 May 2015).

Department of Health (DH) (1974) *Health and Safety at Work Act*. London: HMSO.

Department of Health (1997a) *The New NHS: Modern Dependable*. London: Department of Health.

Department of Health (1997b) *Report on the Review of Patient Identifiable Information (The Caldicott Report)*. London: Department of Health.

Department of Health (1998) *A First Class Service: Quality in the New NHS Health Services*. London: The Stationery Office.

Department of Health (1999a) *Health and Safety at Work Act* (revised). London: HMSO.

Department of Health (1999b) *Management of Health and Safety at Work Regulations*. London: HMSO.

Department of Health (2000a) *The NHS Plan*. London: The Stationery Office.

Department of Health (2000b) *An Organisation with Memory*. London: Department of Health.

Department of Health (2001a) *Agenda for Change*. London: Department of Health.

Department of Health (2001b) *Essence of Care*. London: The Stationery Office.

Department of Health (2002) *Learning from Bristol: the Department of Health's Response to the Report of the Public Inquiry in Children's Health Surgery at the Bristol Royal Infirmary 1984–1995 (Kennedy Report)*. London: The Stationery Office.

Department of Health (2004a) *The NHS Knowledge and Skills Framework (NHS KSF) and the Development Review Process*. London: The Stationery Office.

Department of Health (2004b) *Modernising Medical Careers – The Next Steps*. London: The Stationery Office.

Department of Health (2005a) *Taking Health Care to the Patient: Transforming NHS Ambulance Services*. London: Department of Health.

Department of Health (2005b) *Health and Safety Act*. London: HMSO.

Department of Health (2006a) *Our Health, Our Care, Our Say: A New Direction for Community Services*. London: The Stationery Office.

Department of Health (2006b) *Integrated Governance Handbook – A Handbook for Executives and Non-executives in Health Care Organisations.* London: Department of Health.

Department of Health (2006c) *Modernising Nursing Careers – Setting the Direction.* London: The Stationery Office.

Department of Health (2007) *Capacity and Capability: Building the Workforce.* London: The Stationery Office.

Department of Health (Darzi) (2008a) *High Quality Care For All – NHS Next Stage Review Final Report.* London: The Stationery Office.

Department of Health (2008b) *A High Quality Workforce: NHS Next Stage Review.* London: The Stationery Office.

Department of Health (2008c) *The Secretary of State for Health's Response to Aspiring to Excellence: Final Report of the Independent Enquiry into Modernising Medical Careers.* London: The Stationery Office.

Department of Health (2010a) *Equity and Excellence: Liberating the NHS.* London: The Stationery Office.

Department of Health (2010b) *Achieving Equity and Excellence for Children.* London: The Stationery Office.

Department of Health (2010c) *Healthy Lives, Healthy People: Our Strategy For Public Health.* London: The Stationery Office.

Department of Health (2010d) *How to Use Essence of Care.* London: The Stationery Office.

Department of Health (2010e) *Protection of Vulnerable Adults Scheme Record: Retention and Disposal.* London: The Stationery Office.

Department of Health (2012) *Health and Care Social Act.* Available at: www.legislation.gov.uk/ukpga/2012/7/contents/enacted (accessed 11 May 2015).

Department of Health (2014) *Post-Legislative Assessment of The Health and Social Care Act.* London: The Stationery Office.

Department of Health (2015) *No Secrets: Guidance on Developing and Implementing Multi-agency Policies and Procedures to Protect Vulnerable Adults from Abuse.* London: Department of Health.

Department of Health, Social Services and Public Safety (DHSSPS) (2006) *The Quality Standards for Health and Social Care.* Belfast. Available at: www.dhsspsni.gov.uk/qpi_quality_standards_for_health___social_care.pdf (accessed 18 September 2014).

Dilts, R. (2006) *Sleight of Mouth.* Capitola, CA: Meta Publications.

Doherty, C. and Doherty, W. (2005) 'Patients' preferences for involvement in clinical decision-making in secondary care and the factors that influence their preferences', *Journal of Nursing Management,* 13 (2): 119–27.

Donahue, M.P. (2011) *Nursing – The Finest Art* (3rd edn). St Louis, MO: Mosby.

Donebedian, A. (1966) 'Criteria and standards for quality assessment and monitoring', *Quality Rev. Bulletin,* 2 (3): 99–100.

Douglas, S. and Machin, T. (2004) 'A model for setting up interdisciplinary collaborative working in groups: lessons from an experience of action learning', *Journal of Psychiatric and Mental Health Nursing,* 11 (2): 189–93.

Dowding, L. and Barr, J. (2002) *Managing in Health Care: A Guide for Nurses, Midwives and Health Visitors.* London: Pearson Education.

Driscoll, J. (2007) *Practicing Clinical Supervision: A Reflective Approach for Healthcare Professionals.* Philadelphia, PA: Balliere Tindall, Elsevier. www.nottingham.ac.uk/nmp/sonet/rlos/placs/critical_reflection/models/driscoll.html (accessed 20 March 2014).

Drucker, P.F. (1967) 'The effective executive', in H. Flanagan and P. Spurgeon (1996) *Public Sector Managerial Effectiveness*. Milton Keynes: Open University Press.

Drucker, P.F. (1989) *The Practice of Management*. London: Heinemann.

Dunitz, M. (1995) *Clinical Audit*. London: Martin Dunitz Ltd.

Dye, C.F. (2000) 'Leadership in healthcare. Values at the top', in B.L. Marquis and C.J. Huston (2006) *Leadership Roles and Management Functions in Nursing: Theory and Application*. Philadelphia, PA: Lippincott Williams & Wilkins.

Early Intervention Foundation (2014) *Early Intervention in Domestic Violence and Abuse*. Available at: www.eif.org.uk/wp-content/uploads/2014/03/Early-Intervention-in-Domestic-Violence-and-Abuse-Full-Report.pdf_ (accessed 21 October 2014).

Egan, G. (2013) *The Skilled Helper* (10th revised international edn). London: Cengage Learning Inc.

Erickson, M.H. (2002) *The Seminars of Milton H. Erickson: Presentation to the San Diego Society of Clinical Hypnotherapy No. 1 (Seminars of Milton H. Erickson)*. Phoenix, AZ: The Milton H. Erickson Foundation Press.

Espenshade, T. and Radford, A.W. (2009) *No Longer Separate, Not Yet Equal: Race and Class in Elite College Admission and Campus Life* (2nd edn). Woodstock, UK: Princeton University Press.

Etzioni, A. (ed.) (1969) *The Semi-Professions and their Organization*. London: Collier-Macmillan.

European Foundation for Quality Management (EFQM) (2014) *The EFQM Excellence Model: Public and Voluntary Sectors*. Brussels: EFQM. Available at: www.efqm.org/the-efqm-excellence-model (accessed 11 May 2015).

Eyler, J. and Giles, D.E. Jr (1999) *Where's the Learning in Service-Learning?* San Francisco, CA: Jossey-Bass.

Farrell, G. (2001) 'From tall poppies to squashed weeds: why don't nurses pull together more?', *Journal of Advanced Nursing*, 35 (1): 26–33.

Fayol, H. (1925) *General and Industrial Management*. London: Pitman and Sons.

Fiedler, F.E. (1967) *A Theory of Leadership Effectiveness*. New York: McGraw-Hill.

Firth-Cozens, J. (1998) 'Celebrating teamwork', *Quality in Health Care*, 7: S3–S7.

Flaum, S.A. (2009) *Big Shoes Leadership: How Successful Leaders Grow Into New Roles*. New York: Leadershape Publishing.

Fleming, N. (2010) VARK: A Guide to Learning Styles. Available at: www.vark-learn.com/home (accessed 11 May 2015).

Fletcher, L. and Buka, P. (1999) *A Legal Framework for Caring*. London: Macmillan.

Flin, R. and Maran, N. (2004) 'Identifying and training non-technical skills for teams in acute medicine', *Quality and Safety in Health Care* 13(1): i80–i84.

Flynn, J.R. (2009) *What is Intelligence?: Beyond the Flynn Effect* (expanded paperback edn). Cambridge: Cambridge University Press.

Foot, M. and Hook, C. (1996) *Introducing Human Resource Management*. London: Longman.

Ford, J. (2006) 'Discourses of leadership: gender, identity and contradiction in a UK public sector organisation', *Leadership*, 2 (1): 77–99.

Forsyth, D.R. (2010) *Group Dynamics* (5th edn). California: Wadsworth Cengage Learning.

Foucault, M. (1995) *Discipline and Punish: The Birth of the Prison*. New York: Vantage Books.

Francis, R. (2013) *Report of the Mid-Staffordshire NHS Foundation Trust Public Enquiry: Executive Summary*. Chaired by Robert Francis QC. Available at: http://books.google.co.uk/books?hl=en&lr=&id=5K89wKY3RoMC&oi=fnd&pg=PA3&dq=francis+report+201

3&ots=B8Ptebd48O&sig=d3T23CGcEwd6gkMc4Z697xLGNsk#v=onepage&q=fran cis%20report%202013&f=false (accessed 22 November 2014).

Freidson, E. (1970) *Profession of Medicine: A Study of the Sociology of Applied Knowledge.* Chicago, IL: University of Chicago Press.

French, W.L. and Bell, C.H. (1990) *Organization Development: Behavioural Science Interventions for Organization Improvement* (4th edn). London: Prentice Hall.

Freshwater, D. (2014) 'Board editorial: the challenge of global leadership: managing change, leading movement', *Journal of Research in Nursing*, 19 (2): 93–7.

Freud, S. (1911) *Interpretation of Dreams* (3rd edn) (trans. A.A. Brill). USA: Plain Label Books.

Frew, D.R. (1977) 'Leadership and followership', *Personnel Journal*, 54 (2): 90–7.

Full Gospel Businessman's Training (2014) www.fgbt.orgLeadership-Principles/the-6-c-s-of-decision-making.html (accessed 26 June 2014).

Galbraith, J.R. (2001) *Designing Organisations: An Executive Guide to Strategy, Structure and Process* (2nd rev. edn). San Francisco, CA: Jossey-Bass.

Garbett, R. (1998) 'Clinical governance?' *Nursing Times Learning Curve*, 2 (7): 15.

Gardner, H. (1983) *Frames of Mind*. New York. Basic Books.

Gardner, H. (1990) *Leading Minds*. London: Harper Collins.

Gibbs, G. (1988) *Learning by Doing: A Guide to Teaching and Learning Methods*. Oxford: Further Education Unit, Oxford Polytechnic.

Giger, J.N. and Davidhizar, R.E. (2004) *Transcultural Nursing, Assessment and Intervention* (4th edn). Baltimore, MD: Mosby.

Gilbert, T. (1995) 'Nursing: empowerment and the problem of power', *Journal of Advanced Nursing*, 21 (5): 865–71.

Giuliani, R.W. (2002) *Leadership*. New York: Hyperion.

Glasper, A. (2014) 'CQC develops new criteria for quality and safety of care', *British Journal of Nursing*, 23 (2): 110–11.

Goetch, D.L. and Davis, S. (2014) *Quality Management for Organizational Excellence: Introduction to Total Quality* (7th edn). Harlow: Pearson Education.

Goldman, S. and Kahnweiller, W.M. (2000) 'A collaborator profile for executives for non-profit organisation', *Non-profit Management and Leadership*, 10: 435–50.

Goleman, D. (1995) *Emotional Intelligence*. New York: Bantam.

Goodwin, D. (2014) 'Decision-making and accountability: differences of distribution', *Sociology of Health & Illness*, 36 (1): 44–59.

Gopee, N. and Galloway, J. (2009) *Leadership and Management in Healthcare*. London: Sage.

Gopee, N. and Galloway, J. (2014) *Leadership and Management in Healthcare* (2nd edn). London: Sage.

Green, C. (2012) 'Nursing intuition: a valid form of knowledge', *Nursing Philosophy*, 13 (2): 98–111.

Greenhalgh, T., Glenn, R., Bale, P., Kyriakidou, O., Macfarlane, F. and Peacock, R. (2004) *How to Spread Good Ideas*. London. NCCSDU.

Greenleaf, R.K. (1977) *Servant Leadership: A Journey in the Nature of Legitimate Power and Greatness*. New York: Paulist.

Greenleaf, R.K. (1998) *Power of Servant Leadership*. San Francisco, CA: Berrett-Koehler Publishing Inc.

Greaves, F., Ramirez-Cano, D., Millett, C., Darzi, A. and Donaldson, L. (2012) 'Harnessing the cloud of patient experience: using social media to detect poor quality healthcare', *British Medical Journal Quality and Safety* doi:10.1136/bmjqs-2012-001527.

Griffiths, S. (2014) 'Perspective: global challenges for public health: dilemmas for leadership', *Journal of Research in Nursing*, 19 (2): 163–6.

Grohar-Murray, M.E. and DiCroce, H.R. (2002) *Leadership and Management in Nursing* (3rd edn). London: Prentice Hall.

Grohar-Murray, M.E., DiCroce, H.R. and Langan, J.C. (2010) *Leadership and Management in Nursing* (4th edn). London: Prentice Hall.

Grossman, S. and Valiga, T.M. (2012) *The New Leadership Challenge: Creating the Future of Nursing* (4th edn). Philadelphia, PA: FA Davis.

Gulick, L. (1937) 'Notes on the theory of the organisation', in L. Gulick and L. Urwick (eds) *Papers on the Science of Administration*. New York: Institute of Public Administration.

Hackman, M. (2006) Communicating for Leadership Success. Synopsis by Rod Cox. The 26th Management Forum Series. Available at: www.executiveforum.com (accessed 11 June 2014).

Haddad, A.M. (1992) 'Ethical problems in home health care', *Journal of Nursing Administration*, 22 (3): 46–51.

Hague, G., Malos, E. and Dear, W. (1996) *Multi-agency Work and Domestic Violence: A National Study of Inter-agency Initiatives*. Bristol: The Policy Press.

Hamer, S. and Collinson, G. (2005) *Achieving Evidence-based Practice* (2nd edn). London: Ballière Tindall Elsevier.

Handy, C.B. (1985) *Understanding Organisations* (3rd edn). Oxford: Oxford University Press.

Handy, C.B. (1993) *Understanding Organisations* (4th edn). Oxford: Oxford University Press.

Hargie, O. and Tourish, D. (eds) (2009) *Auditing Organisational Communication – A Handbook of Research, Theory and Practice*. Hove: Routledge.

Harmer, M. (2005) The case of Elaine Bromiley www.chfg.org/wp-content/uploads/2010/11/ElaineBromileyAnonymousReport.pdf (accessed 18 September 2014).

Harrison, S. (2004) 'Racism and the NHS', *Nursing Standard*, 19 (6): 12–14.

Hartley, P. (1997) *Group Communication*. London: Routledge.

Hartman, R.L. and Crume, A.L. (2014) 'Educating nursing students in team conflict communication', *Journal of Nursing Education and Practice*, 4 (11): 107–18.

Haslam, S.A. and Reicher, S.D. (2011) *The New Psychology of Leadership: Identity, Influence and Power*. Hove: Psychology Press.

Havelock, R.G. (1973) *The Change Agent's Guide to Innovation in Education*. Englewood Cliffs, NJ: Educational Technology.

Hawkins, P. and Shohet, R. (2012) *Supervision in the Helping Professions* (4th edn). Maidenhead: Open University Press/McGraw-Hill Education.

Health and Care Professions Council (HCPC) (2013a) *How to Complete your CPD Profile*. London: HPC. Available at www.hpc-uk.org (accessed 16 June 2014).

Health and Care Professions Council (HCPC) (2013b) *Standards of Conduct, Performance and Ethics*. London: HPC. Available at www.hpc-uk.org (accessed 16 June 2014).

Health Education England (Lord Willis) (2015) *Raising the Bar*. London, HEE.

Hein, S. (2003) History and Definition of Emotional Intelligence. Available at www.eqi.org/history.htm (accessed 2 March 2011).

Hersey, P. and Blanchard, K. (1977) *Management of Organisational Behaviour: Utilising Human Resources* (3rd edn). Englewood Cliffs, NJ: Prentice Hall.

Herzberg, F. (1966) *Work and the Nature of Man*. London: Staples Press.

Hewison, A. and Stanton, A. (2003) 'From conflict to collaboration? Contrasts and convergence in the development of nursing and management theory (2)', *Journal of Nursing Management*, 11 (1): 15–24.

Hibbard, J.H. and Peters, E. (2003) 'Supporting informed consumer health care decisions: data presentation approaches that facilitate the use of information in choice', *Annual Review of Public Health*, 24: 413–33.

Hill, K.S. (2004) 'Defy the decades with multigenerational teams', *Nursing Management (USA)*, 35 (1): 32–5.

HM Government (2013) *Working Together to Safeguard Children: A Guide to Inter-agency Working to Safeguard and Promote the Welfare of Children*. London: HMSO.

Hofsted, G. (1980) *Culture's Consequences*. Beverley Hills: Sage, in Open University (1985) *International Perspectives Unit 16, Block V, Wider Perspectives, Managing in Organisations*. Milton Keynes: Open University Press.

Honey, P. (1988) *Improve your People Skills* (2nd edn). London: The Chartered Institute of Personnel and Development.

Honey, P. and Mumford, A. (1982) *The Manual of Learning Styles*. Maidenhead: Peter Honey Publications.

Horsburgh, M., Lamdin, R. and Williamson, E. (2001) 'Multiprofessional learning: the attitudes of medical, nursing and pharmacy students to shared learning', *Medical Education*, 35 (9): 876–83.

Howarth, M. and Haigh, C. (2007) 'The myth of patient centrality in integrated care: the case of back pain services', *Journal of Integrated Care*, 7 (11 July 2007). Available at: www.ncbi. nlm.nih.gov/pmc/articles/PMC1919416/pdf/ijic2007–200727.pdf (accessed 1 June 2011).

Howatson-Jones, I.L. (2004) 'The servant leader', *Nursing Management*, 11 (3): 20–4.

Huber, D. (2014) *Leadership and Nursing Care Management* (5th edn). St Louis, MO: Elsevier Saunders.

Humphries, J. (1998) *Managing Successful Teams: How to Get the Results You Want by Working Effectively With Others*. Oxford: How To Books.

Hunt, J. (2001) 'Research into practice: the foundation for evidence based care', *Cancer Nursing*, 24: 78–87.

Iles, V. and Sutherland, K. (2001) *Organisational Change: Managing Change in the NHS*. London: The National Co-ordinating Centre for NHS Service Delivery, Organization, Research and Development.

Ishikawa, K. (1985) *What is Total Quality Control?* Englewood Cliffs, NJ: Prentice-Hall.

Jackson, S.E. (1996) *The Consequences of Diversity in Multidisciplinary Work Teams*. Cited in M.A. West (1996) *Handbook of Work Group Psychology*. Chichester: Wiley & Sons, pp. 53–75.

Janis, I.L. (1982) *Groupthink* (2nd edn). Boston, MA: Houghton Mifflin.

Jasper, M. (2011) 'Experience of leadership in nursing management', *Journal of Nursing Management*, 19 (4): 419–20.

Jeffery, A.D. (2013) The Art of Nursing Leadership. www.nurseleader.com (accessed 27 August 2014).

Johns, C. (1995) 'Framing learning through reflection within Karper's fundamental ways of knowing in nursing', *Journal of Advanced Nursing*, 22 (2): 226–34.

Johnson, G. and Scholes, K. (1989) *Exploring Corporate Strategy*. London: Prentice Hall.

Juran, J.M. (1986) 'The quality trilogy', *Quality Progress*, 19 (8): 9–24.

Kagawa-Singer, M. and Chung, R. (1994) 'A paradigm of culturally based care in ethnic minority populations', *Journal of Community Psychology*, 22 (3): 192–208.

Kanter, R.M. (1983) *The Change Masters*. London: George Allen.

Kanter, R.M. (1991) 'Change Master skills: what it takes to be creative', in J. Henry and D. Walker (eds) *Managing Innovation*. London: Sage/Open University.

Kanter, R.M. (1993) *Men and Women of the Corporation* (2nd edn). New York: Basic Books.

Keighley, T. (1989) 'Developments in quality assurance', *Senior Nurse*, 9: 7–10.

Kelly-Heidenthal, P. (2004) *Essentials of Nursing Leadership and Management*. New York: Thomson Delmar Learning.

Keogh, B. (2013) *Review into the Quality of Care and Treatment Provided by 14 Hospital Trusts in England:* Overview Report. London: HMSO.

Kets de Vries, M.F.R. and Mead, C. (1992) 'The development of the global leader within the multinational corporation', in V. Pucik, N.M. Tichy and C.K. Barnett (eds) *Globalizing Management, Creating and Leading the Competitive Organization*. New York: John Wiley & Sons.

Kilner, T. (2004) 'Desirable attributes of the ambulance technician, paramedic, and clinical supervisor: findings from a Delphi study', *Emergency Medicine Journal*, 21: 374–8.

King, I.M. (1981) *A Theory for Nursing: Systems, Concepts, Process*. New York. Delmar Publishers.

King's Fund (2012) *Will Hourly Rounds Help Nurses to Concentrate More on Caring?* London: The King's Fund Organisation.

Kipling, R. (1902) 'The elephant's child', in R. Kipling (2006) *Just So Stories for Little Children*. China: OUP.

Kite, N. and Kay, F. (2012) *Understanding Emotional Intelligence: Strategies for Boosting your EQ and Using It in the Workplace*. London: Kogan Page.

Kitson, A. (1988) in WMHA (1990) *Quality and Standard Setting Workshop*. Directorate of Nursing and Quality. Birmingham: WMHA.

Klagsbrun, J. (2011) *Listening and Focussing: Holistic Health Care Tools for Nurses*. Available at: www.focusing.org/klagsbrun.html (accessed 4 May 2011).

Kotter, J.P. (2008) *A Sense of Urgency*. Boston, MA: Harvard Business Press.

Kotter, J.P. and Schlesinger, L.A. (1979) 'Choosing strategies for change', *Harvard Business Review*, March/April, in J. Hayes (2002) *The Theory and Practice of Change Management*. Basingstoke: Palgrave.

Kouzes, J.M. and Posner, B.Z. (2007) *The Leadership Challenge* (4th edn). San Francisco, CA: Jossey-Bass.

Kramer, M. (1974) *Reality Shock – Why Nurses Leave Nursing*. St Louis, MO: Mosby.

Kubler-Ross, E. (1970) *On Death and Dying*. London: Tavistock Publications.

Lancaster, J. (1999) *Nursing Issues in Leading and Managing Change*. Charlottesville, VA: Mosby.

Landsberg, M. (2003) *The Tao of Motivation: Inspire Yourself and Others*. London: Profile Books.

Laschinger, H.K.S. (2010) 'Towards a comprehensive theory of nurse/patient empowerment applying Kanter's empowerment theory to patient care', *Journal of Nursing Management*, 18 (1): 4–13.

Laurenson, M. and Brockelhurst, H. (2011) 'Interprofessionalism, personalization and care provision', *British Journal of Community Nursing*, 16 (4): 184–90.

Lave, J. and Wenger, E. (1991) *Situated Learning: Legitimate Peripheral Participation*. Cambridge: Cambridge University Press.

Laverack, G. (2005) *Public Health: Power and Professional Practice*. London: Palgrave Macmillan.

Learner, S. (2010) 'Raising the bar', *Nursing Standard*, 25 (10): 24–5.

Leavitt, H.J. (1965) 'Applied organisational change in industry: structural, technological and humanistic approaches', in J.G. March (ed.) *Handbook of Organisations*. Chicago, IL: Rand McNally.

Leavitt, H.J. (1978) *Managerial Psychology* (4th edn). Chicago, IL: University of Chicago Press.

Leavitt, H.J. (2005) *Top Down: Why Hierarchies are Here to Stay and How to Manage them More Effectively*. Boston, MA: Harvard Business School Press.

Leininger, M. (1997) 'Transcultural nursing research to transform nursing education and practice: 40 years image', *Journal of Nursing Scholarship*, 29: 341–7.

Levitt, T. (1972) 'Production-line approach to service', *Harvard Business Review*, 50 (5): 41–52.

Lewin, K. (1951) *Field Theory in Social Sciences*. New York: Harper & Row.

Lewin, K., Lippitt, R. and White, R.K. (1939) 'Patterns of aggressive behaviour in experimentally created social climates', *Journal of Social Psychology*, 10: 271–99.

Lilley, R. (1999) *Making Sense of Clinical Governance*. Oxford: Radcliffe Medical Press.

Lilley, R. and Lambden, P. (1999) *Making Sense of Risk Management: A Workbook for Primary Care*. Oxford: Radcliffe Medical Press.

Lindblom, C. (1959) 'The science of muddling through', *Administrative Science Review*, 19: 79–99.

Linstead, S., Fulop, L. and Lilley, S. (2004) *Management and Organization: A Critical Reader*. Basingstoke: Palgrave Macmillan.

Lippet, R., Watson, J. and Wesley, B. (1958) *The Theory of Planned Change*. New York: Harcourt Brace Jovanovich.

Littlejohn, P. (2012) 'The missing link: using emotional intelligence to reduce workplace stress and workplace violence in our nursing and other health care professions', *Journal of Professional Nursing*, 28 (6): 360–8.

Lobel, S.A. (1990) 'Global leadership competencies: managing to a different drumbeat', *Human Resource Management*, 29 (1) Spring: 39–47.

Lucas, S. (1999) *The Passionate Organisation*. New York: American Management Association.

Luft, J. and Ingham, H. (1955) '"The Johari Window" a graphic model of interpersonal awareness', *Proceedings of the Western Training Laboratory in Group Development*. Los Angeles: UCLA.

Lugon, M. and Secker-Walker, J. (2006) *Clinical Governance in a Changing NHS*. London: The Royal Society of Medicine Press.

Lynn, R. (2008) *The Global Bell Curve: Race, IQ, and Inequality Worldwide*. Augusta, GA: Washington Summit Publishers.

MacPheem, M. and Suryaprakash, N. (2012) 'First-line nurse leaders health-care change management initiatives', *Journal of Nursing Management*, 20: 249–59.

Malby, R. (1994) *The Challenges for Nursing and Midwifery in the 21st Century: A Briefing Document*. Leeds: University of Leeds.

Malloch, K. and Porter-O'Grady, T. (2005) *The Quantum Leader Applications for the New World of Work*. London: Jones and Bartlett Publishers.

Mansour, M. (2014) 'Factor analysis of nursing students' perception of patient safety education', *Nurse Education Today* http://dx.doi.org/10.1016/j.nedt.2014.04.020 (accessed 28 August 2014).

Markham, G. (2005) 'Gender in leadership', *Nursing Management*, 3 (1): 18–19.

Marquis, B.L. and Huston, C.L. (2006) *Leadership Roles and Management Functions in Nursing: Theory and Application* (5th edn). Philadelphia, PA: Lippincott.

Marquis, B.L. and Huston, C.L. (2008) *Leadership Roles and Management Functions in Nursing: Theory and Application* (6th edn). Philadelphia, PA: Lippincott.

Marquis, B.L. and Huston, C.L. (2011) *Leadership Roles and Management Functions in Nursing: Theory and Application* (7th edn). Philadelphia, PA: Lippincott.

Marquis, B.L. and Huston, C.L. (2014) *Leadership Roles and Management Functions in Nursing: Theory and Application* (8th international edn). Philadelphia, PA: Wolters Kluwer.

Marriner Tomey, A. (2008) *Guide to Nursing Management and Leadership* (8th edn). St Louis, MO: Mosby.

Martin, C.A. (2003) 'Transitional timelines', *Nursing Management (USA)*, 34 (4): 25–6, 28.

Martin, V. (2001a) 'Mapping the service', *Nursing Management*, 7 (9): 32–6.

Martin, V. (2001b) 'Service planning and governance', *Nursing Management*, 8 (3): 33–7.

Maslow, A. (1987) *Motivation and Personality* (3rd edn). Harlow: Addison Wesley.

Mathieu, J.E., Maynard, T.S., Rapp, T. and Gilson, L. (2008) 'Team effectiveness 1997–2007: A review of recent advancements and a glimpse into the future', *Journal of Management*, 34(3): 410–76.

Maxwell, J.C. (1999) *The 21 Indispensable Qualities of a Leader*. Nashville, TN: Thomas Nelson.

Maxwell, R.J. (1984) 'Quality assurance in health', *British Medical Journal*, 288: 1470–2.

Mayer, J.D., Salovey, P., Caruso, D.R. and Sitarenios, G. (2001) 'Emotional intelligence as a standard intelligence', *Emotion*, 1: 232–42.

Mays, N. (2013) 'Evaluating the Labour Government's English NHS health system reforms: the 2008 Darzi reforms', *Journal of Health Service Research and Policy* 18 (2): 1–10.

McAlpine, A. (2000) *The New Machiavelli: The Art of Politics in Business*. New York: John Wiley.

McCallum, J., Duffy, K., Hastie, E., Ness, V. and Price, L. (2013) 'Developing nursing students' decision making skills: are early warning scoring systems helpful?' *Nurse Education in Practice* 13 (1): 1–3.

McCaughan, D. and Kaufman, G. (2013) 'Patient safety: threats and solutions', *Nursing Standard*, 27 (44): 48–55.

McClelland, D.C. (1984) *Human Motivation*. New Jersey: Longman Higher Education.

McCrae, N. (2011) 'Whither nursing models: the value of nursing theory in the context of evidence based practice and multidisciplinary care', *Journal of Advanced Nursing*, 68 (1): 222–9.

McCutcheon, H. and Pincombe, J. (2001) 'Intuition: an important tool in the practice of nursing', *Journal of Advanced Nursing*, 35 (3): 342–8.

McDaniel, K. and Stumpf, L. (1993) 'The organisational culture: implications for nursing service', *Journal of Nursing Administration*, 23 (4): 54–60.

McElhaney, R. (1996) 'Conflict management in nursing administration', *Nursing Management*, 24: 65–6, in P.E.B. Valentine (2001) 'A gender perspective on conflict management strategies of nurses', *Journal of Nursing Scholarship*, 33 (1): 69–74.

McGregor, D. (1987) *The Human Side of Enterprise*. London: Penguin.

McMullen, B. (2003) 'Emotional Intelligence', *BMJ Career Focus*, 326: 7381.

McNeese-Smith, D.K. and Crook, M. (2003) 'Nursing values and a changing nurse workforce: values, age, and job stages', *Journal of Nursing Administration*, 33 (5): 260–70.

McSherry, R. and Pearce, P. (2011) *Clinical Governance: A Guide to Implementation for Health Care Professionals* (3rd edn). Chichester: Wiley Blackwell.

Mead, M. (1970) 'Culture and commitment: a study of the generation gap', in Z. Sardar and B. Van Loon (1997) *Cultural Studies for Beginners*. Cambridge: Icon Books Ltd.

Mears, P. and Voehl, F. (1994) *Team Building: A Structured Learning Approach*. Delray Beach, FL: St Lucie Press.

Miller, W.R. and Rollnick, S. (2002) *Motivational Interviewing: Preparing People to Change*. London: Guilford Press.

Millward, L.J. and Bryan, K. (2005) 'Clinical leadership in health care: a position statement', *International Journal in Health Care Quality Assurance*, 18 (2/3): xiii–xxv.

Miner, J.B. (2005) *Organisational Behaviour 1: Essential Theories of Motivation and Leadership*. New York: M.E. Sharpe.

Mintzberg, H. (1998) '5 Ps for strategy', in H. Mintzberg, J. Quinn and S. Ghoshal (eds) (2003) *The Strategy Process* (Revised European edn). Englewood Cliffs, NJ: Prentice Hall.

Mintzberg, H. (1989) *Mintzberg on Management: Inside Our Strange World of Organisations*. New York: Free Press.

Mintzberg, H., Lampel, J., Quinn, J.B. and Ghoshal, S. (2003) *The Strategy Process: Concepts, Context, Cases* (2nd edn). New York: Prentice Hall/Financial Times Management.

Moller, J. (2013) 'Leadership accountability and patient safety', *Journal of Gynaecology and Neonatal Nurses (AWHONN)*, 42 (5): 506–7.

Mollon, D. (2014) 'Feeling safe during an inpatient hospitalization: a concept analysis', *Journal of Advanced Nursing* 70 (8): 1727–37.

Moore, A. (2014) 'Seven-day challenge', *Nursing Standard*, 28 (29): 20–2.

Moran, R.T. and Riesenberger, J.R. (1994) *The Global Challenge: Building the New Worldwide Enterprise*. London: McGraw-Hill.

Mosadeghrad, A.M. (2014) 'Why TQM programmes fail? A pathology approach', *TQM Journal*, 26 (2): 160–87.

Moullin, M. (2002) *Delivering Excellence in Health and Social Care*. Buckingham: Open University Press.

Muir Gray, J.A. (1997) *Evidence-Based Healthcare: How to Make Health Policy and Management Decisions*. London: Churchill Livingstone.

Muir Gray, J.A. (2007) *How to Get Better Value Health Care*. Oxford: Offox Press.

Muir, N. (2004) 'Clinical decision-making: theory and practice', *Nursing Standard*, 18 (36): 47–52.

Mukamel, D.B., Cai, S. and Temkin-Greener, H. (2009) 'Cost implications of organising nursing home workforce in teams', *Health Services Research*, 44: 1309–25.

Mulholland, J. (1995) 'Nursing, humanism and trans-cultural theory: the bracketing out of reality', *Journal of Advanced Nursing*, 22 (5): 442–9.

Mullaly, S. (2001) 'Leadership and politics', *Nursing Management*, 8 (4): 21–7.

Mullins, L.J. (1999) *Management and Organisational Behaviour* (5th edn). New York: Prentice Hall/Financial Times.

Mullins, L.J. (2005) *Management and Organisational Behaviour* (7th edn). New York: Prentice Hall/Financial Times.

Mullins, L.J. (2013) *Management and Organisational Behaviour* (10th edn). New York: FT Publishing International.

Mumford, A. (1997) *How to Manage Your Learning Environment*. London: Peter Honey Publications.

Myers-Briggs, I. (1995) *Gifts Differing: Understanding Personality Type*. Palo Alto, CA: Davies-Black Publishing.

National Audit Office (NAO) (2007) *Improving Quality and Safety – Progress in Implementing Clinical Governance: Lessons for the New Primary Care Trusts*. London: NAO.

National Nursing Research Unit (NNRU) (2013) *Does NHS Staff Wellbeing Affect Patient Experience of Care?* Policy Plus 39. London: Kings College In The Kings Fund (2014) *Reading List: Improving Patients' Experience*. London: The Kings Fund.

National Patient Safety Agency (NPSA) (2004) *Seven Steps to Patient Safety*. London: NHS.

National Professional Qualification for Headship (NPQH) (2005) *Securing the Commitment of Others to the Vision (D1.2) in National College for School Leadership*. London: NPQH.

Nelson, S., Wild, D. and Szczepura, A. (2009) 'Innovation in residential care homes: an inreach nursing team project', *Primary Health Care*, 19 (1): 31–4.

NHS Employers (2014) *Women in the NHS Infographic*. Available at: www.nhsemployers.org/case-studies-and-resources/2014/03/women-in-the-nhs-infographic (accessed 11 May 2015).

NHS England (2012) www.6cs.england.nhs.uk (accessed 26 June 2014).

NHS Institute for Innovation and Improvement (NHS III) (2009a) *Access of BME Staff to Senior Position in the NHS*. Coventry: NHS Institute.

NHS Institute for Innovation and Improvement (2009b) *Inspiring Change in the NHS: Introducing the Five Frames*. London: NHS III.

NHS Jobs (2014) www.jobs.nhs.uk/about_nhs.html (accessed 29 August 2014).

NHS Leadership Academy (2011) *Leadership Framework*. Coventry: NHS Institute for Innovation and Improvement.

Northcott, J. (1991) *Britain in 2010: The PSI Report*. London: Policy Studies Institute.

Northouse, P.G. (2012) *Introduction to Leadership: Concepts and Practice* (2nd edn). London: Sage.

Nursing and Midwifery Council (NMC) (2006) *Preceptorship Guidelines*. Circular 21/2006. London: NMC.

Nursing and Midwifery Council (NMC) (2008) *The Prep Handbook*. London: NMC.

Nursing and Midwifery Council (NMC) (2010) *Midwives' Rules and Standards*. London: NMC.

Nursing and Midwifery Council (NMC) (2015) *The Code: Professional Standards of Practice and Behaviour for Nurses and Midwives*. London: NMC.

Orchard, C.A. (2010) 'Persistent isolationist or collaborator? The nurse's role in interprofessional collaborative practice', *Journal of Nursing Management*, 18: 248–57.

Osland, J.S., Bird, A., Mendenhall, M.E. and Osland, A. (2006) 'Developing global leadership capabilities and global mindset: a review', in G.K. Sthal and I. Bjorkman (eds), *Handbook of Research in International Human Resource Management*. Cheltenham: Edward Elgar, pp. 197–22.

Ouchi, W. (1981) *Theory Z: How American Business Can Meet the Japanese Challenge*. Harlow: Addison Wesley.

Øvretveit, J. (1992) *Health Service Quality*. London: Blackwell Scientific Publications.

Owen, J. (2009) *How to Lead* (2nd edn). London: Pearson Business Ltd.

Owen, J. (2011) *How to Lead* (3rd edn). London: Pearson Business Ltd.

Palfrey, C. (2000) *Key Concepts in Health Care Policy and Planning*. London: Macmillan.

Parkin, C. and Bullock, I. (2005) 'Evidence-based healthcare: development and audit in clinical standard for research and its impact on an NHS Trust', *Journal of Clinical Nursing*, 14 (4): 418–25.

Pau, A. and Croucher, R. (2003) 'Emotional intelligence and perceived stress in dental undergraduates', *Journal of Dental Education*, 67: 1023–8.

Pearson, A., Borbasi, S., Fitzgerald, M., Kowanko, I. and Walsh, K. (1997) 'Evidence based nursing: an examination of nursing within the international evidence based health care practice movement', RCNA Discussion Document No. 1, Nursing Review. Sydney: RCNA.

Peters, T. and Waterman, R.H. (2004) *In Search of Excellence*. London: Profile Books.

Pollard, K.C., Thomas, J. and Miers, M. (2010) *Understanding Interprofessional Working in Health and Social Care: Theory and Practice*. London: Palgrave Macmillan.

Pondy, L.R. (1992) 'Reflections on organisational conflict', *Journal of Organizational Behaviour*, 13 (3): 257–61.

Power, M., Stewart, K. and Brotherton, A. (2012) 'What is the NHS Safety Thermometer?' *Clinical Risk*, 18 (5): 163–9.

Pucik, V., Tichy, N.M. and Barnett C.K. (eds) (1992) *Globalizing Management, Creating and Leading the Competitive Organization*. New York: John Wiley & Sons.

Pyzdek, T. and Keller, P. (2014) *The Six Sigma Handbook* (4th edn). London: McGraw Hill Professional.

Radcliffe, S. (2012) *Leadership: Plain and Simple*. Harlow: Pearson Education Ltd.

Rafferty, A. (1993) *Leading Questions: A Discussion Paper on the Issues of Nurse Leadership*. London: King's Fund Centre.

Rahim, M.A. (1983) 'A measure of styles of handling interpersonal conflict', *Academy of Management Journal*, 26: 368–75.

Rahim, M.A. (2011) *Managing Conflict in Organizations*. New Jersey: Transaction Publishers.

Rank, J., Nelson, N.E., Allen, T.D. and Xian, X. (2009) 'Leadership predictors of innovation and task performance: subordinates' self-esteem and self-presentation as moderators', *Journal of Occupational and Organizational Psychology*, 82 (3): 465–89.

Rankin, B. (2013) 'Emotional intelligence: enhancing values-based practice and compassionate care in nursing', *Journal of Advanced Nursing*, 69 (12): 2717–25.

Rayner, D., Chisholm, H. and Appleby, H. (2002) 'Developing leadership through action learning', *Nursing Standard*, 16 (29): 37–971.

Reddin, W.J. (1970) *Managerial Effectiveness*. New York: McGraw Hill.

Reeves, S., MacMillan, K. and van Soren, M. (2010) 'Leadership of interprofessional health and social care teams: a socio-historical analysis', *Journal of Nursing Management*, 18 (3): 258–64.

Reid, J. and Bromiley, M. (2012) 'Clinical human factors: the need to speak up to improve patient safety', *Nursing Standard*, 26 (35): 35–40.

Revens, R. (2011) *A B C of Action Learning*. Farnham: Gower.

Rhinesmith, S.H. (1993) 'A managers' guide to globalisation: six keys to success in a changing world', *Human Resource Development Quarterly*, (Autumn) 6 (3): 323–7.

Ringrose, D. (2013) 'Development of an organizational excellent framework', *The TQM Journal*, 25 (4): 441–52.

Rippon, S. (2001) 'Nurturing nursing leadership – How does your garden grow?', *Nursing Management*, 8 (7): 11–15.

Robertson, C. (1997) *The Wordsworth Dictionary of Quotations*. London: Wordsworth Editions Ltd.

Robinson, S. and Griffiths, P. (2009) *Scoping Review: Preceptorship for Newly Qualified Nurses: Impacts, Facilitators and Constraints*. London: King's Fund National Nursing Research Unit.

Robotham, A. and Frost, M. (2005) *Health Visiting Specialist Community Public Health Nursing* (2nd edn). London: Elsevier.

Rock, D. (2008) 'SCARF: a brain based model for collaborating with and influencing others', *NeuroLeadership Journal*, 1: 44–52.

Rock, D., Tang, Y. and Dixon, P. (2009) 'Neuroscience of engagement', *NeuroLeadership Journal*, 2: 1–9.

Rogers, E. and Shoemaker, F. (1971) *Communication of Innovations: A Cross-cultural Report*. New York: Free Press.

Rogers, E.M. (1983) *Diffusion of Innovations* (3rd edn). New York: Free Press.

Rogers, M. (1997) *Canadian Nursing in the Year 2020: Five Futures Scenarios*. New York: Canadian Nurses Association.

Rolfe, G., Freshwater, D. and Jasper, M. (2001) *Critical Reflection in Nursing and the Helping Professions: A User's Guide*. Basingstoke: Palgrave Macmillan.

Roper, N., Logan, W.W. and Tierney, A. (1980) *The Elements of Nursing*. London: Churchill Livingstone.

Roper, N., Logan, W.W. and Tierney, A. (2000) *The Roper, Logan & Tierney Model of Nursing: Based on Activities of Living*. Edinburgh: Elsevier Health Services.

Rosener, J. (1990) 'Ways women lead Harvard Business Review', in G. Markham (1996) 'Gender in leadership', *Nursing Management*, 3 (1): 18–19.

Rothschild, J.M., Hurley, A.C., Landrigan, C.P., Cronin, J.W., Martell-Waldrop, K., Foskett, C., Burdick, E., Czeisler, C.A. and Bates, D.W. (2006) 'Recovery from medical errors: the critical care nursing safety net', *Joint Commission Journal on Quality and Patient Safety*, 32 (2): 63–72.

Royal College of Nursing (RCN) (2005) *Working with Care: Improving Working Relationships in Healthcare*. London: RCN.

Rushmer, R. (2005) 'Blurred boundaries damage inter-professional working', *Nurse Researcher*, 12 (3): 74–85.

Sadler, P. (2003) *Leadership* (2nd edn). London: Kogan Page.

Salovey, P. and Mayer, J.D. (1990) 'Emotional intelligence', *Imagination, Cognition and Personality*, 9: 185–211.

Sardar, Z. and Van Loon, B. (1997) *Cultural Studies for Beginners*. Cambridge: Icon Books Ltd.

Scally, G. and Donaldson, L. (1998) 'Clinical governance and the drive for quality improvement in the new NHS in England', *British Medical Journal*, 317: 61–5.

Schein, E.H. (1985) *Organizational Culture and Leadership*. San Francisco, CA: Jossey-Bass.

Schein, E.H. (1992) 'Coming to a new awareness of organizational culture', in G. Salaman (ed.), *Human Resource Strategies*. London: Sage.

Schmalenburg, C. and Kramer, M. (1979) *Coping with Reality Shock*. Wakefield, MA: Nursing Resources.

Schön, D. (1987) *Educating the Reflective Practitioner: Towards a New Design for Teaching and Learning in the Professions*. San Francisco, CA: Jossey-Bass.

Scott, G. (2014) 'Proposed changes to the Code affect every nurse', *Nursing Standard*, 28 (39): 3.

Scott, I. (1998) 'Challenging the future', *Nursing Management*, 4 (9): 18–21.

Scrivener, R., Hand, T. and Hooper, R. (2011) 'Accountability and responsibility: principle of nursing practice B', *Nursing Standard*, 25 (29): 35–6.

Seligman, M.E.P. and Csikszentmihalyi, M. (2000) 'Positive psychology', *American Psychology*, 5 (1): 5–14.

Senge, P. (1990) *The Fifth Discipline: The Art and Practice of the Learning Organisation*. New York: Doubleday.

Shannon, C.E. and Weaver, W. (1954) *The Mathematical Theory of Communication*. Urbana-Champaign, IL: University of Illinois Press.

Shanta, L. and Connolly, M. (2013) 'Using King's Interacting Systems Theory to link emotional intelligence and nursing practice', *Journal of Professional Nursing* 29 (3): 174–80.

Shorten, A. and Wallace, M. (1997) 'Evidence based practice: the future is clear', *Australian Nursing Journal*, 4 (6): 22–4, in B.J. Taylor (2000) *Reflective Practice: A Guide for Nurses and Midwives*. Buckingham: Open University Press.

Shapiro, F., Punwani, N. and Urman, R. (2013) 'Putting the patient into Patient Safety Checklists', *AORN Journal* 98 (4): 413.

Simon, H.A. (1960) 'The corporation: will it be managed by machines?', in H. Leavitt and L.R. Pondy (1964), *Readings in Managerial Psychology*. Chicago, IL: University of Chicago Press.

Simon, H.A. (1977) *The New Science of Management Decision* (revised edn). London: Prentice Hall.

Simon, H.A. (1994) 'Administrative behaviour: how organisations can be understood in terms of decision processes', Conference Presentation, 11 March 1994, Department of Computer Science, Roskilde University.

Simon, H.A. (1980) 'Cognitive science: the newest science of the artificial', *Cognitive Science*, 4: 33–46.

Smith, G. (1995) *Managing to Succeed*. Hemel Hempstead: Prentice Hall.

Snape, D., Kirkham J., Preston J., Popay, J., Britten, N., Collins, M., Froggatt, K., Gibson, A., Lobban, F., Wyatt, K. and Jacoby, A. (2014) Exploring areas of consensus and conflict around values underpinning public involvement in health and social care research: a modified Delphi study, *British Medical Journal Open* 4 (1) e00427.

Snell, M. (2009) 'Factors that increase the incidence of groupthink in hospitals: the perception of nurses and managers' (DBA Dissertation), Arizona ProQuest LLC.

Snow, J. (2001) 'Looking beyond nursing for clues to effective leadership', *Journal of Nursing Administration*, 31 (9): 440–3.

Sofarelli, D. and Brown, D. (1998) 'The need for nursing leadership in uncertain times', *Journal of Nursing Management*, 6: 201–7.

Sommerfeldt, S.A. (2013) 'Articulating nursing in an interprofessional world', *Nurse Education in Practice*, 13: 519–23.

Spector, R. (2002) 'Cultural diversity in health and illness', *Journal of Transcultural Nursing*, 13 (3): 197–9.

Stanley, D. (2010) 'Mulitgenerational workforce issues and their implications for leadership in nursing', *Journal of Nursing Management*, 18: 846–52.

Stanley, D. and Sherratt, A. (2010) 'Lamp light on leaderships: clinical leadership and Florence Nightingale', *Journal of Nursing Management*, 18: 115–21.

Starns, P. (2000) *Nurses at War: Women in the Frontline 1939–45*. Stroud: Sutton Publishing Ltd.

Steffaleno, A. and Carlson, E. (2010) 'Providing direct care nurses research and evidence based practice information: an essential component of nursing leadership', *Journal of Nursing Management*, 18 (1): 84–9.

Stewart, I.M. (1918) 'Popular fallacies about nursing education', *The Modern Hospital*, 18 (1), in M.P. Donahue (2011) *Nursing – The Finest Art*. St Louis, MO: Mosby.

Stewart, R. (1996) *Leading in the NHS: A Practical Guide* (2nd edn). London: Macmillan Business.

Stoddart, K., Ciccu-Moore, R., Grant, F., Niven, B.A., Paterson, H. and Wallace, A. (2014) 'Care comfort rounds', *Nursing Management*, 20 (9): 18–23.

Storey, J. and Holti, R. (2013) *Towards a New Model of Leadership for the NHS* London: NHS Leadership Academy and Open University Business School.

Stott, K. (1992) *Making Management Work*. London: Prentice Hall.

Stott, K. and Walker, A. (1995) *Making Management Work: A Practical Approach*. London: Prentice Hall.

Studer Group (2007) 'Best practices: Sacred Heart Hospital, Pensicola, Florida. Hourly rounding supplement. Gulf Breeze', cited in *Policy+*, National Nursing Research Unit, Kings College London, Issue 35, April 2012.

Sullivan, E.J. and Garland, G. (2010) *Practical Leadership and Management in Nursing.* Harlow: Pearson Education Ltd.

Swansburg, R.C. and Swansburg, R.J. (1998) *Introductory Management and Leadership for Nurses* (2nd edn). Boston, MA: Jones and Bartlett.

Tannenbaum, R. and Schmidt, W.H. (1958) 'How to choose a leadership pattern', *Harvard Business Review*, 36: 95–101.

Tappen, R., Weiss, S. and Whitehead, D. (2004) 'Tools for leadership and management problem solving', in D. Whitehead, S. Weiss and R. Tappen (2009), *Essentials of Nursing Leadership and Management* (5th edn). Philadelphia, PA: FA Davis.

Taylor, B.J. (2010) *Reflective Practice for Health Care Professionals: A Practical Guide* (3rd edn). Maidenhead: Open University Press.

Taylor, F.W. (1947) *Scientific Management.* New York: Harper & Row.

The Equality Act (2010) London: The Stationery Office. Available at www.legislation.gov.uk (accessed 5 June 2011).

The Health Foundation (2013) Inspiring Improvements. www.health.org/areas-of-work/top-ics/person-centred-care/person-centred-care/_ (accessed 17 April 2014).

Thomas, K.W. (1976) 'Conflict and conflict management', in M.D. Dunnette (ed.), *Handbook of Industrial and Organisational Psychology.* Chicago, IL: Rand McNally.

Thomas, K.W. (1977) 'Towards multidimensional values in teaching: the example of conflict behaviours', *Academy of Management Review*, July: 487.

Thomas, S.P. (2003) 'Horizontal hostility', *American Journal of Nursing*, 103 (10): 87.

Thompson, P. and Hyrkas, K. (2014) 'Global nursing leadership' (editorial) *Journal of Nursing Management*, 22 (1) 1–3.

Thorndike, E.L. (1932) *The Fundamentals of Learning.* New York: Teachers College Press.

Tuckman, B.C. and Jensen, M.A. (1977) 'Stages of small group development revisited', *Group and Organization Studies*, 2 (4): 419–27.

Tuckman, B.W. (1965) 'Developmental sequence in small groups', *Psychological Bulletin*, 63: 384–99.

Tylor, E.B. (1871) 'Primitive cultures', in Z. Sardar and B. Van Loon (1997) *Cultural Studies for Beginners.* Cambridge: Icon Books Ltd.

UNISON (2011) *Duty of Care Handbook.* London: UNISON.

University of Salford (2009) *Salford Student Becomes First Deaf Male Nurse.* Available at: http://staff.salford.ac.uk/newsitem/1247 (accessed 29 August 2014).

Upton, T. and Brooks, B. (NAHAT) (1995) *Managing Change in the NHS.* London: Kogan Page.

Valentine, P.E.B. (2001) 'A gender perspective on conflict management strategies of nurses', *Journal of Nursing Scholarship*, 33 (1): 69–74.

Van Seters, D.A. and Field, R.H.G. (1990) 'The evolution of leadership theory', *Journal of Organisational Change Management*, 3: 3.

VanGundy, A.B. (1988) *Techniques of Structured Problem Solving* (2nd edn). London: Van Nostrand Reinhold.

Virani, T. (2013) *Interprofessional Collaborative Teams.* Ontario: Canadian Health Services Research Foundation (CHSRF).

Vitello-Cicciu, J.M. (2002) 'Exploring emotional intelligence: implications for nurse leaders', *JONA*, 32 (4): 203–9.

Vroom, V.H. and Yetton, P.W. (1973) *Leadership and Decision Making.* Pittsburgh: University of Pittsburgh.

Vroom, V.H. and Yetton, P.W. (1976) *Leadership and Decision Making.* Pittsburg, PA: University of Pittsburg Press.

Vroom, V.H. and Jago, A.G. (1988) *The New Leadership.* Englewood Cliffs, NJ: Prentice Hall.

Waite, R. and McKinney, N.S. (2014) 'Enhancing conflict competency', *Association Black Nursing Faculty Journal*, 25 (4): 123–8.

Walker, L.O. and Avant, K.C. (2010) *Strategies for Theory Construction in Nursing* (5th edn). Englewood Cliffs, NJ: Prentice Hall.

Walmsley, J., Reynolds, J., Shakespeare, P. and Woolfe, R. (1997) *Health, Welfare and Practice: Reflecting on Relationship*. London: Sage/Open University.

Wanless, D. (2002) *Securing Good Health: Taking a Long Term View*. London: Department of Health.

Wanless, D. (2004) *Securing Good Health for the Whole Population*. London: Department of Health.

Warner, M., Longley, M., Gould, E. and Picek, A. (1998) *Healthcare Futures 2010*. Pontypridd: University of Glamorgan/Welsh Institute for Health and Social Care.

Waterlow, J. (2005) *The Waterlow Pressure Prevention Manual*. Available at: judy-waterlow. co.uk (accessed 14 August 2014).

Weaver, H. (2013) Determined and Dedicated. www.nursingtimes.net (accessed 30 August 2014).

Weberg, D. (2012) 'Complexity leadership: a healthcare imperative', *Nursing Forum*, 47 (l4): 68–77.

Weightman, J. (1999) *Introducing Organisational Behaviour*. Harlow: Addison Wesley Longman.

Weisbord, M. (1976) 'Organisational diagnosis: six places to look with or without a theory', *Group and Organisational Studies* 1: 430–47, in V. Iles and K. Sutherland (2001) *Organisational Change: Managing Change in the NHS*. London: The National Co-ordinating Centre for NHS Service Delivery, Organisation, Research and Development.

Weitz, R., Brinkerhoft, D., White, L.K. and Ortega, S.T. (2011) *Essentials of Sociology* (9th edn). California: Wadsworth Cengage Learning.

West, A. (2002) 'Sparkling fountains or stagnant ponds: an integrative model of creativity and innovation implementation in work groups', *Applied Psychology: An International Review*, 51: 355–87.

West, M.A., Borrill, C.S., Dawson, J.F., Scully, J., Carter, M., Anelay, S., Patterson, M. and Waring, J. (2002) 'The link between the management of employees and patient mortality in acute hospitals', *International Journal of Human Resource Management*, 13: 1299–310.

West, M.A., Borrill, C.S., Dawson, J.F., Brodbeck, F., Shapiro, D.A. and Haward, B. (2003) 'Leadership clarity and team innovation in health care', *The Leadership Quarterly*, 14: 393–410.

Wheelan, S. (1994) 'Group process: a developmental perspective', in P. Hartley (1997) *Group Communication*. London: Routledge.

White, N. (2012) 'Understanding the role of non-technical skills in patient safety', *Nursing Standard*, 26 (26): 43–8.

White, R.K. and Lippitt, R. (1960) 'Autocracy and democracy: an experimental inquiry', in B.L. Marquis and C.J. Huston (2006), *Leadership Roles and Management Functions in Nursing: Theory and Application* (5th edn). Philadelphia, PA: Lippincott.

Whitehead, D. (2006) 'Workplace health promotion: the role and responsibilities of health care managers', *Journal of Nursing Management*, 14 (1): 59–68.

Whitehead, D., Weiss, S. and Tappen, R. (2009) *Essentials of Nursing Leadership and Management* (5th edn). Philadelphia, PA: F.A. Davis Company.

Wilkinson, G. and Miers, M. (1999) *Power and Nursing Practice*. London: Macmillan.

Wood, J.T. (2012) *Gendered Lives: Communication, Gender and Culture* (10th edn). Cincinnati, OH: Wadsworth.

World Health Organization (WHO) (1977) *Health For All*. Geneva: WHO.

World Health Organization (WHO) (1983) *The Principles of Quality Assurance*. Copenhagen: WHO (report on a WHO meeting).

World Health Organization (WHO) (2008a) *Guidance on Developing Quality and Safety Strategies with a Health System Approach*. Geneva: WHO.

World Health Organization (WHO) (2008b) *Primary Health Care – Now More Than Ever*. Geneva: WHO.

World Health Organization (2011) *Patient Safety Curriculum Guide: Multi-professional Edition*. Available at: http://whqlibdoc.who.int/publications/2011/9789241501958_eng.pdf (accessed 18 September 2014).

World Health Organization (2014) *Health Policy*. Available at: www.who.int/topics/health_policy/en/ (accessed 11 May 2015).

Wright, T. (2000) 'The phantom menace', *Nursing Management*, 6 (5): 5.

Yukl, G., Goron, A. and Taber, T. (2002) 'A hierarchical taxonomy of leadership behaviour. Integrating a half century of behaviour research', *Journal of Leadership and Organizational Studies*, 9 (1): 15–32.

Zydziunaite, V., Suominen, T., Astedt-Kurki, P. and Lepaite, D. (2010) 'Ethical dilemmas concerning decision making within healthcare leadership: a systematic literature review', *Medicina* (Kaunas), 46 (9): 596–603.

INDEX